Color Atlas & Synopsis of Clinical Ophthalmology

WILLS EYE HOSPITAL

GLAUCOMA

COLOR ATLAS AND SYNOPSIS OF CLINICAL OPHTHALMOLOGY SERIES

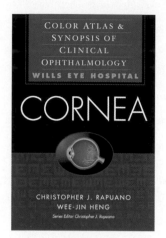

CORNEA
Christopher J. Rapuano, MD
Wee-Jin Heng, MD
0-07-137589-9

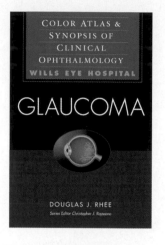

GLAUCOMA
Douglas J. Rhee, MD
0-07-137597-X

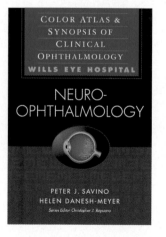

NEUROOPHTHALMOLOGY
Peter J. Savino, MD
Helen Danesh-Meyer, MD
0-07-137595-3

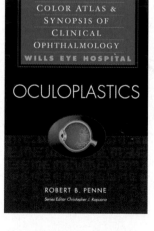

OCULOPLASTICS
Robert B. Penne, MD
0-07-137594-5

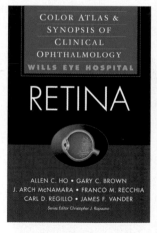

RETINA
Allen C. Ho, MD
Gary C. Brown, MD
J. Arch McNamara, MD
Franco M. Recchia, MD
Carl D. Regillo, MD
James F. Vander, MD
0-07-137596-1

COLOR ATLAS & SYNOPSIS OF CLINICAL OPHTHALMOLOGY

WILLS EYE HOSPITAL

GLAUCOMA

Douglas J. Rhee, M.D.

Assistant Professor of Ophthalmology
Wills Eye Hospital
Assistant Professor of Pathology, Anatomy, and Cell Biology
Jefferson Medical College
Thomas Jefferson University
Philadelphia, Pennsylvania

McGraw-Hill
MEDICAL PUBLISHING DIVISION

New York   Chicago   San Francisco   Lisbon   London
Madrid   Mexico City   Milan   New Delhi   San Juan   Seoul
Singapore   Sydney   Toronto

Glaucoma: Color Atlas and Synopsis of Clinical Ophthalmology

Copyright © 2003 by The **McGraw-Hill** Companies, Inc. All rights reserved. Printed in the United States of America. Except as permitted under the United States Copyright Act of 1976, no part of this publication may be reproduced or distributed in any form or by any means, or stored in a data base or retrieval system without the prior written permission of the publisher.

1234567890   IMP IMP   098765432

ISBN 0-07-137597-X

This book was set in Times Roman by TechBooks.
The editors were Darlene Cooke, Kathleen McCullough, and Regina Y. Brown.
The production supervisor was Richard Ruzycka.
The cover designer was Mary Belibasakis.
The index was prepared by Robert Swanson.
Quebecor/Spain was the printer and binder.

This book is printed on acid-free paper.

Library of Congress Catalog-in-Publication Data

Rhee, Douglas J.
    Glaucoma : color atlas and synopsis of clinical ophthalmology / Douglas Rhee.
        p.;   cm.—(Color atlas and synopsis of clinical ophthalmology series)
    Includes bibliographical references and index.
    ISBN 0-07-137597-X
    1. Glaucoma—Handbooks, manuals, etc. 2. Glaucoma—Atlases.   I. Title.   II. Series.
    [DNLM: 1. Glaucoma—Atlases.   WW 17 R469g 2003]
    RE871 .R48   2003
    617.7´41—dc21

                                                                                  2002075386

DEDICATION

To my lovely wife, Tina, for your patience and support for this endeavor. To my father and mother, Dennis and Serena Rhee, in appreciation for your endless love and dedication. Also to Susan Rhee for her understanding and kindness. Finally, to all my families—Rhee, Chang, Kim, and Chomakos—and especially my grandparents for their guidance and encouragement.

CONTENTS

Section 4

IMAGING TECHNOLOGIES   363

Introduction (General Principles and Uses)

CONTRIBUTORS

Augusto Azuara-Blanco, M.D., Ph.D.

Consultant Ophthalmic Surgeon
Aberdeen Royal Infirmary
Honorary Clinical Senior Lecturer
University of Aberdeen
Aberdeen, United Kingdom

Oscar Beaujon-Rubin, M.D., Ph.D.

Clinica Luis Razetti and Metropolitan
Center of Ophthalmology
Francisco Risquez Hospital
Caracas, Venezuela

Oscar Beaujon Balbi, M.D.

Clinica Luis Razetti and Metropolitan
Center of Ophthalmology
Hospital F.A. Risquez. Caracas Venezuela.
Caracas, Venezuela

Ronald Buggage, M.D.

Director, Uveitis Fellowship Program
National Eye Institute
National Institutes of Health
Bethesda, Maryland

Mary Jude Cox, M.D.

Glaucoma Fellow, Wills Eye Hospital
Jefferson Medical College
Thomas Jefferson University
Philadelphia, Pennsylvania

Erin C. Doe, M.D.

Director, Glaucoma Service
Brooke Army Medical Center
San Antonio, Texas

Francisco F. Fantes, M.D.

Associate Professor of Ophthalmology
Bascom Palmer Eye Institute
University of Miami School of Medicine
Miami, Florida

Alon Harris, M.S., Ph.D.

Director, Glaucoma Research and
Diagnostic Center
Letzter Professor of Ophthalmology
Professor of Physiology and Biophysics
Indiana University School of Medicine
Indianapolis, Indiana

Hiroshi Ishikawa, M.D.

Assistant Professor
Director, Ocular Imaging Center
The New York Eye and Ear Infirmary
New York, New York

John B. Jeffers, M.D.

Director, Residency Program
Wills Eye Hospital
Jefferson Medical College
Thomas Jefferson University
Philadelphia, Pennsylvania

L. Jay Katz, M.D., F.A.C.S.

Co-Director, Glaucoma Service
Wills Eye Hospital
Professor of Ophthalmology
Jefferson Medical College
Thomas Jefferson University
Philadelphia, Pennsylvania

Jeffrey M. Liebmann, M.D., F.A.C.S.

Associate Director, Glaucoma Service
Professor of Clinical Ophthalmology
The New York Eye and Ear Infirmary
New York, New York

Michele C. Lim, M.D.

Assistant Professor of Ophthalmology
University of California, Davis
Sacramento, California

Marlene M. Moster, M.D.

Professor of Clinical Ophthalmology
Wills Eye Hospital
Jefferson Medical College
Thomas Jefferson University
Philadelphia, Pennsylvania

Jonathan S. Myers, M.D.

Associate Professor of Ophthalmology
Jefferson Medical College
Thomas Jefferson University
Philadelphia, Pennsylvania

Jamie E. Nicholl, BFA

Ophthalmic Photographer
Wills Eye Hospital
Philadelphia, Pennsylvania

Paul F. Palmberg, M.D., Ph.D.

Professor of Ophthalmology
Bascom Palmer Eye Institute
University of Miami School of Medicine
Miami, Florida

Douglas J. Rhee, M.D.

Assistant Professor of Ophthalmology
Wills Eye Hospital
Assistant Professor of Pathology, Anatomy, and Cell Biology
Jefferson Medical College
Thomas Jefferson University
Philadelphia, Pennsylvania

Robert Ritch, M.D., F.A.C.S., FICS, FRC OPHTH

Surgeon Director
Chief, Glaucoma Service
Professor of Clinical Ophthalmology
The New York Eye and Ear Infirmary
New York, New York

Joel S. Schuman, M.D.

Director, Glaucoma Service
New England Eye Center
Professor of Ophthalmology
Tufts University School of Medicine
Boston, Massachusetts

Louis W. Schwartz, M.D.

Clinical Associate Professor
Jefferson Medical College
Thomas Jefferson University
Philadelphia, Pennsylvania

Geoffrey P. Schwartz, M.D.

Resident, Wills Eye Hospital
Jefferson Medical College
Thomas Jefferson University
Philadelphia, Pennsylvania

Clinton Sheets

Medical Student
Indiana University School of Medicine
Indianapolis, Indiana

Rajesh K. Shetty, M.D.

Glaucoma Fellow
Wills Eye Hospital
Philadelphia, Pennsylvania

George L. Spaeth, M.D.

Director, Glaucoma Service
Wills Eye Hospital
Professor of Ophthalmology
Jefferson Medical College
Thomas Jefferson University
Philadelphia, Pennsylvania

Celso Tello, M.D.

Clinical Assistant Professor of Ophthalmology
Glaucoma Associates of New York
The New York Eye and Ear Infirmary
New York, New York

Tara A. Uhler, M.D.

Glaucoma Fellow
Wills Eye Hospital
Philadelphia, Pennsylvania

Hoai Viet Tran, M.D.

Research Fellow
Director, Ultrasound Biomicroscopy
Laboratory
The New York Eye and Ear Infirmary
New York, New York

Zinaria Y. Williams

Medical Student
Tufts University School of Medicine
Boston, Massachusetts

ABOUT THE SERIES

The beauty of the atlas/synopsis concept is the powerful combination of illustrative photographs and a summary approach to the text. Ophthalmology is a very visual discipline which lends itself nicely to clinical photographs. While the five ophthalmic subspecialties in this series, Cornea, Retina, Glaucoma, Oculoplastics, and Neuroophthalmology, employ varying levels of visual recognition, a relatively standard format for the text is used for all volumes.

The goal of the series is to provide an up-to-date clinical overview of the major areas of ophthalmology for students, residents, and practitioners in all the healthcare professions. The abundance of large, excellent quality photographs and concise, outline-form text will help achieve that objective.

Christopher J. Rapuano, M.D.
Series Editor

FOREWORD

I would like to thank the many authors and contributors who participated in this endeavor. I believe that the diversity of representations is one of the strengths of this text.

PREFACE

Glaucoma: Color Atlas & Synopsis of Clinical/Ophthalmology attempts to cover as many of the glaucoma syndromes as possible. No condition appears identical in all cases. Therefore, many different representative images are presented for the more common conditions in an attempt to reflect the diversity of presentations. I hope that you will find this atlas to be a useful reference and an aid to your clinical endeavors.

Douglas J. Rhee, M.D.

GLAUCOMA DIAGNOSIS

Douglas J. Rhee, MD

INTRODUCTION

The term *glaucoma* is from the Greek *glaukos,* which means "watery blue." It is first mentioned in the Hippocratic Aphorisms around 400 BC. However, it was considered a disease of the crystalline lens for several hundred years following. "The scientific history of glaucoma began the day on which cataracts were put in their correct place" (Albert Terson, 1867–1935, French ophthalmologist). The correct anatomic location of cat 1894, German ophthalmologist) and its subsequent use by Edward Jaeger (1818–1884) led to the belief that the optic nerve was also involved. Cupping of the optic nerve as a sign of glaucoma was confirmed by anatomist Heinrich Muller in the late 1850s. Von Graefe is credited as having first described contraction of the visual field and paracentral defects in glaucoma in 1856.

In recent history, glaucoma had been defined by having an intraocular pressure (IOP) above 21 mm Hg (i.e., more than 2 standard deviations above the mean IOP from a population-based survey of IOP). Later research indicated that the majority of people with IOPs above 21 mm Hg do not develop glaucomatous visual field loss. Additionally, up to 40% of patients with documented glaucomatous visual field loss never achieve IOPs higher than 21 mm Hg. Our modern concept of primary open-angle glaucoma (POAG) is a description of the constellation of signs frequently seen in "glaucoma" that incorporate IOP, optic nerve appearance, and characteristic visual field changes. The hallmark of the diagnosis of glaucoma is progressive change in the optic nerve or visual field, or both, over time. Many glaucoma specialists believe that POAG probably represents many diseases with a final common pathway. I am sure that our definition of glaucoma will continue to evolve as our understanding of the disease increases.

A more modern definition for glaucoma is as follows: a pathologic condition in which there is a progressive loss of ganglion cell axons causing visual field damage that is related to IOP. Currently, we look to evaluate the following components when making the diagnosis of glaucoma: history, presence or absence of risk factors, IOP, optic nerve examination, and visual field testing.

The chapters in this section describe the various methods for obtaining the information we use for both diagnosing glaucoma and following the adequacy of treatment.

BIBLIOGRAPHY

Blodi FC. Development of our concept of glaucoma. In: *Basic and Clinical Science Course, Section 10.* San Francisco: American Academy of Ophthalmology; 1996.

Kronfeld PC. Glaucoma. In: *History of Ophthalmology.*

Mikelberg FS, Drance SM. Glaucomatous visual field defects. In: Ritch R, Shields MB, Krupin T, eds. *The Glaucomas.* St. Louis, MO: Mosby-Year Book; 523–537, 1996.

Sommer A, Tielsch JM, Katz J, Quigley HA, Gottsch JD, Javitt JC, Singh K. Relationship between intraocular pressure and primary open angle glaucoma among white and black Americans: The Baltimore eye survey. *Arch Ophthalmol* 109:1090–1095, 1991.

Chapter 1

BASICS OF AQUEOUS FLOW AND OPTIC NERVE

Douglas J. Rhee, MD

THE IMPORTANCE OF INTRAOCULAR PRESSURE

Having a basic understanding of the physiology of the eye is helpful to understanding the pathophysiology, diagnosis, and management of glaucoma. Many clinicians and scientists now believe that several factors are involved in the pathogenesis of glaucoma, such as apoptosis, altered blood flow to the optic nerve, and possible autoimmune reactions. However, intraocular pressure remains one of the most important risk factors for the disease syndromes. Additionally, lowering of the intraocular pressure is the only rigorously proven treatment for glaucoma. Although we have some understanding of the physiology of intraocular pressure, we do not yet fully understand how the eye regulates intraocular pressure at the cellular and molecular level. With each passing year, more is learned about this physiologic process. Some day, we may have the answer to what many patients have asked—what causes my eye pressure to be too high?

BRIEF SUMMARY OF AQUEOUS PHYSIOLOGY AND INTRAOCULAR PRESSURE

Aqueous is formed in the ciliary processes (pars plicata region of the retina) (Figure 1-1A–C). The epithelial cells of the inner nonpigmented layer are felt to be the site of aqueous production (Figure 1-2). Aqueous is produced by a combination of active secretion, ultrafiltration, and diffusion. Many of the intraocular pressure–lowering agents work by decreasing aqueous secretion in the ciliary body.

Aqueous then flows through the pupil and into the anterior chamber nourishing the lens, cornea, and iris (Figure 1-3). Aqueous drains

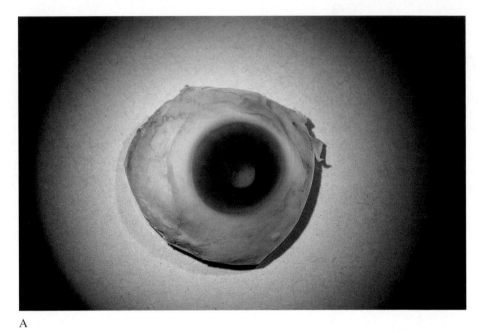

A

Figure 1-1A,B,C   Gross dissection of a cadaver eye   **A.** *Anterior segment from a cadaver eye.*

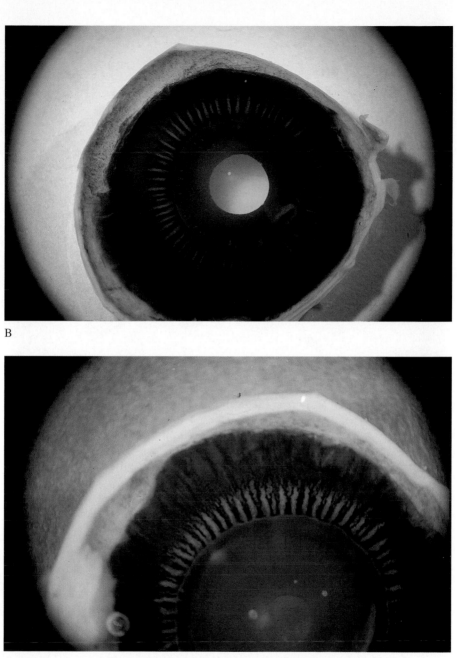

B

C

Figure 1-1A,B,C Gross dissection of a cadaver eye *(continued)* **B.** *Same anterior segment turned over, looking from behind the lens. The lens is still supported by the zonular fibers extending from the ciliary body processes.* **C.** *Higher magnification view of the ciliary body process. This region is called the pars plicata. The pars plana is peripheral to the pars plana.*

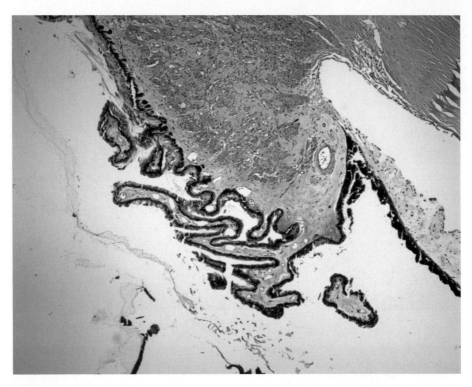

Figure 1-2 Hemotoxylin and eosin (H&E)–stained section of the ciliary body *The multiple folds help increase the overall surface area.*

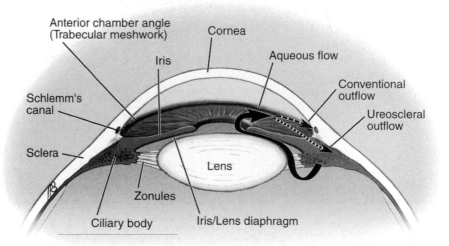

Figure 1-3 Route of aqueous flow *Schematic diagram showing the route of aqueous from the ciliary body to the outflow tract. (From Rhee DJ, Budenz DL. Acute angle-closure glaucoma. In:* Atlas of Office Procedures. *Philadelphia: Saunders, 3(2):267–279, 2000.)*

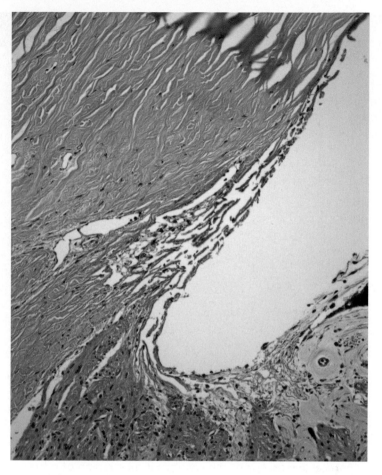

Figure 1-4   H&E-stained section of the anterior chamber angle showing the outflow tracts of the eye   *The conventional outflow pathway consists of seven layers of trabecular meshwork beams (corneoscleral and uveal trabecular meshwork), the juxtacanalicular region, Schlemm's canal, collecting channels, and episcleral veins. The uveoscleral pathway consists of the uveal face, with flow eventually moving into the choroidal space. This pathway is not well understood. There is evidence to show that the aqueous drains out the vortex veins and through the scleral wall.*

through the anterior chamber angle, which contains the trabecular meshwork and ciliary body face (Figure 1-4).

Between 80% and 90% of aqueous outflow is through the trabecular meshwork (TM)—the so-called conventional pathway—with the remaining 10% to 20% through the ciliary body face—the so-called uveoscleral or alternative pathway. The TM is thought to be the region where regulation of aqueous humor outflow takes place. Within the TM, especially under conditions of elevated intraocular pressure, the juxtacanalicular area appears to have the highest resistance to outflow (Figure 1-5).

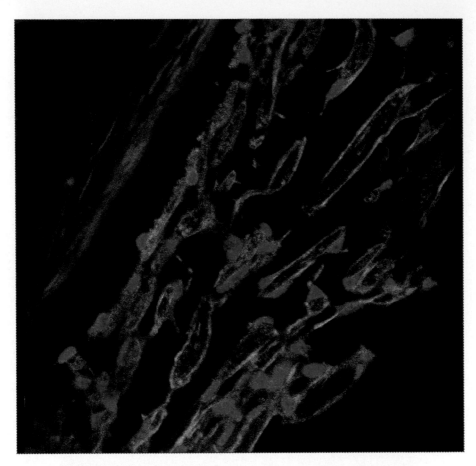

Figure 1-5   Confocal microscopy of the juxtacanalicular region of trabecular meshwork (TM)   *The green (fluorescein labeled) indicates staining for a nonspecific secreted matricellular protein. The red (Texas red labeled) indicates staining for smooth muscle actin (within the TM endothelial cells), whereas the blue (DAPI) stains for nuclear material. These smaller, bubble-shaped nuclei correspond to the cells of the inner wall of Schlemm's canal, whereas the elongated nuclei correspond to the TM endothelial cells. One can see that the uveal and corneoscleral TM consists of endothelial cell–lined beams, whereas the juxtacanalicular region is an amorphous area of extracellular matrix and TM endothelial cells.*

Intraocular pressure is physiologically determined by the rate of aqueous production in the ciliary body, resistance to outflow through the conventional outflow tract (trabecular meshwork and Schlemm's canal), resistance to outflow through the unconventional outflow tract (uveoscleral outflow), and episcleral venous pressure. In the Goldmann equation $[P_0 = (F/C) + P_v]$, P represents the intraocular pressure, F is the rate of aqueous formation, and C is the facility of outflow, which roughly corresponds to the inverse of the total resistance to outflow. As one can imagine, elevations of episcleral venous pressure can result in an elevated intraocular pressure (Figure 1-6A–E).

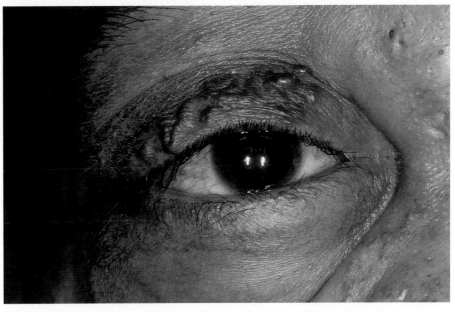

A

Figure 1-6A–E   Composite figure showing an extreme example of neglected bilateral carotid cavernous sinus fistula   A–C. *The chronic elevation of venous pressure has resulted in dilation of all the downstream venous channels with lid involvement. The patient had elevated intraocular pressure with moderate generalized cupping in the right optic nerve* (**D**) *and inferior notch in the left optic nerve* (**E**).

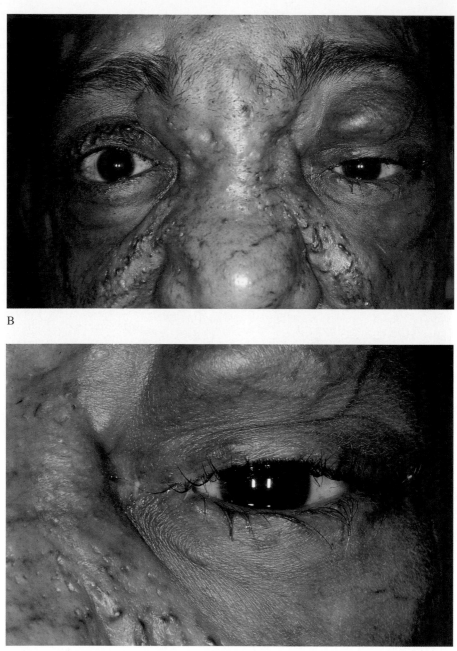

B

C

Figure 1-6A–E *(continued)*

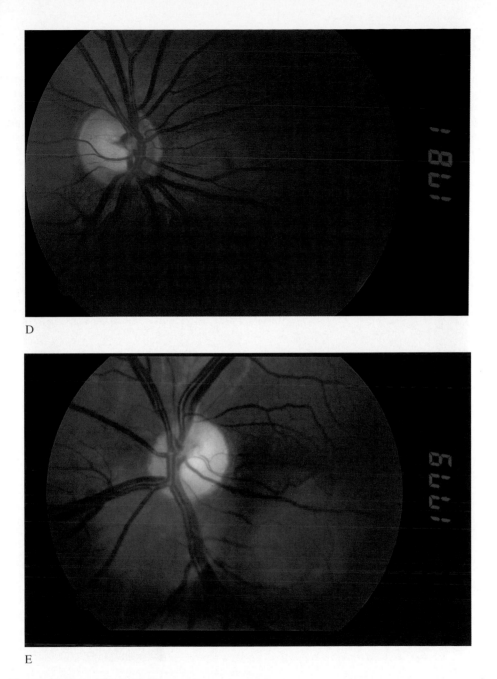

D

E

Figure 1-6A–E *(continued)*

OPTIC NERVE

The optic nerve consists of all the axons from the ganglion cell layer of the retina. The optic nerve is the site of damage in glaucoma (Figures 1-7 and 1-8A,B). Functionally, optic nerve damage causes visual field changes. Without treatment, an elevated intraocular pressure can result in progressive loss of the visual field, eventually leading to blindness. The various patterns of optic nerve change and means of measuring the functional status of the optic nerve are described in more detail in subsequent chapters.

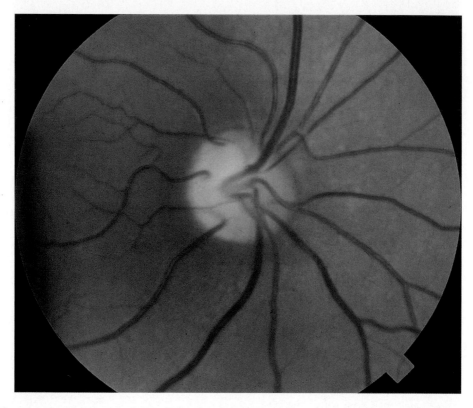

Figure 1-7 *Photograph of the optic nerve showing an inferior notch from a patient with glaucoma. Note the relative absence of pallor. (Contributed by L. Jay Katz, MD, Wills Eye Hospital, Philadelphia, PA.)*

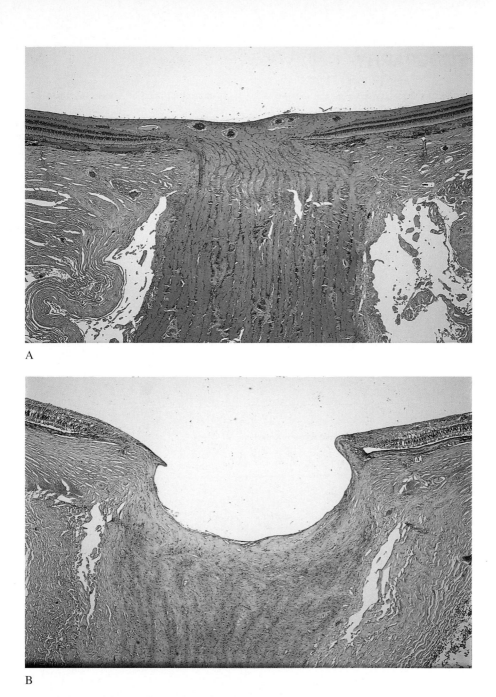

A

B

Figure 1-8A,B   H&E-stained histopathologic section of optic nerves   A. *Normal optic nerve.* **B.** *Optic nerve from advanced glaucoma (bean pot cup). (Contributed by Ralph J. Eagle, MD, Wills Eye Hospital, Philadelphia, PA.)*

BIBLIOGRAPHY

Bill A. The drainage of aqueous humor. *Invest Ophthalmol Vis Sci* 14:1–3, 1975.

Bill A, Phillips CI. Uveoscleral drainage of aqueous humour in human eyes. *Exp Eye Res* 12:275–281, 1971.

Grant WM. Further studies on facility of flow through the trabecular meshwork. *Arch Ophthalmol* 60:523–533, 1958.

Maepea O, Bill A. Pressures in the juxtacanalicular tissue and Schlemm's canal in monkeys. *Exp Eye Res* 54:879–883, 1992.

Maepea O, Bill A. The pressures in the episcleral veins, Schlemm's canal and trabecular meshwork in monkeys: Effects of changes in intraocular pressure. *Exp Eye Res* 49:645–663, 1989.

Moses RA, Grodzki WJ, Etheridge EL, Wilson CD. Schlemm's canal: The effect of intraocular pressure. *Invest Ophthalmol Vis Sci* 20:61–68, 1981.

Pederson JE, Gaasterland DE, MacLellan HM. Uveoscleral aqueous outflow in the rhesus monkey: Importance of uveal reabsorption. *Invest Ophthalmol Vis Sci* 16:1008–1017, 1977.

Seiler T, Wollensak J. The resistance of the trabecular meshwork to aqueous humor outflow. *Graefes Arch Clin Exp Ophthalmol* 223:88–91, 1985.

Chapter 2

TONOMETRY

Rajesh K. Shetty, MD

Tonometry is the measurement of the intraocular pressure (the pressure within the eye). The instruments used in tonometry rely on deforming an area of the cornea with a small amount of force that is used to calculate the intraocular pressure.

Tonometers can be divided into types that applanate, or flatten, the cornea and those that indent it. The accuracy of either type of tonometer assumes that all eyes have a similar ocular rigidity, corneal thickness, and ocular blood flow.

GOLDMANN APPLANATION TONOMETER (FIGURE 2-1)

Applanation tonometry is based on the Imbert-Fick Law that the intraocular pressure is equal to the amount of force needed to flatten a spherical surface divided by the applanated area. Goldmann applanation, the "gold-standard" and most commonly used form of tonometry, was introduced in 1954. This technique can be used only in patients seated at the slit lamp. The cornea is viewed through a prismatic doubling device in the center of a cone-shaped head that is obliquely illuminated with a cobalt blue light. While the patient's head is held steady, the applanation head is gently placed against a fluorescein-stained, anesthetized cornea (Figure 2-2). The examiner sees a split image of the tear film meniscus around the tonometer head. These fluorescein rings just overlap when the pressure at the head equals the intraocular pressure. The

graduated dial on the side measures the force in grams and is converted to millimeters of mercury by multiplying by ten.

With a circular applanation surface of 3.06 mm in diameter, the surface tension of the tear film counteracts the force needed to overcome the rigidity of the cornea, allowing the amount of force applied to equal the intraocular pressure. The tip flattens the cornea less than 0.2 mm, displaces 0.5 μL of aqueous, increases the intraocular pressure by 3%, and provides a reliable measurement of ±0.5 mm Hg. In corneas with high astigmatism (greater than 3 diopters), the flattest corneal meridian should be placed at 45 degrees to the axis of the cone. This can be done simply by placing the red line on the tonometer tip at the same axis of the minus cylinder of the eye.

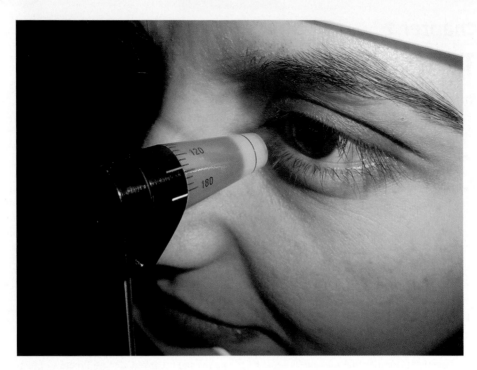

Figure 2-1 Goldmann tonometer *Example of a Goldmann tonometer mounted on a Haag-Streit slit lamp. The red lines on the cone can be aligned to the axis of negative cylinder in patients with high astigmatism.*

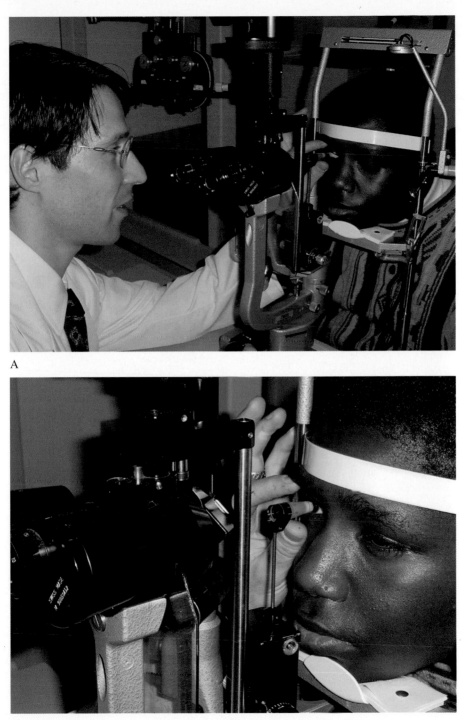

A

B

Figure 2-2A,B Applanation technique *A. An individual demonstrating blepharospasm on attempted applanation. B. Successful contact between the tonometer tip and the cornea, with the examiner demonstrating proper technique of placing supporting traction only on the orbital rims, not on the globe itself.*

SCHIÖTZ TONOMETER (FIGURE 2-3)

Introduced in 1905, the Schiötz tonometer is the classic indentation tonometer, and requires the patient to be supine. As opposed to applanation tonometry, the amount of indentation of the cornea by the Schiötz tonometer is proportionate to the intraocular pressure. This deformation, however, creates an unpredictable and relatively large intraocular volume displacement. The 16.5-g Schiötz tonometer has a base weight of 5.5 g that is attached to the plunger. This weight may be increased to 7.5, 10, or 15 g for higher ocular pressures. The calibrated footplate of the tonometer is placed gently on the anesthetized cornea, and the free vertical movement of the attached plunger determines the scale reading. To estimate intraocular pressure, conversion tables are available based on empirical data from both human cadaver eyes and in vivo studies. The tables assume a standard ocular rigidity such that in eyes with altered scleral rigidity (e.g., after retinal detachment surgery), the Schiötz measurement may not be accurate.

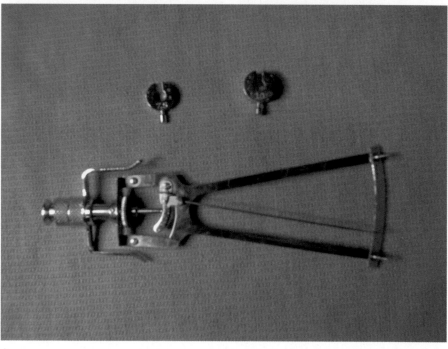

A

Figure 2-3A,B Schiötz tonometer *A. Image of the Schiötz tonometer with the 7.5- and 10-g weights shown.*

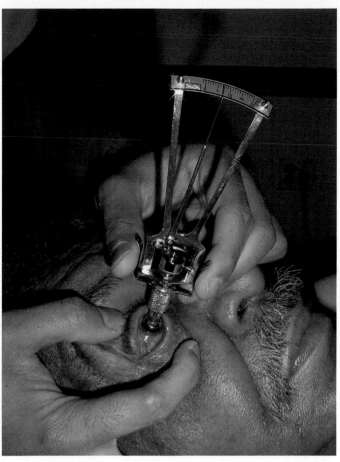

B

Figure 2-3A,B Schiötz tonometer *(continued)* ***B.*** *Schiötz indentation tonometry can be used only on patients in a supine position.*

PERKINS TONOMETER (FIGURE 2-4)

This handheld Goldmann-type applanation tonometer is especially useful in infants and children. The light source is battery powered, and the instrument can be used in either a vertical or a supine position. The force of corneal applanation varies by rotating a calibrated dial with the same measuring device as the Goldmann tonometer.

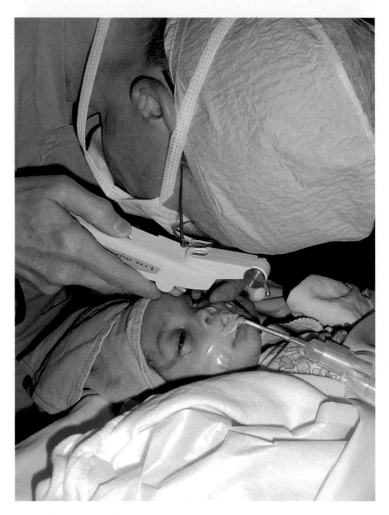

Figure 2-4　Perkins tonometer　*Perkins tonometry is commonly used in the examination of infants under anesthesia.*

TONO-PEN© (FIGURE 2-5)

The handheld Tono-Pen© (Mentor Ophthalmics, Santa Barbara, CA) can measure intraocular pressure in either a seated or a supine patient. This technique is especially useful in patients with scarred or edematous corneas, those unable to be examined at a slit lamp, or pediatric patients. With a Mackay-Marg–type of tonometer such as the Tono-Pen©, the effects of corneal rigidity are transferred to a surrounding sleeve so that the central plate measures only the intraocular pressure. A microprocessor in the Tono-Pen© that is connected to a strain-gauge transducer measures the force of the 1.02-mm diameter central plate as it applanates the corneal surface. Measurements of four to ten readings will give a final readout with a variability between the lowest and highest acceptable readings of less than 5%, 10%, 20%, or greater than 20%.

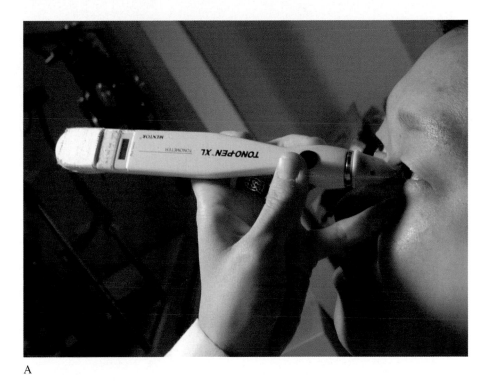

A

Figure 2-5A,B   Tono-Pen©   *A. The Tono-Pen XL© is a handheld device that does not require a slit lamp.*

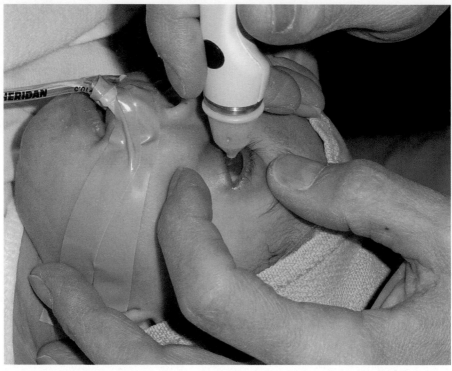

B

Figure 2-5A,B **Tono-Pen©** *(continued)* ***B.*** *Proper placement of the Tono-Pen© is 90 degrees perpendicular to the surface of the cornea. The small diameter of the Tono-Pen© makes it also useful in children.*

PNEUMOTONOMETER

This handheld device can also be used without a slit lamp, with the patient seated or supine, and on eyes with irregular corneal surfaces. Like the Tono-Pen©, this Mackay-Marg–type tonometer has its sensing surface in the center, with an adjacent surrounding rim that transfers the force needed to overcome corneal rigidity.

The central sensing area is a silastic diaphragm that caps an air-filled plunger. When this flexible diaphragm is applied to the cornea, gas escape from the plunger is impeded, allowing the air pressure to rise until it balances the intraocular pressure. An electronic transducer measures the air pressure in the chamber.

Chapter 3

GONIOSCOPY

Oscar V. Beaujon-Balbi, MD

Oscar Beaujon-Rubin, MD

Gonioscopy is an examination of great importance for the evaluation, diagnosis, and treatment of the patient with glaucoma. Its main purpose is visualization of the configuration of the anterior chamber angle. Under normal circumstances, the structures of the anterior angle cannot be seen directly through the cornea because of the optical phenomenon known as total internal reflection. Briefly, this phenomenon refers to optical physics whereby light that is reflected from the anterior chamber angle is bent internally within the cornea at the cornea-air interface. The gonioscopy lens (or goniolens) eliminates this effect by placing the lens-air interface at a different angle, making it possible to observe the light reflected from the structures of the angle.

Gonioscopy can be direct or indirect, depending on the lens employed, with a magnification of 15 to 20 times normal.

DIRECT GONIOSCOPY

The Koeppe lens is an example of a direct gonioscopy instrument (Figure 3-1A,B). It requires a magnification device (microscope) and a separate light source. The patient needs to be in a supine position.

Advantages

- Direct gonioscopy is useful in patients with nystagmus and irregular corneas.

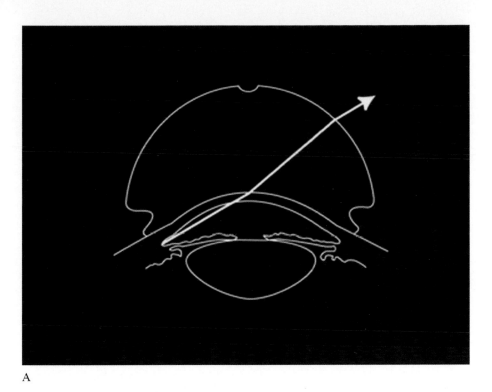

A

Figure 3-1A,B   Direct Gonioscopy instruments   *A. Direct gonioscopy.*

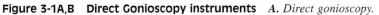

- It is useful for examination in children at the office under topical anesthesia. If necessary they can be sedated as usual, and the Koeppe lens allows examination of both the angle and the posterior pole.
- It allows a wide and panoramic evaluation of the angle that enables comparison between the different sectors and between both eyes if two lenses are placed simultaneously.
- It allows retroillumination, which is of great importance in differentiating congenital and acquired abnormalities of the angle (Figure 3-2).

Disadvantages

- Direct gonioscopy requires that the patient be in the supine position.
- It is technically more difficult to perform.
- It requires a separate light source and magnification device (microscopy) with less optic quality than the examination made at the slit lamp (Figure 3-3).

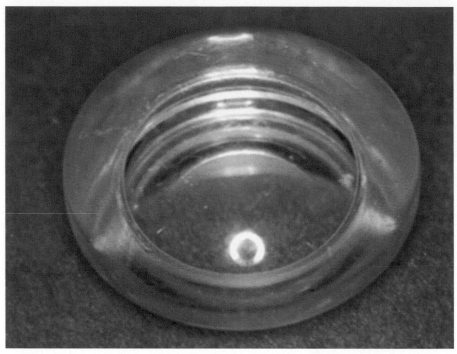

B

Figure 3-1A,B *B. Koeppe lens. (continued)*

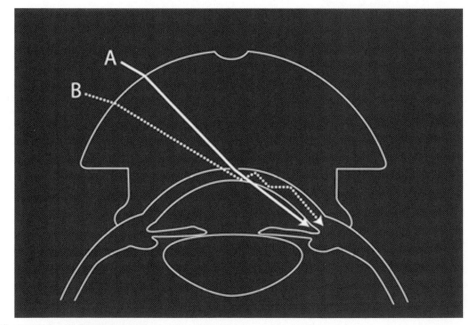

Figure 3-2 **Retroillumination** *Retroillumination with the Koeppe lens.*

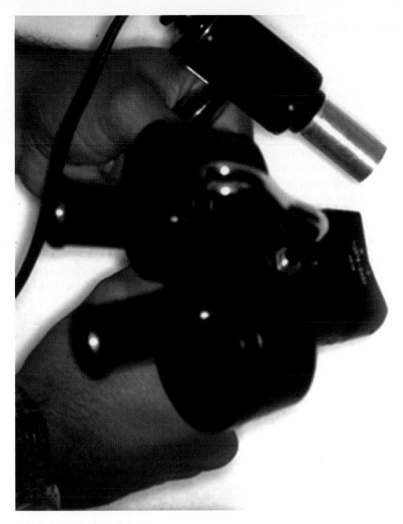

Figure 3-3 Barkan's device *Barkan's optical and illumination device.*

INDIRECT GONIOSCOPY

The angle is visualized with a lens that has one or more mirrors, allowing the evaluation of the structures opposite to the mirror employed. For evaluating the nasal quadrant, the mirror is placed temporally, but the superior and inferior orientation of the image is maintained. The examination is performed using the slit lamp. Since the introduction of Goldmann's indirect concept with the one-mirror goniolens, multiple lenses have been developed (Table 3-1). Lenses are available with two mirrors that enable examination of all quadrants with rotation of 90 degrees of the lens. Other lenses, with four mirrors, allow evaluation of the entire angle without rotation. The Goldmann and similar lenses have a contact surface with a curvature radius and diameter higher than the cornea, requiring the use of a viscous coupling substance. Zeiss and similar lenses do not require any coupling substance, because the radius of curvature is similar to that of the anterior cornea. These lenses also have a smaller contact surface diameter, and the tear film fills the cornea-lens space (Figure 3-4A–C).

Proper selection of the type of goniolens is crucial to perform an effective gonioscopy. To aid this selection, some aspects should be considered. Without using a goniolens, the anterior chamber depth can first be estimated using Van Herick Shaffer's method. If a wide-open angle is suspected, any lens could be employed because there is no element that would prevent visualization of the angle (Figure 3-5).

TABLE 3-1   CHARACTERISTICS OF GONIOLENSES

Lens	Corneal Diameter (mm)	Radius (mm)	Peripheral Curve (mm)	Distance to Center (mm)	Mirror Height (mm)
Goldmann, 3 mirrors	12	7.4	3	7	12
Goldmann, 1 mirror	12	7.4	1.5	3	17
Zeiss, 3 mirrors	11	7.7	3.5	7	20
Zeiss, 4 mirrors	9	7.85	—	5	12
Allen Thorpe	10	8.15	—	5	7
Sussman OS4M	9	—	—	—	15

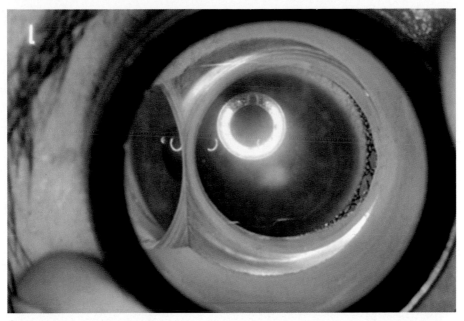

A

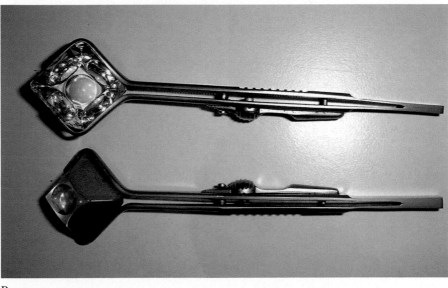

B

Figure 3-4A–C Types of goniolenses *A. Indirect gonioscopy using a Goldmann one-mirror lens. **B.** Zeiss four-mirror type of indirect goniolens, which uses a handle.*

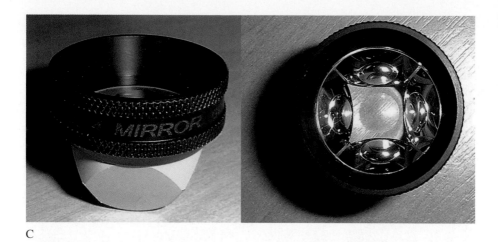

C

Figure 3-4A–C Types of goniolenses *(continued)* *C. Sussman four-mirror type of indirect goniolens, which is handheld.*

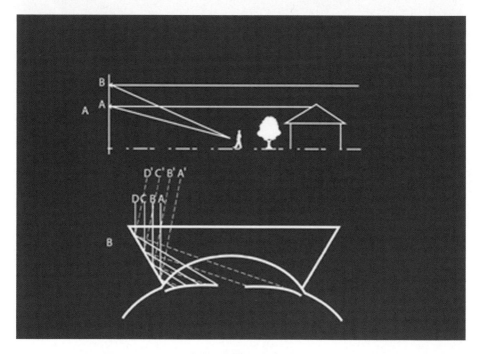

Figure 3-5 Diagram of an open-angle configuration *This figure shows that with an open angle, you can view any object in a reflective mirror, no matter the height or distance from the center, because you do not have any interference.*

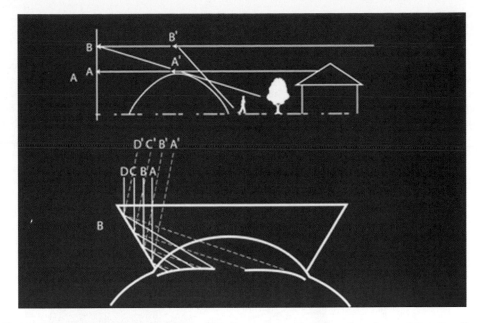

Figure 3-6   Observer and obstacle   *This figure shows that when there is an obstruction (in this example, the hill; with gonioscopy, the convex iris of a narrow angle), it is better to be higher and closer to the center. This is analogous to using a goniolens whose mirrors are higher and closer to the center.*

On the other hand, if a shallow angle is suspected, it is preferable to use a one- or two-mirror Goldmann or a Zeiss lens. The mirrors of these goniolenses are higher and closer to the center, enabling visualization of the structures that would be otherwise occluded by the anterior displacement of the lens-iris diaphragm. To better explain this concept, see Figure 3-6. Imagine an observer standing at point A who wants to see a house that is placed behind a hill. The hill in this example resembles the iris convexity. To solve the problem, the observer could go to a higher point, B, that enables him to see the house, or move closer to the center (top of the hill), point A', or even better, go to point B', which allows complete observation of the house and surrounding elements.

ESTIMATING THE ANTERIOR CHAMBER DEPTH

Before evaluating the anterior chamber angle configuration, the Van Herick-Shaffer technique is used to estimate the anterior angle depth. The procedure is performed while evaluating the patient with the slit lamp. With the thinnest slit beam possible, the cornea is illuminated perpendicularly near the temporal limbus (creating an optical section) and viewed at 50 to 60 degrees from the slit incidence. To estimate the anterior chamber depth, the ratio between the cornea-iris distance and corneal thickness is observed. If the separation of the cornea-iris is more than 50% of the corneal thickness, the anterior chamber is most likely deep with a wide-angle configuration (Figure 3-7A,B). On the other hand, if it is less than 50%, a narrow angle is suspected (Figure 3-7C,D).

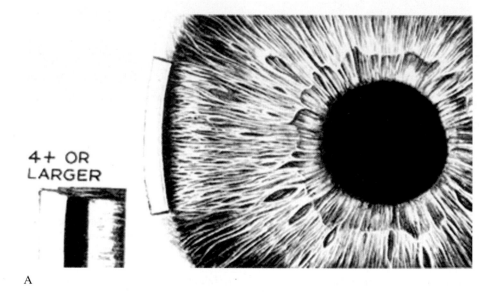

4+ OR
LARGER

A

Figure 3-7A,B Van Herick's technique for angle depth estimation *A. Schematic showing proper placement of the slit beam; magnified view shows the depth of the anterior chamber (AC) (black) is greater than 50% of the corneal slit beam (white), estimating a wide angle.*

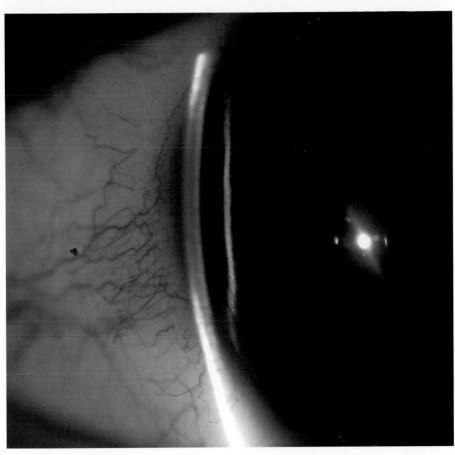

B

Figure 3-7A,B   Van Herick's technique for angle depth estimation   *(continued)*
B. Demonstration of the preceding placement in a live patient. In this example, the AC depth is approximately 90% of the corneal slit beam.

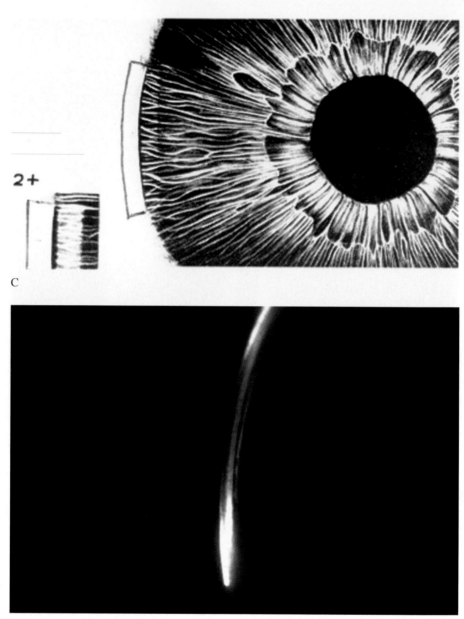

C

D

Figure 3-7C,D   Van Herick's technique   *C. Schematic showing proper placement of the slit beam; magnified view shows the AC depth (black) is less than 50% of the corneal slit beam (white), estimating a narrow angle. **D**. Demonstration of the preceding placement in a live patient. In this example, the AC depth is approximately 10% to 15% of the corneal slit beam.*

The angle can be graded as follows:

Grade 0 (closed)—when the iris is contacting the corneal endothelium

Grade I—when the space between the iris and cornea is less than 25% of corneal thickness

Grade II—when the space is 25%

Grade III—when it is 25% to 50%

Grade IV—when it is higher than 50%

This technique does not substitute gonioscopy, but it can be of great help in estimating the amplitude of the anterior chamber, especially in patients with opacities or cloudy corneas.

GONIOSCOPY

Technique

A drop of anesthetic is administered to both eyes, and the examination is performed at the slit lamp. Depending on the lens employed, a viscous coupling substance may be required. The goniolens must be placed gently on the eye, while trying to avoid distortion of the intraocular elements (Figures 3-8A,B,C and 3-9). To obtain a good view of the angle, the incidence of the light beam must be perpendicular to the mirror of the goniolens. Some adjustments on the slit lamp have to be made as the evaluation

is performed:

- To evaluate the superior and inferior angles, the patient is asked to look at the light source.
- To evaluate the nasal and temporal angles, the illumination source is inclined forward and the goniolens is shifted slightly downward, and the patient is asked to look to the side being evaluated.

These simple technical details are vital to enable evaluation of narrow angles and to identify the different elements of the angle, especially Schwalbe's line.

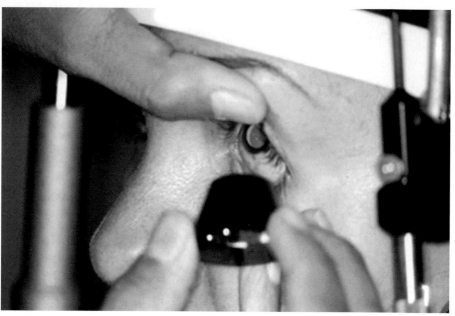

A

Figure 3-8A,B,C Goldmann goniolens *Placing of a Goldmann one-mirror–type goniolens.*

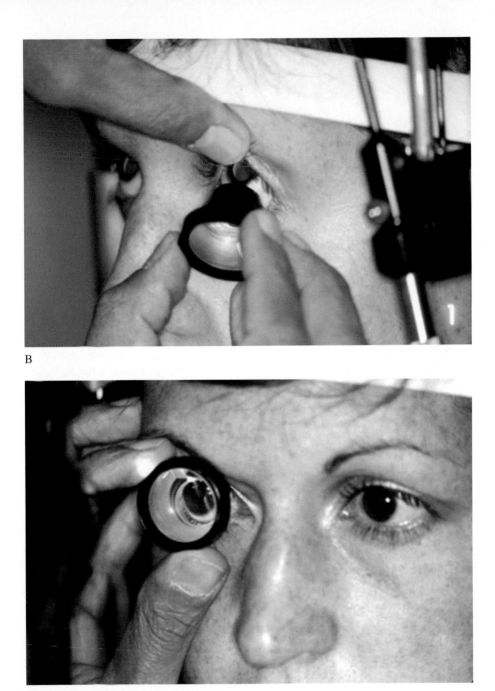

B

C

Figure 3-8A,B,C   *(continued)*

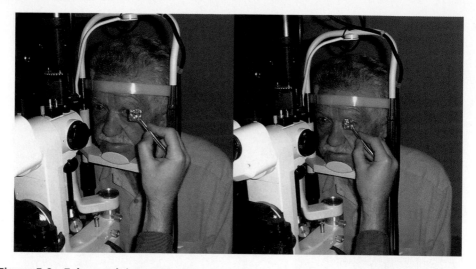

Figure 3-9   Zeiss goniolens   *Placing of a Zeiss-type goniolens.*

Elements of the Angle Structure

In Figure 3-10A,B, the different elements to be identified during gonioscopy are illustrated. The angle extends from the last iris fold to Schwalbe's line. The angle structures can be divided into two groups:

1. A fixed portion that includes Schwalbe's line, the trabecular meshwork, and the scleral spur.
2. A mobile portion that includes the anterior-superior face of the ciliary body and the iris insertion, with its last fold.

The examiner must make a general inspection in order to identify some important aspects:

Iris plane—this can be planar on wide angles and very convex on narrow angles.

Last iris fold and its distance from Schwalbe's line—these two elements are used to estimate the amplitude of the angle. The superior angle portion is generally narrower than the other portions.

Iris root—this represents the insertion on the ciliary body. It is the thinnest portion, and the most easily displaced with elevation of the posterior chamber pressure. In myopic eyes, the iris is larger and thinner, with numerous crypts, and is usually inserted more posterior on the ciliary body. On the other hand, in hyperopic eyes, the iris tends to be thicker and its insertion is more anterior than in emetopic eyes, resulting in a narrower angle configuration.

Iris nodules, cysts, nevi, or foreign bodies (Figure 3-11).

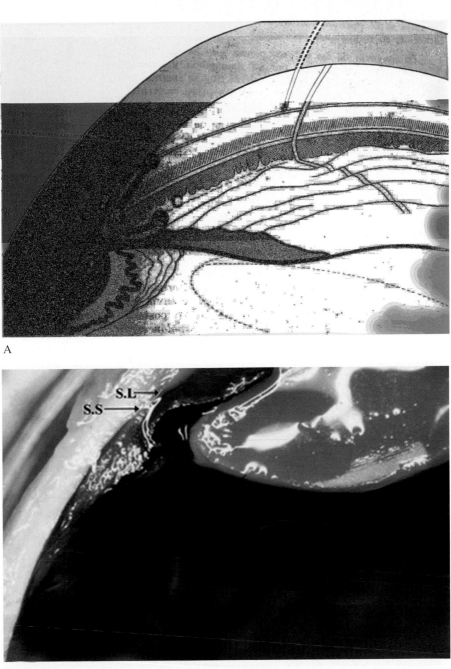

Figure 3-10A,B   Angle structure elements   *A. Schwalbe's line (S), scleral spur*
(E), and ciliary body (C). **B.** *Angle structure elements in a human cadaver eye.*
S.L. = Schwalbe's line; S.S. = scleral spur.

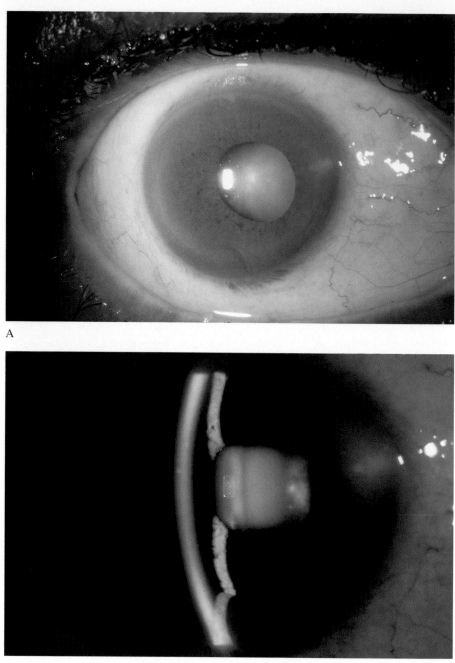

A

B

Figure 3-11A–C Iris cyst *A. Slit-lamp photograph showing an iris mass inferiorly. B. Slit beam showing the same.*

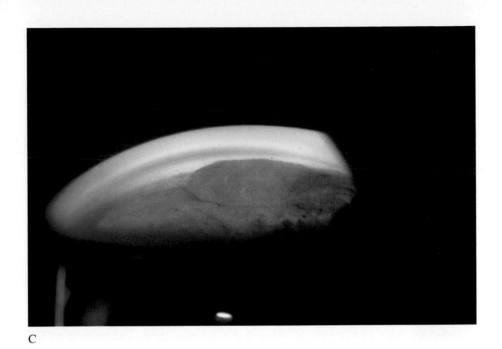

C

Figure 3-11A–C Iris cyst *(continued)* *C. Gonioscopic view of the inferior angle showing the cystic mass. The cystic nature of this mass was confirmed by ultrasound biomicroscopy (UBM) (not shown).*

Most of the time, it is easy to identify one element, making it possible to discern the others. For example, Figure 3-12 shows Schlemm's canal filled with blood. This is a frequent observation in patients with low intraocular pressure or those with increased pressure in the episcleral veins. *An elevation on episcleral venous pressure can occur* when the examiner presses the lens too strongly onto the sclera during gonioscopy. Pathologically, it can occur in cases of secondary glaucoma such as those caused by increased episcleral venous pressure, Sturge-Weber syndrome, carotid cavernous fistula, or in some cases of iridocyclitis in which the venous pressure of congestive eyes could be elevated, causing a passage of the blood from the venous system to Schlemm's canal.

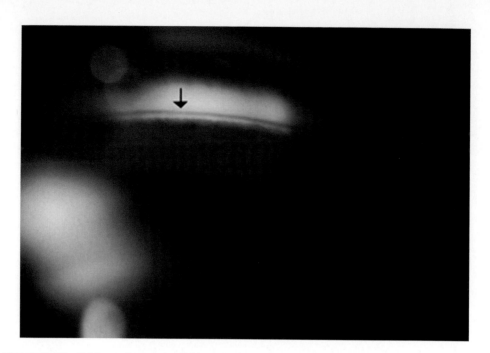

Figure 3-12   Schlemm's canal   *Schlemm's canal filled with blood* (arrow).

Identification of Angle Elements

Schwalbe's line represents the end of Descemet's membrane and marks the anterior limit of the angle. In some patients, Schwalbe's line can be thickened with protrusion to the anterior chamber, which has been termed posterior embryotoxon (Figure 3-13A,B).

Pigment frequently deposits around Schwalbe's line, because it marks the transition between the corneal and scleral curvatures. This change of curvature produces a step that facilities deposition of pigment and other material. If Schwalbe's line is not visible, it can easily be localized by aiming a thin slit beam on the angle. This beam gives reflexes on both the anterior and the posterior surfaces of the cornea. The inner reflection line corresponds to the posterior surface of the cornea and is contiguous with the angle structures and iris surface. The outer, corresponding to the anterior cornea, ends just where the Schwalbe's line is located, at the point where both light beams are joined (see Figures 3-10A and 3-14A,B). This maneuver is very important for evaluating a narrow angle and differentiating it from a closed angle (Figure 3-15).

In Figure 3-16, the following elements can be observed:

- Trabecular meshwork that extends from the scleral spur to Schwalbe's line.
- Schlemm's canal, situated just anterior to the scleral spur. The scleral spur has a grayish appearance in young patients and becomes more pigmented with age. In the figure, a pigment band is evident, corresponding to the pigmented trabecular meshwork.
- Scleral spur, a whiter line just inferior to the trabecular meshwork. This serves as the insertion to the longitudinal portion of the ciliary muscle.

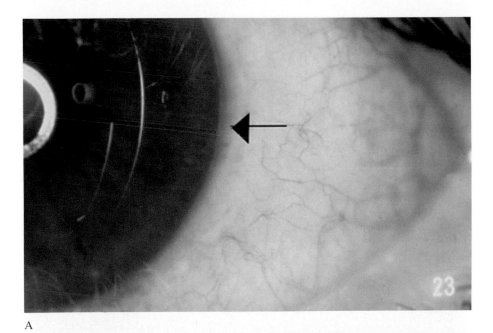

A

B

Figure 3-13A,B Schwalbe's line *A. Posterior embryotoxon* (arrow). *B. Schwalbe's line in gonioscopy* (arrow).

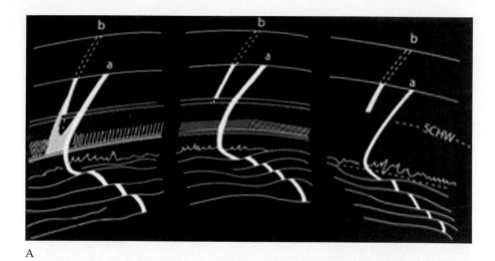

A

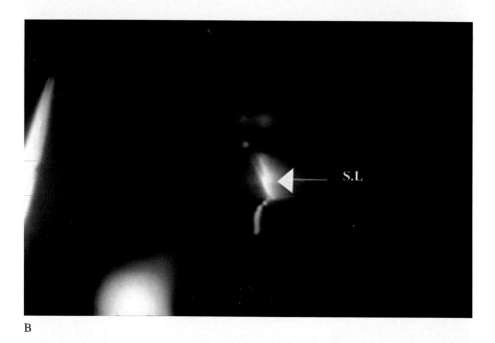

B

Figure 3-14A,B   Schwalbe's line   *A. Schwalbe's line localization using the edges of the corneal slit beam. The different beam reflexes are shown; "b" corresponds to anterior cornea and "a" to posterior cornea. **B.** Gonioscopic view demonstrating that Schwalbe's line is located where the anterior and posterior light reflexes of the corneal slit beam converge. S.L = Schwalbe's line* (arrow). *(A, Reproduced with permission from Beaujon-Rubin O, ed.* Glaucoma Primario: Diagnostico & Tratamiento. *Caracas, Venezuela: Venezuelan Society of Ophthalmology, 1983.)*

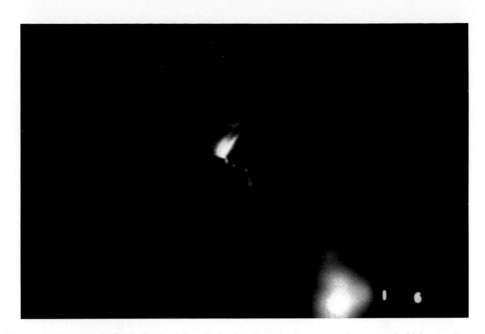

Figure 3-15 Schwalbe's line *Schwalbe's line localization using the corneal slit beams in a narrow angle.*

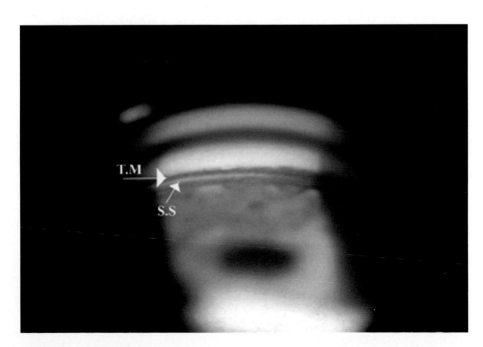

Figure 3-16 Gonioscopy *Open angle. T.M. = trabecular meshwork; S.S. = scleral spur.*

• Last iris fold, and anterior insertion of the ciliary body. The position where it is inserted determines in major part the amplitude of the chamber angle. The visible portion of the ciliary body extends from its insertion to the scleral spur and is covered anteriorly by trabecular meshwork, termed *uveal meshwork.*

Sometimes, this tissue is formed of wide and multiple bands that insert on the scleral spur, but they may also extend over the trabecular meshwork. These last are called *iris processes* (Figure 3-17). Iris processes can overpass the trabecular meshwork, coating the angle, and insert onto Schwalbe's line, representing a minor manifestation of abnormal embryologic development (Figure 3-18).

It is important to avoid confusing iris processes with peripheral anterior synechiae, which are products of adherence of the peripheral iris to any of the angle structures, most often Schwalbe's line or the peripheral cornea. Peripheral anterior synechiae are observed as tents passing over the angle (Figure 3-19A,B).

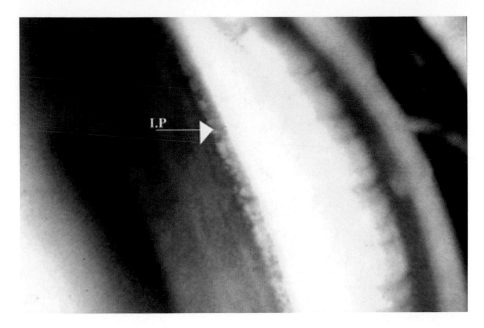

Figure 3-17 **Iris processes** *Gonioscopic view of the anterior chamber angle demonstrating iris prcoesses (I.P.;* arrow*).*

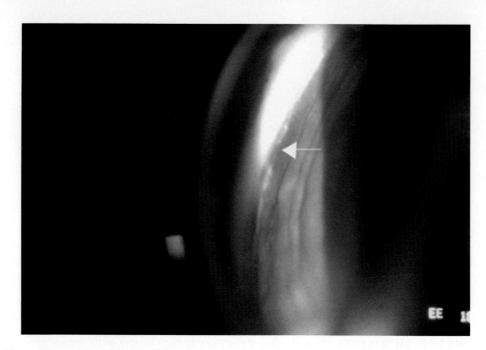

Figure 3-18   Iris processes   *Iris processes inserting onto Schwalbe's line* (arrow).

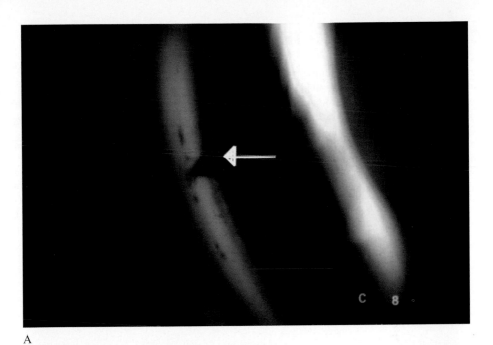

A

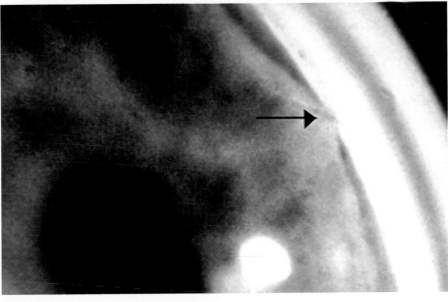

B

Figure 3-19A,B **Peripheral anterior synechiae** *Examples of peripheral anterior synechiae* (arrow).

CLASSIFICATION OF THE ANGLE

Among the objectives of gonioscopy is to determine the amplitude of the angle, and to determine whether the glaucoma is of the open-angle or closed-angle type. Each type has a different epidemiology, physiopathology, treatment, and prevention. Shaffer's classification (Figure 3-20) estimates the angle amplitude between the last iris fold and the trabecular meshwork–Schwalbe's line, as follows:

Grade IV—45 degrees.
Grade III—30 degrees.

Grade II—20 degrees; angle closure is possible.
Grade I—10 degrees; angle closure is likely.
Slit—angle is less than 10 degrees; angle closure is more likely.
Closed—iris is stuck to the meshwork (Figure 3-21).

Spaeth's classification adds detail regarding peripheral iris and the effects of indentation on the configuration of the angle (Figure 3-22).

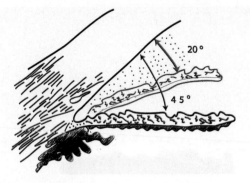

Figure 3-20 Shaffer's classification *Diagram of Shaffer's classification of angle amplitude.*

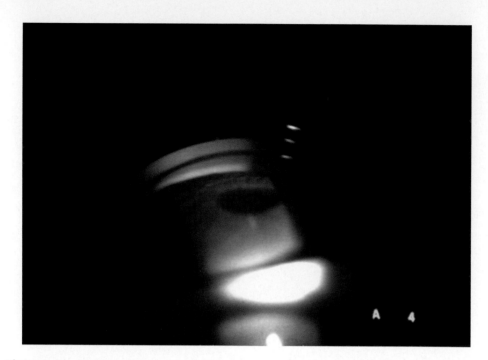

Figure 3-21   Narrow angle   *Aspect of the narrow angle on gonioscopy. Note the marked convexity of the iris, sometimes referred to as iris bowing. The angle structures are difficult to visualize.*

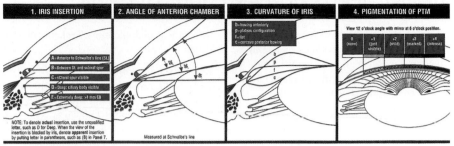

GONIOSCOPIC EVALUATION *(Spaeth Grading System)*

| 1. IRIS INSERTION | 2. ANGLE OF ANTERIOR CHAMBER | 3. CURVATURE OF IRIS | 4. PIGMENTATION OF PTM |

COSOPT is indicated for the reduction of elevated intraocular pressure (IOP) in patients with open-angle glaucoma or ocular hypertension who are insufficiently responsive to beta blockers (failed to achieve target IOP determined after multiple measurements over time). The IOP-lowering effect of COSOPT b.i.d. was slightly less than that seen with the concomitant administration of 0.5% timolol b.i.d. and 2.0% dorzolamide t.i.d.

COSOPT is contraindicated in patients with (1) bronchial asthma; (2) a history of bronchial asthma; (3) severe chronic obstructive pulmonary disease (see WARNINGS); (4) sinus bradycardia; (5) second- or third-degree atrioventricular block; (6) overt cardiac failure (see WARNINGS); (7) cardiogenic shock; or (8) hypersensitivity to any component of this product.

A

GONIOSCOPIC EVALUATION *(Spaeth Grading System)*
Examples

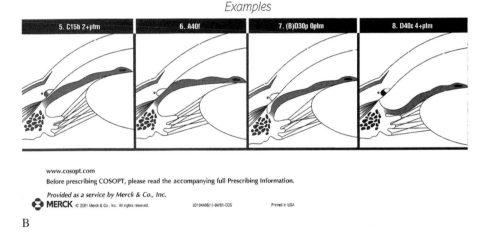

| 5. C15b 2+ptm | 6. A40f | 7. (B)D30p 0ptm | 8. D40c 4+ptm |

B

Figure 3-22 **Spaeth's classification** *Spaeth's classification, which provides additional information and detail. (Courtesy of Dr. George L. Spaeth, Wills Eye Hospital, Philadelphia, PA.)*

PIGMENT DEPOSITION AND GONIOSCOPY

The amount of pigment deposition in the angle varies widely among individuals. Sometimes the pattern can serve as a diagnostic tool to determine the underlying mechanism. Some examples are described next.

Pigmentary Glaucoma In this condition, a high dense band of brown pigment is deposited on the trabecular meshwork in a homogeneous fashion (Figure 3-23A). This pigment is observed on the posterior lens capsule and on the corneal endothelium (Krukenberg spindle) (Figure 3-23B).

Lens Pseudoexfoliation This entity occurs when material of amorphous substance is deposited on and anterior to Schwalbe's line in an undulating pattern known as Sampaolesi's sign (Figure 3-24). The material also deposits on lens zonule and can be observed during gonioscopy (Figure 3-25).

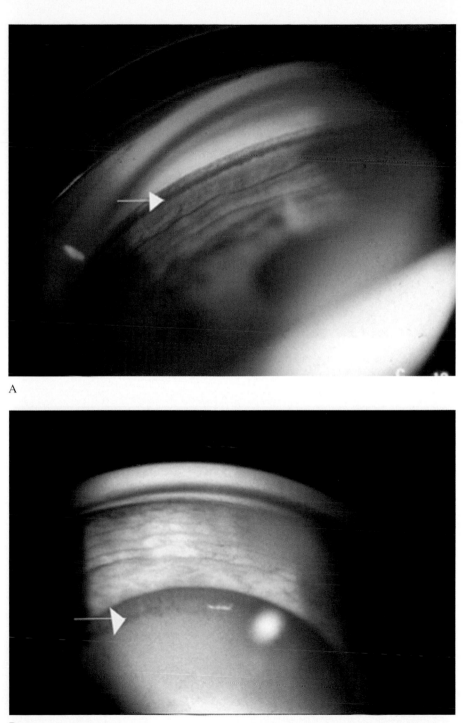

A

B

Figure 3-23A,B   Pigmentary glaucoma   *A. Pigmentary deposition on the trabecular mesh-work* (arrow) *in an eye with pigment dispersion syndrome.* ***B.*** *Pigmentary deposition on the posterior lens capsule (Zentmeyer line,* arrow) *in an eye with pigment dispersion syndrome.*

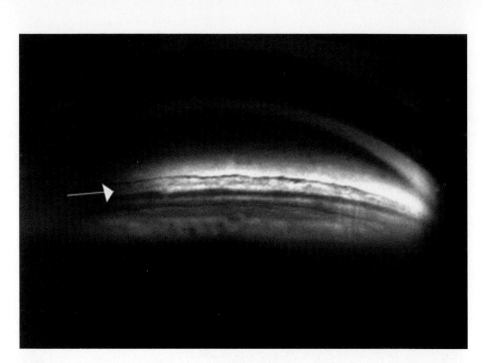

Figure 3-24 **Lens pseudoexfoliation** *Sampaolesi's sign* (arrow).

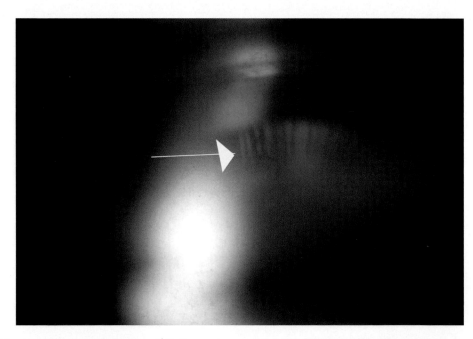

Figure 3-25 **Lens pseudoexfoliation** *Deposit of pseudoexfoliation material on the lens zonule* (arrow).

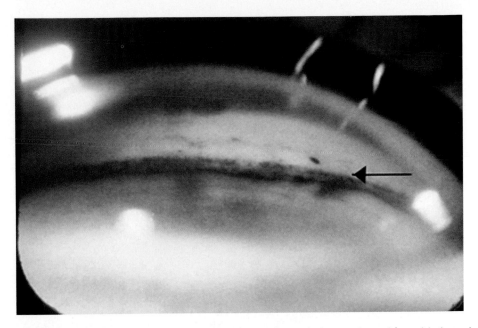

Figure 3-26 **Uveitis** *Irregular pigment deposits on the angle in a patient with uveitis* (arrow).

Uveitis In cases of uveitis, irregular areas of pigment deposits can be observed, giving an appearance of a "dirty" angle (Figure 3-26).

Angle-closure Glaucoma In cases of angle-closure glaucoma, a patchy area of pigment may be observed on any angle structure, an indication that the iris was stuck at that place but a permanent adherence did not develop. The presence of patchy pigment and a narrow angle can be an indication of a previous episode of acute angle-closure glaucoma (Figure 3-27).

Vascularization is usually absent on the angle. Sometimes, small branches of the ciliary body's arterial circle can be observed. These branches are usually covered by the uveal meshwork and form a circumferential serpiginous pattern or can be observed radially toward the iris sphincter. In neovascular glaucoma, abnormal vessels cross over the ciliary body and arborize the trabecular meshwork. Contraction of myofibrils of the fibroblasts that accompany the abnormal vessels causes peripheral anterior synechiae and angle closure (Figure 3-28A,B).

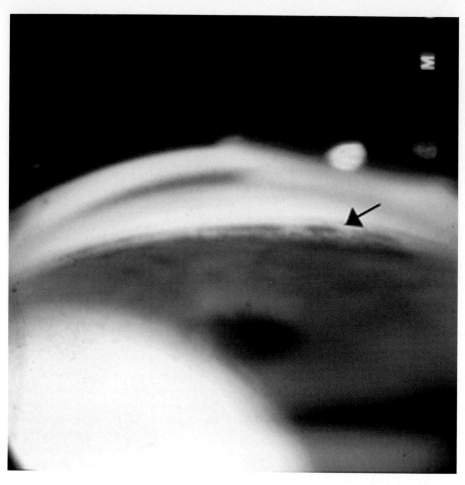

Figure 3-27   Angle-closure glaucoma   *Pigment patches formed after angle-closure crisis* (arrow).

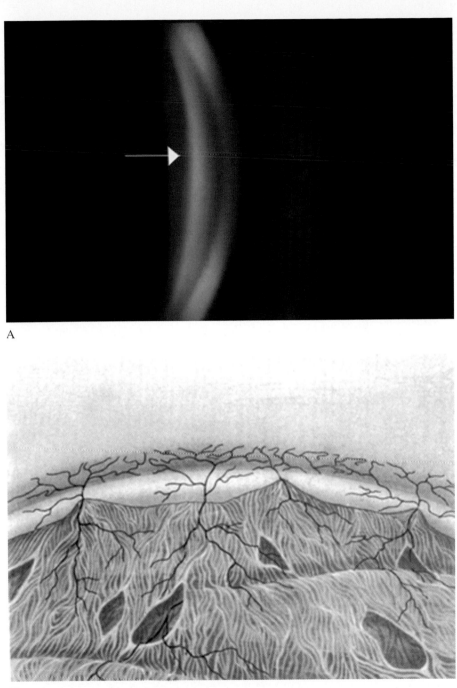

A

B

Figure 3-28A,B   Neovascular glaucoma   *A. Fibrovascular membrane over the angle* (arrow). *At this stage, the angle is open but occluded. There is marked corneal edema, giving a hazy view. B. Diagram of a fibrovascular membrane growing over the angle and causing peripheral anterior synechiae from contraction in neovascular glaucoma.*

ERROR FACTORS ON GONIOSCOPY

When performing gonioscopy, the examiner must be aware that some maneuvers alter the precision of the procedure. The gonioscopy lens can deepen the amplitude of the angle if too much pressure is applied to the sclera by forcing a fluid movement toward the angle (Figure 3-29).

This indentation goniscopy is invaluable in evaluating angle-closure glaucoma, especially in differentiating iris apposition from real synechiae. For this maneuver, the Zeiss type gonioscopy lens is recommended. The procedure, which is called dynamic gonioscopy, employs the mechanical effect on aqueous humor that follows the corneal indentation, enabling the examiner to alter the relative position of the iris in a dynamic way. This maneuver helps to distinguish narrow from closed angles and to determine the risk of closure. An excess of pressure produces folds on Descemet's membrane that makes evaluation of the angle difficult (Figure 3-30A,B).

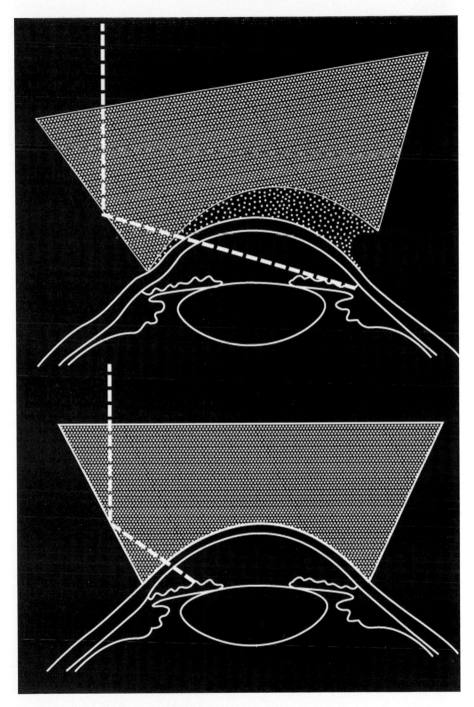

Figure 3-29 Error factors in gonioscopy *Placing obliquely directed pressure on the sclera.*

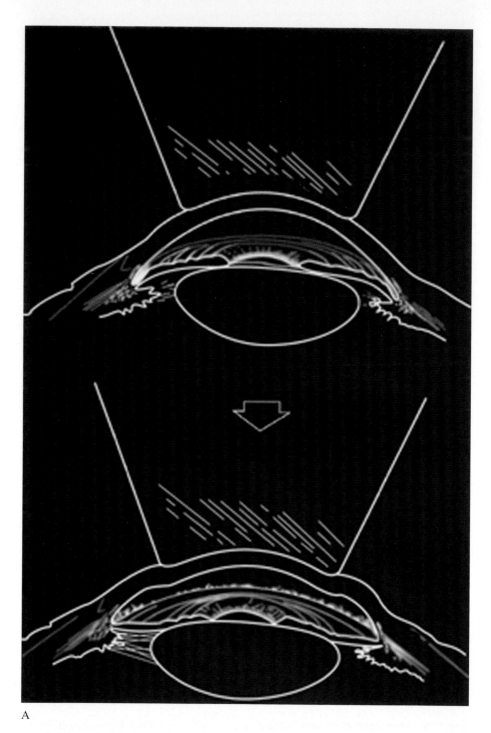

A

Figure 3-30A,B   Dynamic gonioscopy   *A. Schematic demonstrating dynamic, compression, or indentation gonioscopy.*

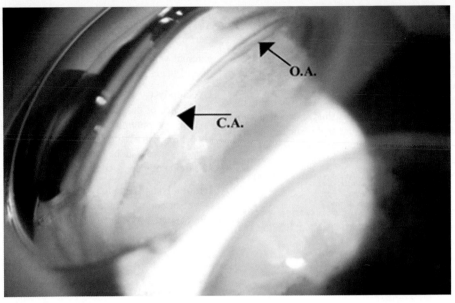

B

Figure 3-30A,B   Dynamic gonioscopy   (continued)   B. *Dynamic gonioscopy demonstrating peripheral anterior synechia formation (C.A. = closed angle) and chronic angle-closure glaucoma in a patient with narrow angles. Part of the angle is still open (O.A. = open angle).*

USE OF GONIOSCOPY IN TRAUMA

Contusion Trauma   When the cornea is hit, a wave of fluid abruptly forms. This wave moves toward the angle because the iris-lens diaphragm acts as a valve, preventing the fluid from going in a posterior direction. This fluid movement can harm the structures of the angle, creating acute lesions that are related to trauma intensity (Figure 3-31). Separation of the iris insertion from the scleral spur, termed *iridodialysis,* is one of these lesions (Figure 3-32).

Angle Recession   Angle recession occurs when the ciliary body is separated, leaving the external wall covered by the longitudinal portion of the ciliary muscle (Figure 3-33).

Cyclodialysis   Cyclodialysis is a completed dehiscence of the ciliary body from the sclera, opening a communication pathway to the suprachoroidal space (Figure 3-34). These gonioscopic patterns can be found in the same patient and frequently are accompanied by hyphema.

Iridodialysis   Iridodialysis occurs when there is separation of the iris insertion from the scleral spur.

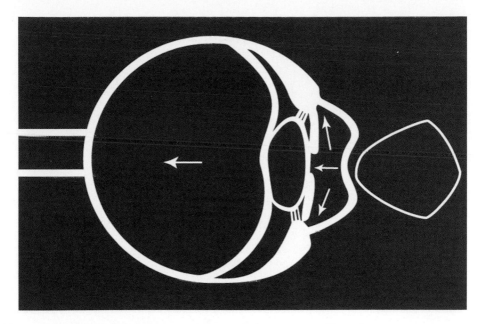

Figure 3-31   Contusion trauma   *Diagram of blunt trauma to the eye.*

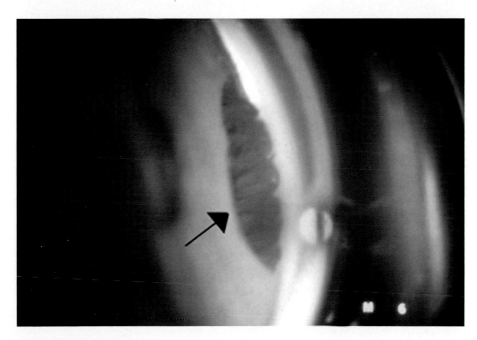

Figure 3-32   Iridodialysis   *The iris root* (arrow) *has fallen, exposing the underlying ciliary body processes.*

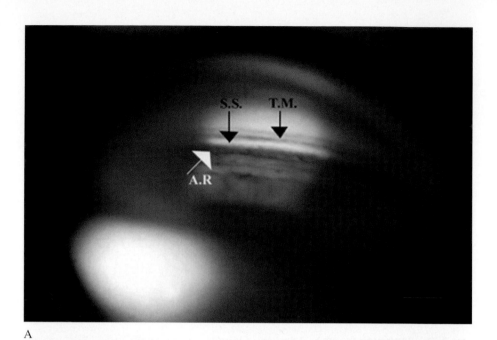

A

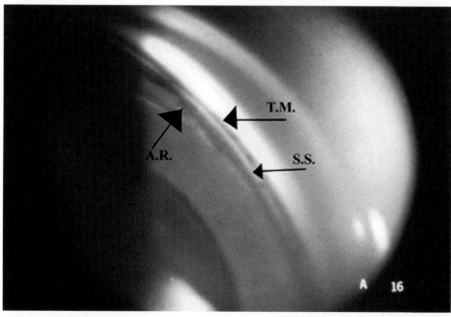

B

Figure 3-33A,B   Angle recession after trauma   *A. Extensive angle recession after trauma. In this example, the normal angle insertion is not visible, which could fool an examiner into thinking that the angle is normal. B. Angle recession after trauma. In this example, there is a smaller degree of angle recession and the border between the recessed angle and the normal angle is seen. A.R. = angle recession; S.S. = scleral spur; T.M. = trabecular meshwork.*

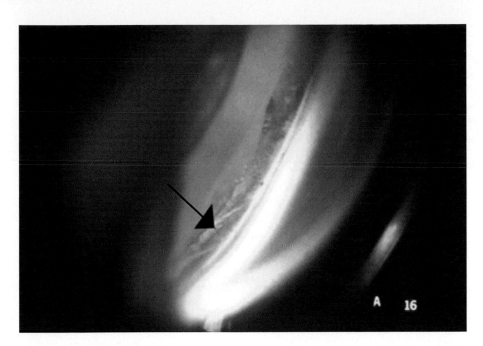

Figure 3-34   Cyclodialysis   *The ciliary body is completely detached, exposing the underlying sclera (arrow).*

Chapter 4

CLINICAL APPEARANCE OF GLAUCOMATOUS OPTIC NEUROPATHY

Tara A. Uhler, MD

THE OPTIC DISC

The optic nerve contains over 1 million axons of the retinal ganglion cells, the cell bodies of which are in the superficial retinal layers. Although normal variations in size and shape exist, the shape of the optic nerve head is usually a vertical oval. In the center of the disc is a depressed region, the cup, which is typically a horizontal oval. The central region is usually pale owing to the absence of axons with exposure of the underlying lamina cribosa. The tissue between the cup and disc margins is referred to as the neuroretinal rim and represents the location of the bulk of the axons of the retinal ganglion cells (Figure 4-1). This tissue, which usually has an orange-red hue because of the associated capillaries, becomes pale in disease states.

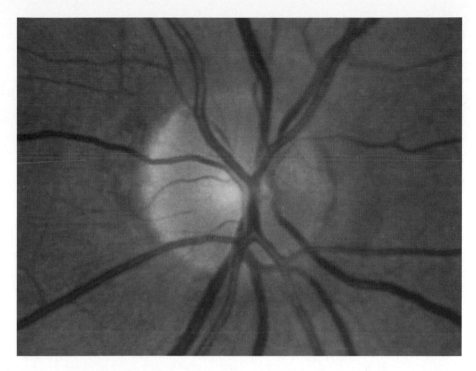

Figure 4-1   Normal optic nerve   *Photograph of a normal optic nerve with vertically oval disc and horizontally oval cup. Notice the healthy, orange-red neuroretinal rim.*

Determination of optic disc size is extremely important in evaluating glaucomatous optic neuropathy. The optic disc size is correlated with the size of the optic cup and neuroretinal rim: the larger the optic disc, the larger the cup and neuroretinal rim. A large cup in a large disc can be normal whereas a small cup in a smaller disc can be pathologic (Figure 4-2A,B). In addition, the depth of the cup is related to the cup area and, indirectly, to cup size in normal eyes.

The area of the neuroretinal rim is positively correlated with the area of the disc; larger discs have larger neural rim areas and smaller discs have smaller neural rim areas.[1] The rim width generally obeys the ISNT rule: the *i*nferior rim is widest followed by the *s*uperior, then *n*asal, and, finally, *t*emporal rims. Preferential loss of the neuroretinal rim, particularly in the inferior and superior disc regions, occurs in the early to medium-advanced stages of glaucoma. Nonglaucomatous optic nerve damage is not usually associated with a loss of neuroretinal rim.

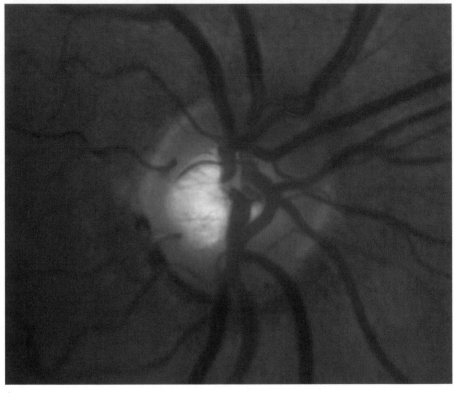

A

Figure 4-2A,B   Variations in optic nerve size   *A. Photograph of a small optic nerve with a relatively large cup in a patient with glaucomatous optic neuropathy. (Courtesy of Dr. George L. Spaeth, Wills Eye Hospital, Philadelphia, PA.)*

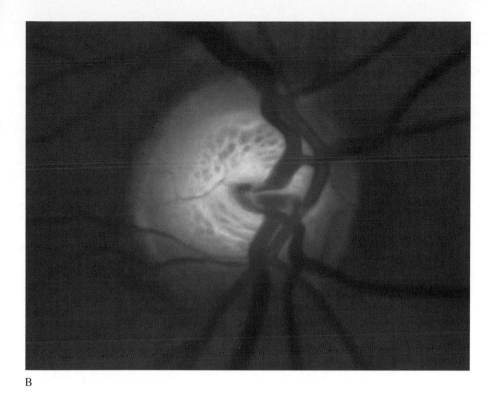

B

Figure 4-2A,B   Variations in optic nerve size   *(continued)*   ***B.*** *Photograph of a large optic nerve with a physiologically large cup in a patient with no evidence of glaucomatous optic neuropathy.*

EVALUATING THE GLAUCOMATOUS OPTIC DISC

Loss of Neuroretinal Rim

Degeneration of retinal ganglion cell axons in glaucoma leads to an increase in cup size with loss of neuroretinal rim tissue. The mean neuroretinal rim area is typically reduced in glaucomatous discs compared with normal discs, and this is a better parameter than cup-to-disc ratio in differentiating early glaucoma from normal physiology. Rim loss may be focal or concentric.

Focal loss of the neuroretinal rim often begins as a small, localized defect in the contour of the inner edge of the cup, leading to narrowing of the rim. This appearance has been referred to as focal notching or pit-like changes.

This defect may enlarge and develop a sharp margin (Figures 4-3A–C and 4-4A–C). When the narrowing reaches the disc margin and there is no rim tissue left, a sharp edge is produced. Vessels crossing this sharpened rim bend abruptly; this is referred to as bayoneting and is helpful when evaluating rim width.[2]

Concentric glaucomatous atrophy with enlargement of the cup in concentric circles may be more difficult to distinguish from a physiologic cup. Remembering the ISNT rule of rim thickness and that the normal cup is typically a horizontally, not vertically, oriented, oval may be helpful.

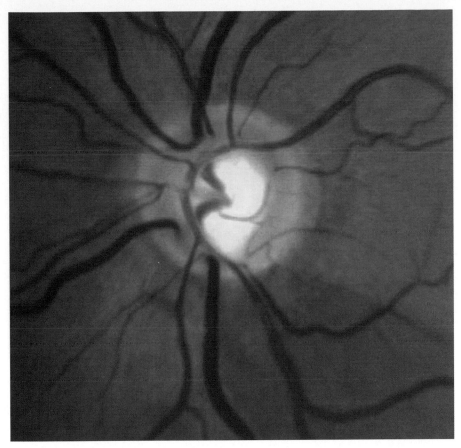

A

Figure 4-3A–C   Glaucomatous optic nerves   *Photograph (A) shows a large focal notch inferiorly. Notice the sharp bending of the vessels as they cross the rim in the region of the notch; this is referred to as bayoneting and is a useful marker of rim loss. There is also an associated nerve fiber layer defect, present as a wedge-shaped area of attenuation of the nerve fiber layer in that region.*

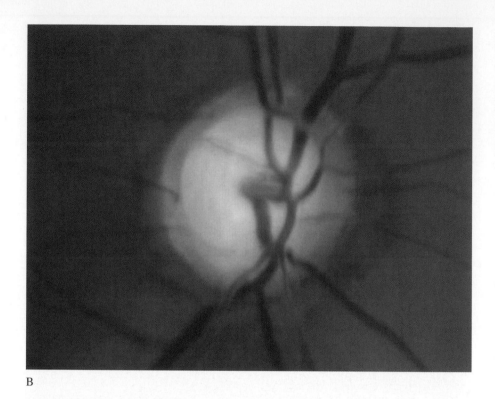

B

Figure 4-3A–C Glaucomatous optic nerves *(continued)* *(**B**) shows more concentric atrophy. Violating the ISNT rule, there is relatively greater loss of tissue inferiorly. Again, notice the bayoneting of the vessels as they cross the rim.*

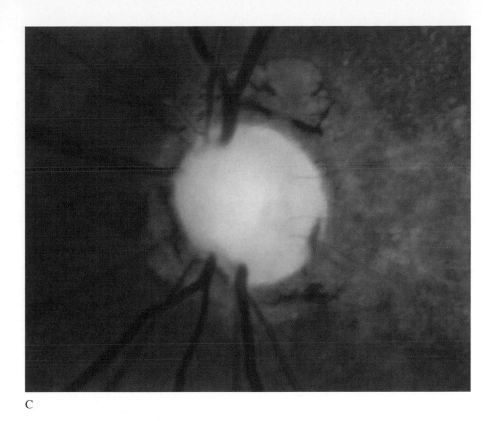

C

Figure 4-3A–C Glaucomatous optic nerves *(continued)* *(C) shows advanced cupping in end-stage glaucoma. Note the absence of rim for a significant portion of the circumference.*

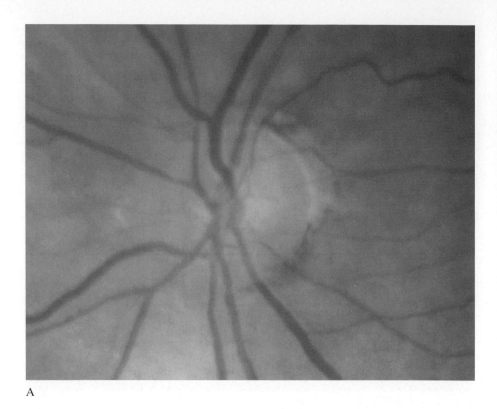

A

Figure 4-4A–C   Focal tissue loss   *Photograph and Heidelberg retinal tomography (HRT) scan of a focal area of notching. (A) shows a disc photograph showing a subtle area of tissue loss superotemporally. One month earlier, a disc hemorrhage had been present in that area.*

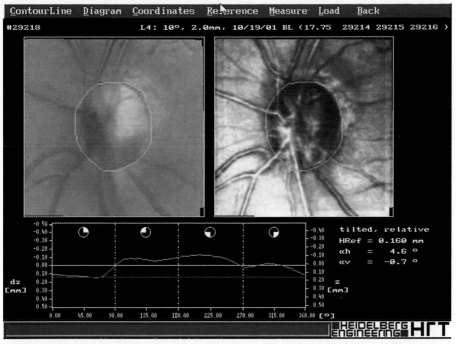

B

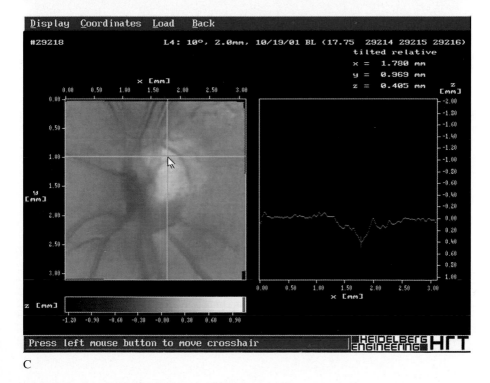

C

Figure 4-4A–C Focal tissue loss *(continued) (B) and (C) are the corresponding HRT scans highlighting the focal area of tissue loss.*

Laminar Dot Sign

At the surface of the nerve head, the axons bend acutely to leave the eye through fenestrated sheets of connective tissue, the lamina cribosa.

Deepening of the optic cup in glaucoma may lead to exposure of the underlying pores of the lamina cribosa. This is referred to as the laminar dot sign[2] (Figure 4-5). It is unclear if deepening of the cup itself has clinical significance.

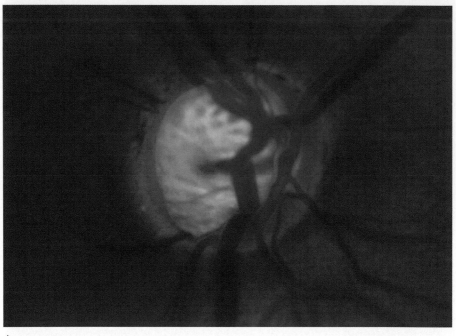

A

Figure 4-5 Laminar dots *Photograph of an optic nerve with a deep cup and prominent laminar dots. Notice the prominent parapapillary atrophy, giving the artificial appearance of thicker, healthier rim tissue (Courtesy of Dr. George L. Spaeth, Wills Eye Hospital, Philadelphia, PA.)*

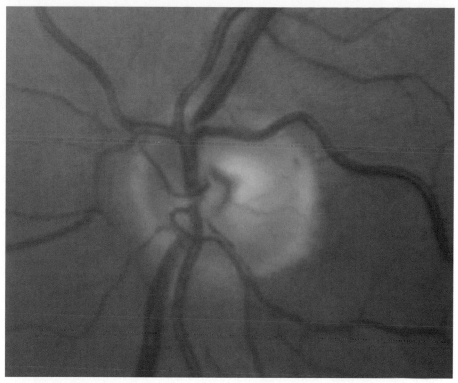

B

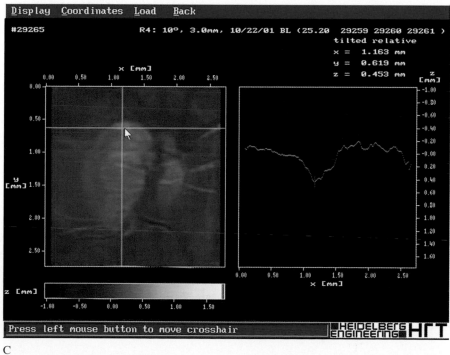

C

Figure 4-5 **Laminar dots** *(continued)*

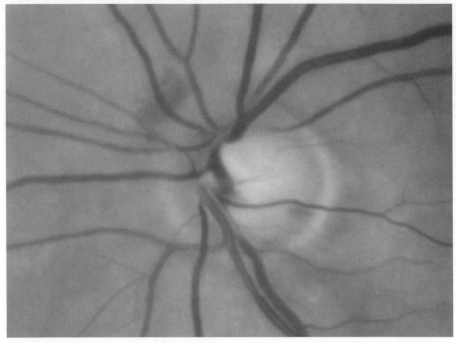

D

Figure 4-5   Laminar dots *(continued)*

Disc Hemorrhages

Splinter- or flame-shaped hemorrhages at the border of the optic disc, termed *Drance hemorrhages,* are considered particularly suspicious for glaucomatous optic neuropathy[3] (Figure 4-6A–D). Drance hemorrhages may be more commonly seen in low-tension glaucoma. They are associated with nerve fiber layer defects, neuroretinal rim notches, and circumscribed scotomas in the visual field.

Nerve Fiber Layer Defects

Striations in the retinal nerve fiber layer are normally seen ophthalmoscopically as light reflexes from bundles of nerve fibers. Loss of retinal ganglion cell axons in glaucoma leads to neuroretinal rim loss and visible nerve fiber layer (NFL) defects. These are attenuations of the retinal nerve fiber layer and

appear ophthalmoscopically as dark, wedge-shaped defects pointing toward or touching the optic disc border (see Figure 4-3A). Nerve fiber layer defects are best detected with red-free or green light. Their presence may be useful in the early detection of glaucomatous damage.[4] However, they are not pathognomonic for glaucomatous damage because they occur in eyes with optic neuropathy due to other causes.

Parapapillary Chorioretinal Atrophy

Parapapillary atrophy, especially beta zone, is more common and of greater size in eyes with glaucomatous damage.[5] It correlates with increasing neuroretinal rim loss. The area of atrophy is greatest in the sector of greatest neuroretinal rim loss (see Figure 4-5). Because parapapillary atrophy occurs less commonly

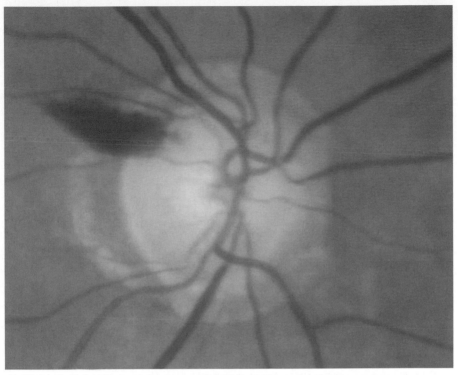

A

Figure 4-6A–D   Drance hemorrhages   *Photograph (A) shows an extremely large, flame-shaped disc hemorrhage located superotemporally. (B) and (C) are the corresponding HRT scans highlighting the focal area of tissue loss in that region. (D) shows the commonly more subtle appearance of a disc hemorrhage located inferotemporally; parapapillary hemorrhage can also be seen superonasally.*

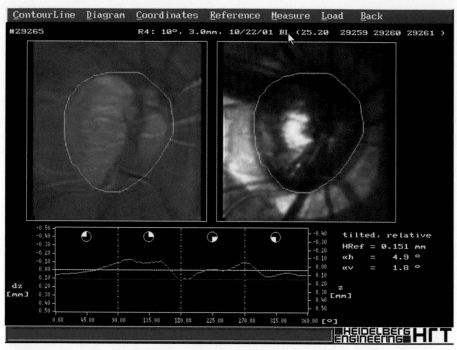

B

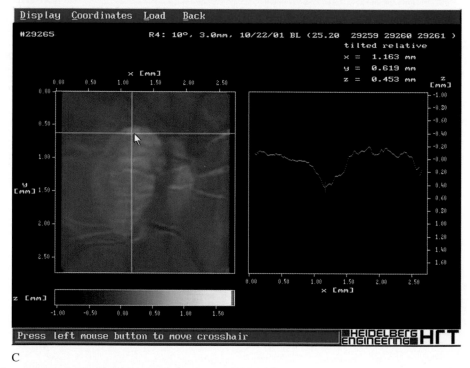

C

Figure 4-6A–D **Drance hemorrhages** *(continued)*

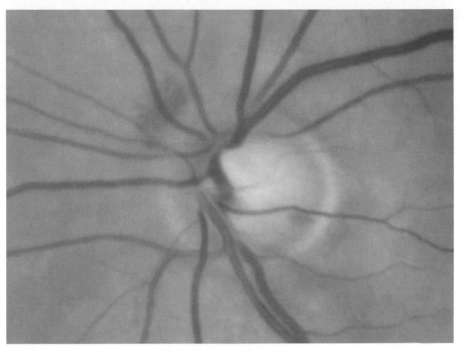

D

Figure 4-6A–D   Drance hemorrhages   *(continued)*

in eyes with nonglaucomatous optic nerve damage, its presence can help to distinguish between glaucomatous and nonglaucomatous optic neuropathy.

Appearance of Vessels

The appearance of the vessels on the optic nerve may be helpful in assessing the presence of glaucomatous nerve damage. Bayoneting of vessels has been mentioned already. In addition, some examiners find the overpass phenomenon useful in detecting glaucomatous damage. Overpass refers to the appearance of vessels bridging a cup that is becoming deeper. With progressive loss of underlying tissue, the vessels lose their support and appear to hang, suspended in the now empty space above the cup.

Many other changes are nonspecific. Focal narrowing of retinal arterioles and diffuse narrowing of retinal vessels, more marked in the area

of greatest rim loss, can be seen in both glaucomatous and nonglaucomatous optic neuropathy.

Nonglaucomatous Optic Neuropathy

Distinguishing between glaucomatous and nonglaucomatous optic neuropathy can be difficult. Pallor out of proportion to cupping, or pallor with intact neuroretinal rim, is a useful characteristic prominent in nonglaucomatous optic neuropathy.[6] Examples of nonglaucomatous optic neuropathy include giant cell arteritis and compressive lesions of the optic nerve. Nonglaucomatous optic nerve damage is not usually associated with a loss of neuroretinal rim. Therefore, the shape of the neuroretinal rim is not dramatically altered. In contrast, with glaucomatous optic neuropathy there is evidence of loss of neuroretinal rim tissue, with pallor increasing due to enlargement of the size of the cup.

Stereophotography

Assessment of changes in the optic nerve over time can be evaluated by using color stereophotographs (Figure 4-7). Stereophotographs can be produced by taking two photographs in sequence, either by manually repositioning the camera or by using a sliding carriage adapter (Allen separator). Alternatively, they can be produced by taking two photographs simultaneously with two cameras that utilize the indirect ophthalmoscopic principle (Donaldson stereoscopic fundus camera) or a twin-prism separator. In general, simultaneous disc photos have better reproducibility.[7]

Other techniques for capturing images and measurements of the nerve for comparison over time include Heidelberg retinal tomography (HRT), GDx laser polarimetry, and optical coherence tomography (OCT). These techniques and their utility are discussed elsewhere.

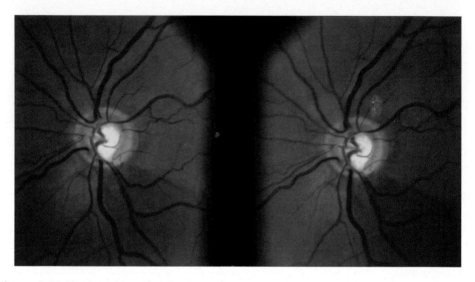

Figure 4-7   Stereophotography   *Photograph of simultaneous disc photos. With the use of a special viewer, stereovision is achieved. Stereophotography is a useful way to assess optic nerve changes over time.*

REFERENCES

1. Jonas JB, Gussek GC, Naumann GOH. Optic disc, cup and neuroretinal rim size, configuration and correlations in normal eyes. *Invest Ophthalmol Vis Sci* 29:1151, 1988.
2. Read RM, Spaeth GL. The practical clinical appraisal of the optic disc in glaucoma: The natural history of cup progression and some specific disc-field correlations. *Trans Am Acad Ophthalmol Otol* 78:255, 1974.
3. Drance SM, Fairclough M, Butler DM, Kottler MS. The importance of disc hemorrhage in the prognosis of chronic open-angle glaucoma. *Arch Ophthalmol* 95:226, 1977.
4. Quigley HA, Katz J, Derick RJ, et al. An evaluation of optic disc and nerve fiber layer examinations in monitoring progression of early glaucoma damage. *Ophthalmology* 99:19, 1992.
5. Jonas JB, Naumann GOH. Parapapillary chorioretinal atrophy in normal and glaucoma eyes. II. Correlations. *Invest Ophthalmol Vis Sci* 30:919, 1989.
6. Rosenthal AR, Kottler MS, Donaldson DD, Falconer DG. Comparative reproducibility of the digital photogrammetric procedure utilizing three methods of stereophotography. *Invest Ophthalmol Vis Sci* 16:54, 1977.
7. Trobe JD, Glaser JS, Cassady J, et al. Nonglaucomatous excavation of the optic disc. *Arch Ophthalmol* 98:1046, 1980.

Chapter 5

PSYCHOPHYSICAL TESTING

Douglas J. Rhee, MD

Tara A. Uhler, MD

L. Jay Katz, MD

The broad term *psychophysical testing* refers to the subjective testing of vision of an eye. In clinical terms for the glaucoma patient, this involves perimetry to assess the peripheral vision of an eye. Because the pathophysiology of glaucoma affects the peripheral vision before affecting central acuity, there are both diagnostic and therapeutic benefits to assessing the patient's visual field. It is important to note that usage of the term *peripheral* vision does not necessarily mean far periphery. In fact, most glaucomatous visual field defects occur paracentrally (within 24 degrees of fixation). Our use of the term *peripheral* refers to anything beyond central fixation (i.e., greater than the central 5 to 10 degrees).

The goal of this chapter is to show representative visual field patterns for glaucoma rather than provide a comprehensive discussion of perimetry. There are several texts dedicated solely to the extended description of perimetry and atlases dedicated to just perimetric findings.

PURPOSE OF TEST

Diagnosis

As part of the initial evaluation of a patient suspected of having glaucoma, automated monochromatic visual field testing is an important aspect of the diagnostic determination of glaucomatous optic nerve damage. Visual field abnormalities have localizing value for lesions along the entire visual tract, which extends from the retina to the occipital lobes. Glaucomatous visual field defects are those that are typically found with lesions localizing to the optic nerve.

It is very important to note that the presence of a so-called optic nerve field (i.e., defects that localize to the optic nerve) is not solely diagnostic of glaucoma. This must occur in the presence of a characteristic optic nerve appearance (covered in Chapter 4) and history. Other findings, such as intraocular pressure, gonioscopic appearance, and anterior segment findings, may help categorize the specific type of glaucoma. All optic neuropathies (e.g., anterior ischemic optic neuropathies, compressive optic neuropathies, etc.) demonstrate "optic nerve" visual fields.

It is also critical to note that the absence of an optic nerve field does not exclude the diagnosis of glaucoma. Although in the year 2002 automated achromatic static visual field (AASVF) testing is the gold standard for the evaluation of optic nerve function, its threshold of sensitivity to detect ganglion cell loss is still limited. Clinicopathologic and experimental evidence indicates that the earliest visual field defect detectable by AASVF corresponds to approximately 40% ganglion cell loss.

Management

Automated achromatic static visual field testing along with serial optic nerve evaluations remain the gold standard for the monitoring of glaucoma. The goal (or target) intraocular pressure is the therapeutic range at which we modify the ocular physiology in an attempt to protect the optic nerve from further barotraumas. However, the determination of the target pressure is empirical, meaning that we estimate what the goal should be. AASVF and serial optic nerve evaluations are the ways in which we determine if that empirically derived pressure range is actually effective at protecting the optic nerve.

DESCRIPTION

Perimetric testing attempts to determine the visual threshold at a particular location in the visual field. The visual threshold is defined as the minimum level of light that can be perceived at a given location in the visual field; this concept is also termed *retinal sensitivity*. This is a different concept from the lowest level of photic energy that will stimulate a photoreceptor cell or area of retina. Perimetric testing relies on the patient to subjectively determine what he or she can see. Therefore, the visual threshold is subject to some level of cognitive and intraretinal processing, hence the name psychophysical testing.

The visual threshold is highest in the fovea, which is defined as the center of the visual field. As the field extends peripherally, the sensitivity decreases. The three-dimensional representation of this is often called the "hill of vision" (Figure 5-1). The visual field for one eye extends 60 degrees superiorly, 60 degrees nasally, 75 degrees inferiorly, and 100 degrees temporally.

There are two main methods of perimetry: static and kinetic (Figure 5-2). Historically, various forms of kinetic testing were developed first, and these are generally performed manu-

ally. Briefly, a visual stimulus of known size and intensity is brought from the far periphery, where it would not be expected to be perceived, toward the center. At some point, it will move into an area where it is perceived; this is the visual threshold at that location. This process is continued with varying stimuli of size and intensities to give a topographic map of the hill of vision. The Goldmann visual field attempts to map the entire visual field (Figure 5-3).

Static visual field testing presents visual stimuli in varying sizes and intensities at fixed locations. Although there are many different strategies for determining the visual threshold, most use the following basic principle. The examiner begins by presenting stimuli of higher intensity and, in measured steps, presents stimuli of lower intensity until the patient no longer perceives the stimulus. Then the test is usually rechecked by presenting a gradually increasing intensity of stimulus in smaller increments until the patient again can perceive the stimulus. That intensity of light is defined as the visual threshold in that region of the visual field. Generally, static visual field testing is automated and presents white-colored stimuli on a white

The Field Analyzer Primer

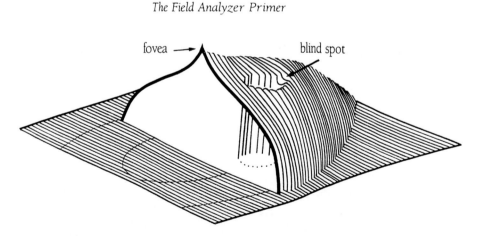

Figure 5-1   The "hill of vision"   *A three-dimensional representation of the visual threshold in various locations within the visual field of a normal eye. (From Haley MJ, ed.* The Field Analyzer Primer. *2nd ed. San Leandro, CA: Humphrey Instruments, 1987, Fig. 1, p 4.)*

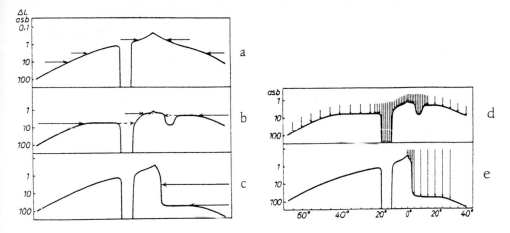

Figure 5-2   Comparison of statis and kinetic perimetry   *Slopes and scotomas are shown better by statis than by kinetic perimetry. Although the normal visual field with its gradual slope and absence of abnormal scotomas is well outlined by kinetic testing (**a**), the presence of field defects makes this method less precise than static testing. In (**b**), the flat temporal slope might yield a response at any point between 40 degrees and 12 degrees if the test object were optimum for testing that zone. Nasally, the best-chosen kinetic test might be reported anywhere between 25 degrees and 7 degrees, and it would miss the relative scotoma between 7 degrees and 12 degrees. When the slope is steep, kinetic perimetry usually outlines the defect well with a few well-chosen test objects, but the choice is often arbitrary and may, as in (**c**), fail to reveal the actual steepness of the slope. Static tests elucidate well the flat slopes and small scotomas in (**d**) and both kinds of slope in (**e**). (From Aulhorn E and Harms H, 1976, with permission from S. Karger.)*

background, hence the name automated achromatic static visual field testing (AASVF). There are many makers of AASVF machines, among them Humphrey (Allergan; Irvine, CA), Octopus, (Figure 5-10) and Dicon. In our practice, we prefer the Humphrey machine.

Various testing algorithms have been developed, such as full threshold, FASTPAC, STATPAC, and Swedish interactive threshold algorithm (SITA), among others. They vary with regard to length of test time and slightly with regard to depth of field defect.

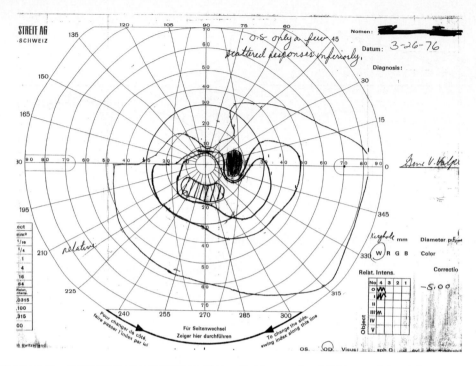

Figure 5-3   Goldmann visual field testing   *Goldmann visual field test of the right eye showing superior nasal step and arcuate defect.*

COMMON OPTIC NERVE VISUAL FIELDS FOUND IN PATIENTS WITH GLAUCOMA

The anatomic location of the defect in glaucoma is in the optic nerve, with focal spots within the lamina cribrosa. On the field test, the visual defects manifest in relatively specific patterns because of the anatomy of the retinal nerve fiber layer (RNFL). The RNFL is primarily comprised of the axons from the ganglion cells projecting through the optic nerve to the lateral geniculate nucleus (Figure 5-4).

Axons from ganglion cells located nasal to the optic disc travel straight into optic disc; defects in the optic nerve affecting fibers from this region produce a temporal wedge defect (Figure 5-5A–C). Axons from ganglion cells located temporal to the optic nerve arc into the optic nerve. A line that intersects the fovea and the optic nerve defines the horizontal raphe. Ganglion cells located superiorly to the horizontal raphe arc superiorly and deliver their fibers to the superotemporal aspect of the optic nerve. The converse is true for ganglion cells located temporal to the optic nerve and inferior to the horizontal raphe.

Defects in the optic nerve affecting fibers from the area temporal to the optic nerve produce both nasal step defects and arcuate defects. The nasal step defect (Figures 5-6 and 5-7A–C) gets its name not only from the nasal location of the field defect but also from the fact that the defect respects the horizontal median. The horizontal raphe is the anatomic basis for this appearance. The arcuate defect gets its name from the appearance of the defect (Figure 5-8A–C). Nasal step and arcuate defects are far more common than temporal wedge defects. As glaucoma progresses, multiple defects can present (Figure 5-9) in a single eye.

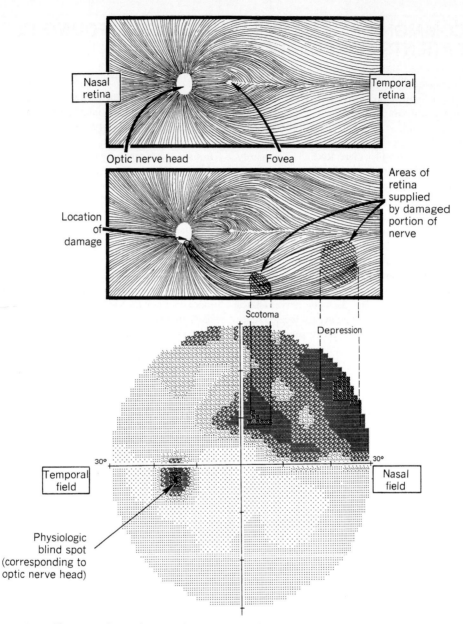

Figure 5-4 Glaucomatous damage to nerve bundles and location of resulting visual abnormalities *Damage at the lower pole of the optic disc causes abnormalities in the visual field as shown (left eye). (From Anderson DR, Patella VM.* Automated Statis Perimetry. *2nd ed. St. Louis, MO: Mosby, 1999, Fig. 4-4, p 51.)*

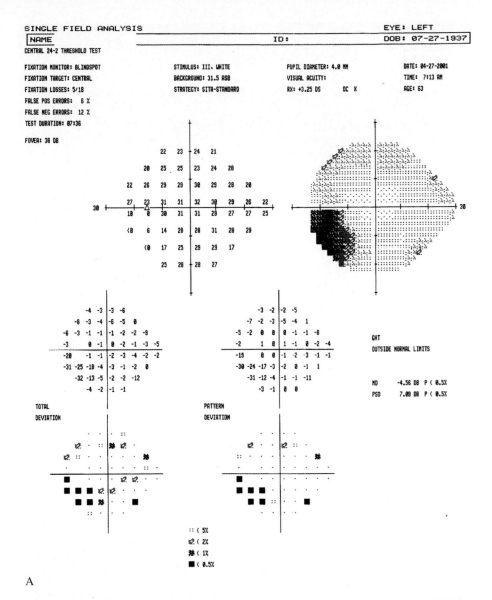

A

Figure 5-5A–C   Temporal wedge   *A. Humphrey automated achromatic static visual field (AASVF) testing. **B.** Corresponding optic nerve photograph showing some nasal thinning. **C.** Corresponding Heidelberg retinal tomography (HRT) scan.*

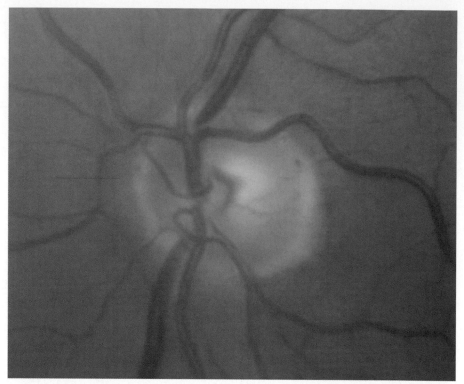

B

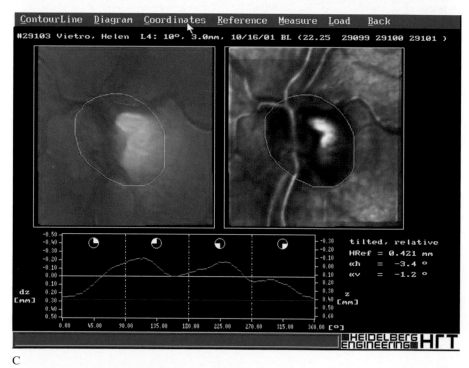

C

Figure 5-5A–C   Temporal wedge   *(continued)*

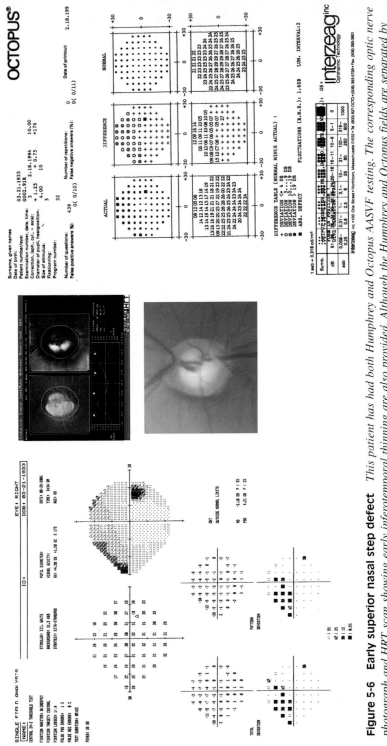

Figure 5-6 Early superior nasal step defect *This patient has had both Humphrey and Octopus AASVF testing. The corresponding optic nerve photograph and HRT scan showing early inferotemporal thinning are also provided. Although the Humphrey and Octopus fields are separated by many years, this patient had no clinical progression of disease, so the fields are roughly comparable.*

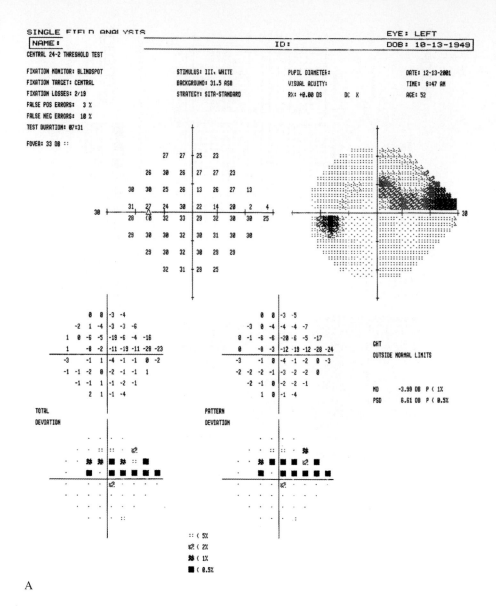

A

Figure 5-7A–C More advanced superior nasal step defect *A. Humphrey AASVF testing.*
B. Corresponding optic nerve photograph showing more advanced inferotemporal thinning.
C. Corresponding HRT scan.

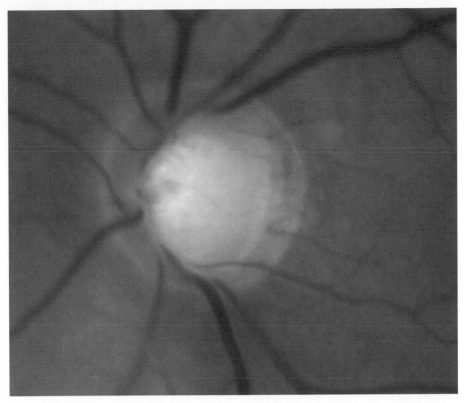

B

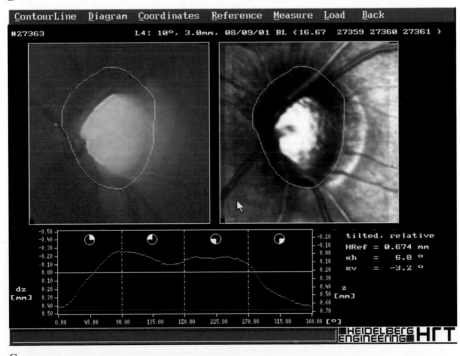

C

Figure 5-7A–C   More advance superior nasal step defect   *(continued)*

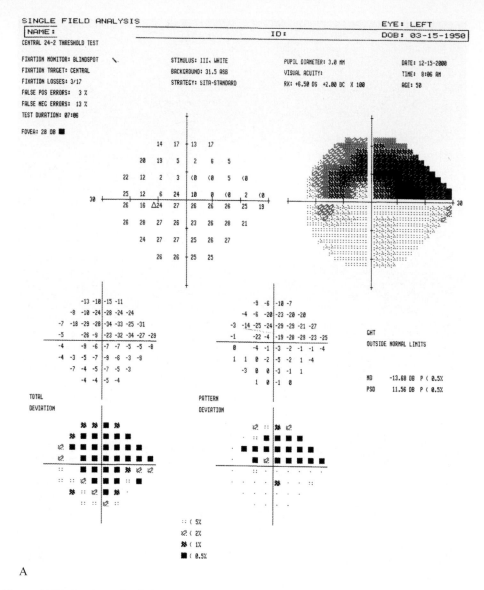

SINGLE FIELD ANALYSIS

NAME :

CENTRAL 24-2 THRESHOLD TEST

EYE : LEFT

ID :

DOB : 03-15-1950

FIXATION MONITOR: BLINDSPOT
FIXATION TARGET: CENTRAL
FIXATION LOSSES: 3/17
FALSE POS ERRORS: 3 %
FALSE NEG ERRORS: 13 %
TEST DURATION: 07:06

FOVEA: 28 DB ■

STIMULUS: III, WHITE
BACKGROUND: 31.5 ASB
STRATEGY: SITA-STANDARD

PUPIL DIAMETER: 3.0 MM
VISUAL ACUITY:
RX: +6.50 DS +2.00 DC X 100

DATE: 12-15-2000
TIME: 8:06 AM
AGE: 50

TOTAL DEVIATION

PATTERN DEVIATION

GHT
OUTSIDE NORMAL LIMITS

MD   -13.68 DB P < 0.5%
PSD   11.56 DB P < 0.5%

:: < 5%
✷ < 2%
✸ < 1%
■ < 0.5%

A

Figure 5-8A–C   Arcuate defect   *A. Humphrey AASVF testing. **B.** Corresponding optic nerve photograph showing some nasal thinning. **C.** Corresponding HRT scan.*

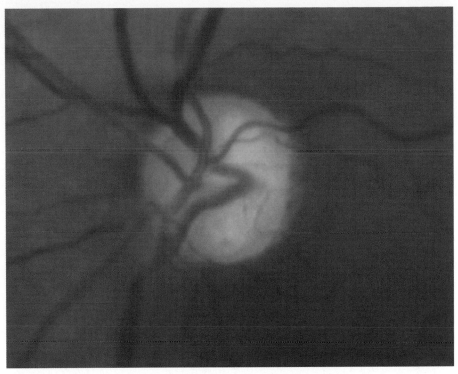

B

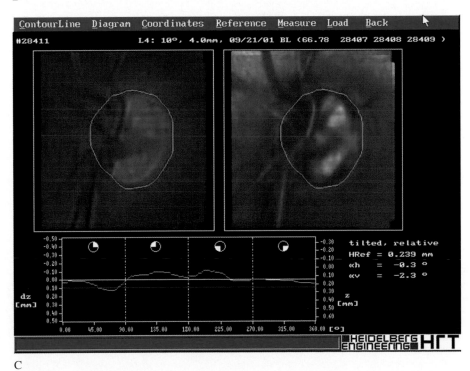

C

Figure 5-8A–C Arcuate defect *(continued)*

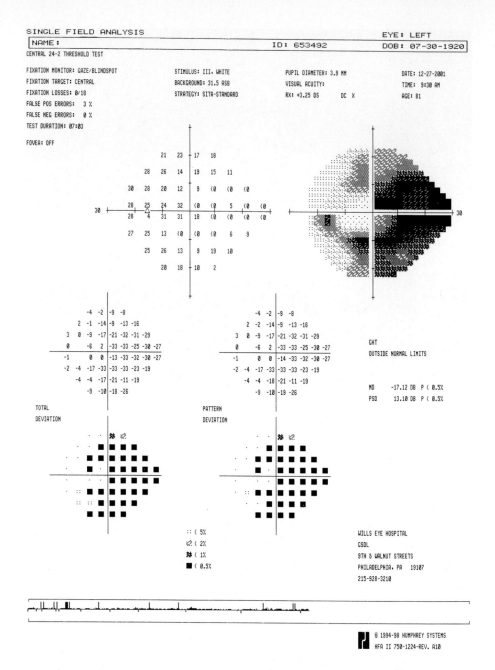

Figure 5-9 *AASVF test from a Humphrey machine demonstrating a combination of defects. There are both superior and inferior nasal steps with both inferior and superior arcuate defects. The inferior arcuate is more prominent than the superior arcuate.*

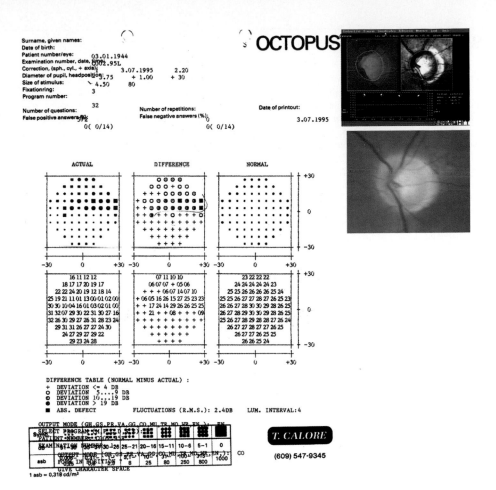

Figure 5-10 *Octopus AASVF test with corresponding optic nerve photograph and HRT scan.*

BIBLIOGRAPHY

Anderson DR, Patella VM. *Automated Static Perimetry.* 2nd ed. St. Louis, MO: Mosby, 1999.

Aulhorn E, Harms H. Early visual field defects in glaucoma. In: *Glaucoma Symposium, Tutzing Castle, 1966.* W Leydhecker, 151–186, 1967.

Budenz DL. *Atlas of Visual Fields.* Philadelphia: Lippincott-Raven; 1997.

Drance SM, Wheeler C, Patullo M. The use of static perimetry in the early detection of glaucoma. *Can J Ophthalmol* 2:249–258, 1967.

Harwerth RS, Carter-Dawson L, Shen F, Smith EL, Crawford MLJ. Ganglion cell losses underlying visual field defects from experimental glaucoma. *Invest Ophthalmol Vis Sci* 40:2242–2250, 1999.

Heijl A. Automatic perimetry in glaucoma visual field screening. A clinical study. *Graefes Archiv Clin Exp Ophthalmol* 200:21–37, 1976.

Heijl A, Lundqvist L. The location of earliest glaucomatous visual field defected documented by automatic perimetry. *Doc Ophthalmol Proceed Series* 35:153–158, 1983.

Katz J, Tielsch JM, Quigley HA, Sommer A. Automated perimetry detects visual field loss before manual Goldmann perimetry. *Ophthalmology* 102:21–26, 1995.

Lynn JR. Examination of the visual field in glaucoma. *Invest Ophthalmol* 8:76–84, 1969.

Quigley HA, Dunlelberger GR, Green WR. Retinal ganglion cell atrophy correlated with automated perimetry in human eyes with glaucoma. *Am J Ophthalmol* 107:453–464, 1989.

Section 2

GLAUCOMA MANAGEMENT

Douglas J. Rhee, MD

INTRODUCTION

What Is the Goal of Treatment?

We currently understand the pathophysiology of glaucoma to be a progressive loss of ganglion cells resulting in visual field damage that is caused by intraocular pressure. The goal of treatment is to retard or halt the ganglion cell loss to prevent symptomatic visual loss while attempting not to cause untoward side effects.

Although many clinicians now feel that there are several factors involved in the pathogenesis of glaucoma, the only rigorously proven method of treatment is the lowering of intraocular pressure. There continues to be a mounting body of evidence that supports this fact.

How Do We Treat Glaucoma?

Glaucoma was first thought of as a surgical disease. The first filtration procedure (not iridectomy) was suggested by Louis de Wecker (1832–1906) in 1869. Although the miotic effects of eserine and pilocarpine had been reported in the early 1860s, they were not used for treatment until later. Adolf Weber (1829–1915) first introduced them as medical treatments of glaucoma in 1876. The first study comparing the two available forms of glaucoma treatment, eserine and iridectomy, was performed at Wills Eye Hospital in 1895 by Zentmayer et al (*Arch Ophthalmol* 24:378–394, 1895). This study showed that both treatments are equivalent and that a patient's visual status could be maintained for periods ranging from 5 to 15 years on chronic medical treatment.

The debate over the best initial therapy continues today. In Europe, many clinicians perform surgery as the initial treatment for glaucoma. Most clinicians in the United States continue to use medications as the initial treatment for glaucoma. In the United States, two large studies were performed to compare medical treatment versus laser trabeculoplasty (Glaucoma Laser Trial [GLT]) and medical treatment versus trabeculectomy (Collaborative Initial Glaucoma Treatment Study [CIGTS]). At 2 years of follow-up in the GLT, eyes that received argon laser trabeculoplasty (ALT) showed a lower mean intraocular pressure (between 1 and 2 mm Hg) compared with eyes started on timolol, but showed no difference in visual field or acuity. At 7 years, eyes that received ALT had a greater reduction in intraocular pressure (1.2 mm Hg) and greater sensitivity in the visual field (0.6 dB). These results seem to indicate that ALT is at least as good as medical treatment for glaucoma.

Interim results of the CIGTS study (i.e., 5 years) show no difference in visual field despite a lower intraocular pressure in the surgical group. Visual acuity and local eye symptoms seem to be worse in the surgical group. To date, the CIGTS results do not yet support changing the current paradigm of medical treatment as initial treatment. However, longer follow-up data are needed to provide more conclusive recommendations for a chronic disease such as glaucoma.

The subsequent chapters in this section describe the different therapies commonly utilized for glaucoma.

BIBLIOGRAPHY

AGIS Investigators. The Advanced Glaucoma Intervention Study (AGIS): 7. The relationship between control of intraocular pressure and visual field deterioration. *Am J Ophthalmol* 130:429–440, 2000.

Bergea B, Bodin L, Svedbergh B. Impact of intraocular pressure regulation on visual fields in open-angle glaucoma. *Ophthalmology* 106:997–1005, 1999.

Collaborative Normal-Tension Glaucoma Study Group. Comparison of glaucomatous progression between untreated patients with normal-tension glaucoma and patients with therapeutically reduced intraocular pressures. *Am J Ophthalmol* 126:487–497, 1998.

Glaucoma Laser Trial Research Group. The Glaucoma Laser Trial (GLT). 2. Results of argon laser trabeculoplasty versus topical medicines. *Ophthalmology* 97:1403–1413, 1990.

Glaucoma Laser Trial Research Group. The Glaucoma Laser Trial (GLT) and glaucoma laser trial follow-up study. 7. Results. *Am J Ophthalmol* 120:718–731, 1995.

Janz NK, Wren PA, Lichter PR, Musch DC, Gillespie BW, Guire KE, Mills RP, CIGTS Study Group. The Collaborative Initial Glaucoma Treatment Study: Interim quality of life findings after initial medical or surgical treatment of glaucoma. *Ophthalmology* 108:1954–1965, 2001.

Lichter PR, Musch DC, Gillespie BW, Guire KE, Janz NK, Wren PA, Mills RP, CIGTS Study Group. Interim clinical outcomes in the Collaborative Initial Glaucoma Treatment Study comparing initial treatment randomized to medications or surgery. *Ophthalmology* 108:1943–1953, 2001.

Mao LK, Steward WC, Shield MB. Correlation between intraocular pressure control and progressive glaucomatous damage in primary open-angle glaucoma. *Am J Ophthalmol* 111:51–55, 1991.

Chapter 6

MEDICATIONS

Douglas J. Rhee, MD

Medical treatment of glaucoma began in the late 1800s with use of eserine and pilocarpine.

In the United States, glaucoma treatment is typically begun with topical medications.

PURPOSE

The short-term goal of medications is to lower intraocular pressure (IOP). The long-term goals are to prevent symptomatic visual loss while minimizing the side effects from the treatments.

DESCRIPTION AND PHYSIOLOGY

Unless there are extreme circumstances, such as an intraocular pressure higher than 40 mm Hg or an impending risk to central fixation, treatment is started using a so-called one-eyed therapeutic trial. Typically, one type of drop is started in only one eye with reexamination in 3 to 6 weeks to check for effectiveness. Effectiveness is determined by comparing the difference in IOP in the two eyes prior to therapy with the difference in IOP after initiating therapy. For example, if IOP is 30 mm Hg OD (*oculus dexter;* in the right eye) and 33 mm Hg OS (*oculus sinister;* in the left eye) prior to treatment, and, following treatment of the right eye, IOP is 20 mm Hg OD and 23 mm Hg OS, the drug is not having any effect. If the IOP after starting treatment is 25 mm Hg OD and 34 mm Hg OS, then the drug is having an effect.

There are several different classes of medications. All medications work to lower IOP through varying pharmacologic mechanisms. Intraocular pressure is determined by the balance between secretion and drainage of aqueous humor. All medications either decrease secretion or increase outflow. In the subsequent sections, the mechanism of action, common side effects, and contraindications for the different classes of medications are presented. Table 6-1 lists the medications within each class that are available in the United States as of 2001–2002.

The side effects and contraindications described in this chapter are not a complete listing. I recommend that all clinicians read the package insert before prescribing any medication. The figures show sample bottles of medications available in the United States.

TABLE 6-1　PHARMACOLOGIC AGENTS ORGANIZED BY PHARMACOLOGIC CLASS

Medication[a]	Available Strengths
Alpha Agonists	
Apraclonidine (*Iopidine*)	0.5%, 1%
Brimonidine (*Alphagan*)	0.2%
Beta-Blockers	
Betaxolol (*Betoptic*)	0.5%
Carteolol (*Ocupress*)	1%
Levobunolol (*Betagan*)	0.25%, 0.5%
Metipranolol (*OptiPranolol*)	0.3%
Timolol hemihydrate (*Betimol*)	0.25%, 0.5%
Timolol maleate (*Timoptic*)	0.25%, 0.5%
Carbonic Anhydrase Inhibitors—Oral	
Acetazolamide (*Diamox*)	125–500 mg
Methazolamide (*Neptazane, Glauctabs*)	25–50 mg
Carbonic Anhydrase Inhibitors—Topical	
Brinzolamide (*Azopt*)	1%
Dorzolamide (*Trusopt*)	2%
Hyperosmolar Agents	
Glycerin (*Osmoglyn*)	50% solution
Isosorbide (*Ismotic*)	4% solution
Mannitol (*Osmitrol*)	5%–20% solution
Miotics	
Physostigmine (*Eserine*)	0.25%
Pilocarpine hydrochloride (*Pilocarpine, Pilocar*)	0.25%, 0.5%, 1%, 2%, 4%, 6%
Pilocarpine nitrate (*Pilagan*)	1%, 2%, 4%
Prostaglandins	
Bimatoprost (*Lumigan*)	0.03%
Latanoprost (*Xalatan*)	0.005%
Travoprost (*Travatan*)	0.004%
Unoprostone isopropyl (*Rescula*)	0.15%
Sympathomimetic Agents	
Dipivefrin (*Propine*)	0.1%
Epinephrine (*Epifrin*)	0.5%, 1%, 2%

[a]Trade names available in the United States are indicated in *italics*.

ALPHA AGONISTS (FIGURE 6-1)

Mechanism of Action   Activation of alpha-2 receptors in ciliary body inhibits aqueous secretion.

Side Effects   Local irritation, allergy, mydriasis, dry mouth, dry eye, hypotension, lethargy.

Contraindications   Monoamine oxidase (MAO) inhibitor use. Brimonidine is not to be used in children younger than 2 years of age; it has been associated with apnea in children.

Comments   Apraclonidine is for short-term use and prophylaxis of postlaser IOP spikes.

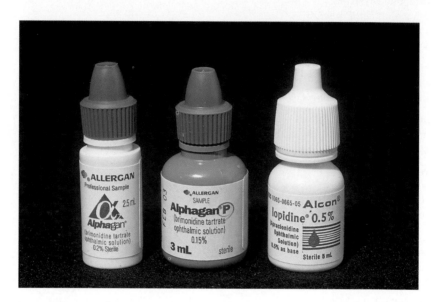

Figure 6-1   Alpha agonists   *All trade-name alpha agonists available in the United States at the time of publication.* From left to right: *Alphagan (Allergan; Irvine, CA), Alphagan-P (Allergan; Irvine, CA), and Iopidine 0.5% (Alcon; Fort Worth, TX). Note: Iopidine 1% is not shown.*

BETA-BLOCKERS (FIGURE 6-2)

Mechanism of Action Blockade of the beta receptors in the ciliary body reduces intraocular pressure by decreasing aqueous humor production.

Side Effects

Local Blurred vision, corneal anesthesia, and superficial punctate keratitis.

Systemic Bradycardia or heart block, bronchospasm, fatigue, mood change, impotence, decreased sensitivity to hypoglycemic symptoms in insulin-dependent diabetics, worsening of myasthenia gravis.

Contraindications Asthma, severe chronic obstructive pulmonary disease (COPD), bradycardia, heart block, congestive heart failure, myasthenia gravis.

Comments Some medications are considered nonselective versus relatively cardioselective (Table 6-2). The relatively cardioselective medications may have fewer pulmonary side effects.

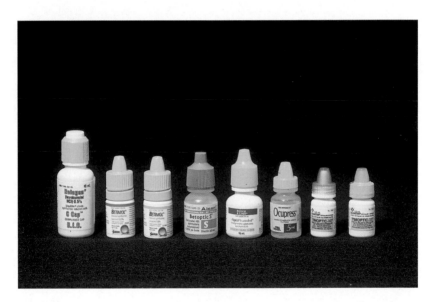

Figure 6-2   Beta-blockers *Nearly all single-agent, trade-name beta-blockers available in the United States at the time of publication; Betagan 0.25% and Betoptic are missing. From left to right: Betagan 0.5% (Allergan; Irvine, CA), Betimol 0.25% and 0.5%, respectively (Santen; Tampere, Finland), Betoptic-S (Alcon; Fort Worth, TX), OptiPranolol (Bausch & Lomb; Claremont, CA), Ocupress (Novartis; Atlanta, GA), and Timoptic XE 0.25% and 0.5%, respectively (Merck; West Point, PA).*

TABLE 6-2   **RELATIVE RECEPTOR SELECTIVITY OF THE VARIOUS BETA-BLOCKER MEDICATIONS**

Drug	Relative Specificity of the Receptor Effect
Betaxolol	Relatively cardioselective
Carteolol	Nonselective; has intrinsic sympathomimetic activity
Levobunolol	Nonselective (long half-life)
Metipranolol	Nonselective (*white* top)
Timolol hemihydrate	Nonselective
Timolol maleate	Nonselective

CARBONIC ANHYDRASE INHIBITORS (CAI) (FIGURES 6-3 AND 6-4)

Mechanism of Action Inhibition of the enzyme carbonic anhydrase decreases aqueous production in the ciliary body. When given parentally, CAIs will also cause dehydration of the vitreous.

Side Effects

Local (with topical therapy): Bitter taste.

Systemic With topical therapy—diuresis, fatigue, gastrointestinal upset, Stevens-Johnson syndrome, theoretical risk of aplastic anemia. With systemic therapy—hypokalemia and acidosis, renal stones, paresthesias, nausea, cramps, diarrhea, malaise, lethargy, depression, impotence, unpleasant taste, aplastic anemia, Stevens-Johnson syndrome.

Contraindications Sulfa allergy, hyponatremia or hypokalemia, recent renal stones, thiazide diuretics, digitalis use.

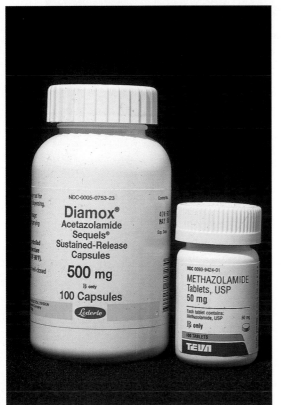

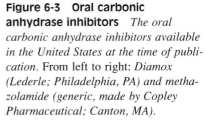

Figure 6-3 Oral carbonic anhydrase inhibitors *The oral carbonic anhydrase inhibitors available in the United States at the time of publication.* From left to right: *Diamox (Lederle; Philadelphia, PA) and methazolamide (generic, made by Copley Pharmaceutical; Canton, MA).*

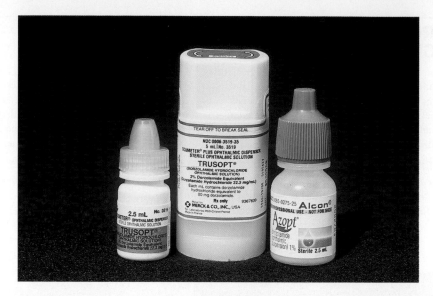

Figure 6-4 Topical carbonic anhydrase inhibitors *All single-agent, trade-name topical carbonic anhydrase inhibitors available in the United States at the time of publication.* From left to right: *Trusopt, old and new bottle, respectively (Merck; West Point, PA), and Azopt (Alcon; Fort Worth, TX)*

HYPEROSMOLAR AGENTS

Mechanism of Action Dehydrates the vitreous and decreases intraocular fluid volume by osmotically drawing fluid into the intravascular space. The agents are given orally or intravenously.

Side Effects

MANNITOL Congestive heart failure (CHF), urinary retention in men, backache, myocardial infarction, headache, and mental confusion.

GLYCERIN Vomiting; less likely to produce CHF than mannitol, otherwise similar to mannitol.

ISOSORBIDE Same as glycerin except perhaps safer in diabetic patients.

Contraindications Congestive heart failure, diabetic ketoacidosis (glycerin), subdural or subarachnoid hemorrhage, preexisting severe dehydration.

MIOTICS (FIGURE 6-5)

Mechanism of Action Direct-acting cholinergics stimulate muscarinic receptors, and indirect-acting cholinergics block acetylcholinesterase (Table 6-3). Miotics cause pupillary muscle constriction, which is believed to pull open the trabecular meshwork to increase trabecular outflow.

Side Effects

DIRECT-ACTING CHOLINERGIC

Local Brow ache, breakdown of blood/aqueous barrier, angle closure (increases pupillary block and causes the lens/iris diaphragm to move anteriorly), decreased night vision, variable myopia, retinal tear or detachment, and possibly anterior subcapsular cataracts.

Systemic Rare.

INDIRECT-ACTING CHOLINERGIC

Local Retinal detachment, cataract, myopia, intense miosis, angle closure, increased bleeding postsurgery, punctal stenosis, increased formation of posterior synechiae in chronic uveitis.

Systemic Diarrhea, abdominal cramps, enuresis, and increased effect of succinylcholine.

Contraindications

DIRECT CHOLINERGIC Peripheral retinal pathology, central media opacity, young patient (increases myopic effect), uveitis.

INDIRECT CHOLINERGIC Succinylcholine administration, predisposition to retinal tear, anterior subcapsular cataract, ocular surgery, uveitis.

TABLE 6-3 MECHANISM OF ACTION OF VARIOUS MIOTIC AGENTS

Drug	Notes
Echothiophate iodide	Indirect; avoid in phakic patients
Physostigmine	Indirect; avoid in phakic patients
Demecarium bromide	Indirect
Acetylcholine	Direct; used during surgery
Carbachol	Direct/indirect
Pilocarpine hydrochloride	Direct
Pilocarpine nitrate	Direct

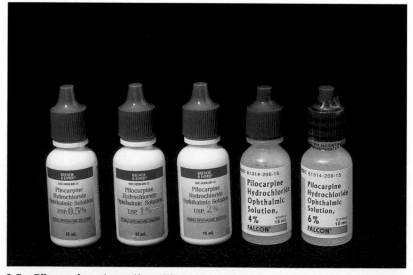

Figure 6-5 Pilocarpine strengths *The various strengths of pilocarpine, from 0.5% to 6%.*

PROSTAGLANDINS (FIGURE 6-6)

Mechanism of Action Prostaglandin $F_{2\alpha}$ analogues increase uveoscleral outflow by increasing extracellular matrix turnover in the ciliary body face.

Side Effects

Local Increase in melanin pigmentation in iris, blurred vision, and eyelid redness; cystoid macular edema and anterior uveitis have been reported.

Systemic Systemic upper respiratory infection symptoms, backache, chest pain, and myalgia.

Contraindications Pregnancy; consider not using in inflammatory conditions.

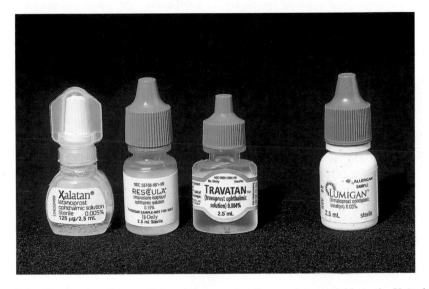

Figure 6-6   Prostaglandin agonists *All prostaglandin agonists available in the United States at the time of publication.* From left to right: *Xalatan (Pharmacia-UpJohn; Kalamazoo, MI), Rescula (Novartis; Atlanta, GA), and Travatan (Alcon; Fort Worth, TX). Separated from the rest of the group is the medication Lumigan (Allergan; Irvine, CA), which is chemically similar to the other drugs but is considered a prostamide.*

SYMPATHOMIMETIC AGENTS (FIGURE 6-7)

Mechanism of Action   In the ciliary body, the response is variable (beta stimulation increases aqueous production, but alpha stimulation decreases aqueous production); in trabecular meshwork, beta stimulation causes increased trabecular outflow and increased uveoscleral outflow; overall effect lowers IOP.

Side Effects

Local   Cystoid macular edema in aphakia (more likely with epinephrine than dipivefrin), mydriasis, rebound hyperemia, blurred vision, adrenochrome deposits, and allergic blepharoconjunctivitis.

Systemic   Tachycardia/ectopy, hypertension, headache.

Contraindications   Narrow angles, aphakia, pseudophakia, soft lenses, hypertension, and cardiac disease.

Comments   Dipivefrin requires 2 to 3 months to obtain the full effect. Epinephrine has mixed alpha- and beta-agonist activity.

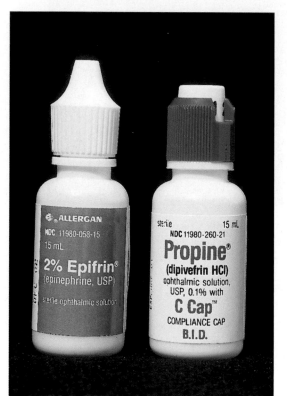

Figure 6-7   Sympathomimetic agents   *All sympathomimetic agents available in the United States at the time of publication. From left to right: Epifrin (Allergan; Irvine, CA) and Propine (Allergan; Irvine, CA).*

COMBINATION AGENT (FIGURE 6-8)

Only one combination agent is currently available, Cosopt, which combines the beta-blocker timolol (0.5%) with the topical CAI dorzolamide. The mechanisms of action, side effects, and contraindications of both beta-blockers and topical CAIs apply to this medication.

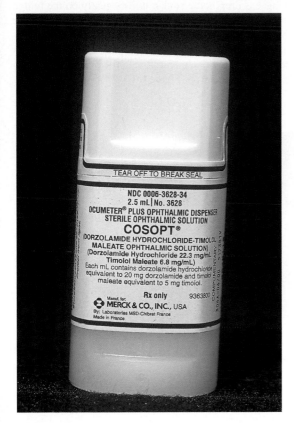

Figure 6-8 Combination agent
The combination agent Cosopt (Merck; West Point, PA).

TECHNIQUE OF DROP INSTILLATION

Self-Administration

In the upright position, drops can be administered in many ways. Briefly, I will describe a two-handed method. First, the patient should tilt the head back so that he or she is looking upward. With the nondominant hand, the patient uses the thumb and forefinger to hold open both upper and lower lids. With the dominant hand, the drop bottle is held over the eye, and a drop is administered (Figure 6-9A,B).

If tremor or generalized weakness makes this technique difficult, an alternate technique using one hand can be utilized. First, the patient should tilt the head back so that he or she is looking upward. The dominant hand holds the drop bottle so that it rests gently on the bridge of the nose. The tip of the drop bottle should be over the eye. Squeezing the bottle will administer the drop. This technique allows the patient's nose to help brace the bottle and assist the aim of the drop (Figure 6-10A,B).

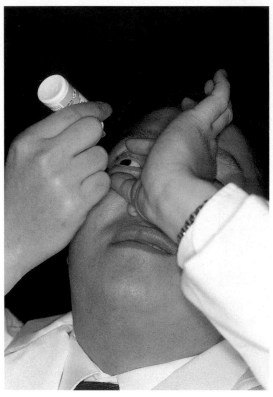

A

Figure 6-9A,B Self-administration of drops: two-handed method
Two-handed method for self-administration of topical drop.
A. Frontal view.

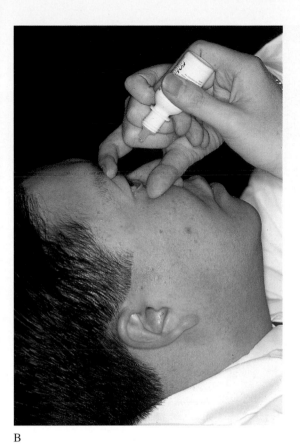

B

Figure 6-9A,B Self-administration of drops: two-handed method *(continued)*
B. Lateral view.

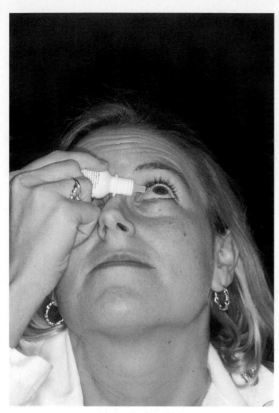

Figure 6-10A,B Self-administration of drops: one-handed method
Using the bridge of the nose to aid with steadiness of the hand for self-administration of topical drop.
A
A. Frontal view.

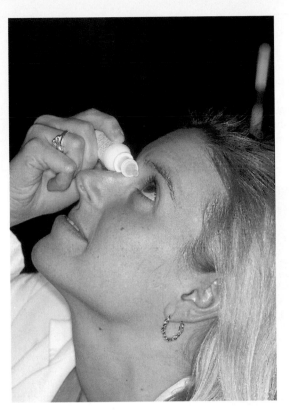

B

**Figure 6-10A,B   Self-administration
of drops: one-handed method**
(continued)   *B. Lateral view.*

Punctal Occlusion

Often, excess drops will drain into the tear drainage system and then into the nose. Absorption of the drug through the nasal mucosa can greatly increase the systemic effect of the medication. This increased systemic absorption does not typically enhance the drug's ocular effects because most drugs penetrate the cornea well and in sufficient quantity to supersaturate the intraocular receptors. However, the increased systemic absorption usually increases the likelihood of undesired systemic side effects.

Manual punctal occlusion minimizes the drug's access to the nasal mucosa. To perform this maneuver, the patient simply holds a finger over the common canaliculi (angle of the nose) (Figure 6-11A,B).

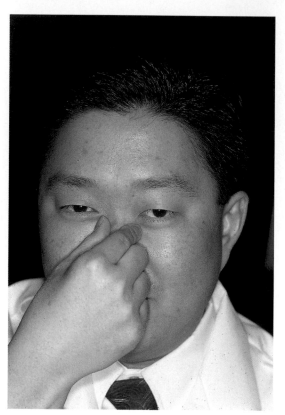

A

Figure 6-11A,B Punctal occlusion
Punctal occlusion to minimize systemic absorption of topically administered medications through the nasolacrimal system. **A.** *Frontal view.*

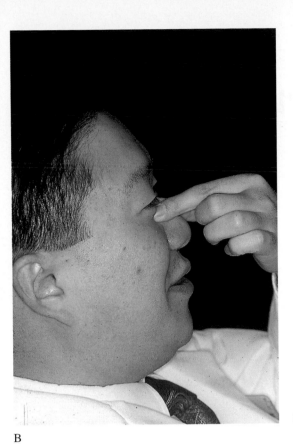

B

Figure 6-11A,B   Punctal occlusion
(continued)   ***B.** Lateral view.*

Chapter 7

LASER TRABECULOPLASTY

L. Jay Katz, MD, FACS

INDICATIONS

For uncontrolled open-angle glaucoma, either primary or secondary, laser trabeculoplasty has been proven to be helpful in lowering the intraocular pressure. Primary open-angle glaucoma, normal-tension glaucoma, pigmentary glaucoma, and pseudoexfoliative glaucoma are the most amenable for a good response. In juvenile glaucoma and secondary glaucomas, such as neovascular and inflammatory glaucomas, results with laser trabeculoplasty are typically poor. Clear media and a good view of the trabecular meshwork are required. Eyes with hazy corneas or extensive peripheral anterior synechiae may prevent proper treatment application with the laser. Mastery of gonioscopy and accurate identification of the angle structures are essential for proper laser trabeculoplasty.

ARGON LASER TRABECULOPLASTY (ALT)

Technique

Since the introduction of ALT in 1979 by Witter and Wise, there has been remarkably little alteration of the technique. A 50-μm spot size is applied to the trabecular meshwork with up to 1000 mW of energy, enough to cause minimal blanching of the pigment. The least amount of energy is employed to attain the tissue endpoint (Figure 7-1).

The laser spot is aimed at the junction of the pigmented and nonpigmented trabecular meshwork. Either a single treatment session of the entire 360 degrees with up to 100 applications, or two sessions of 180 degrees each with 50 shots, may be performed. A single or three-mirrored Goldmann lens or Ritch goniolens is used to apply the laser shots to the target tissue.

A topical alpha agonist (apraclonidine or brimonidine) is given pre- and postlaser treatment to minimize the possibility of a transient intraocular pressure spike (Figure 7-2). A topical corticosteroid is prescribed four times daily for a week to prevent postlaser inflammation.

After the treatment, the patient is examined 1 hour later to measure the eye pressure. If a pressure spike occurs, it is treated with glaucoma medications such as oral carbonic anhydrase inhibitors or oral hyperosmotic agents. The patient is reexamined at 1 week and again 1 month after the treatment. At the last visit, a determination is made as to whether the laser therapy was beneficial.

Mechanism of Action

Theories have been offered, but none verified, as to how laser therapy lowers the eye pressure. The extent of pigmentation of the trabecular

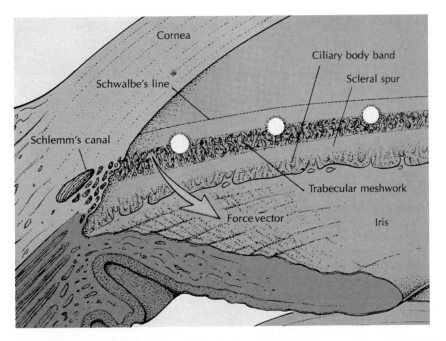

Figure 7-1 Tissue response to laser treatment *The "ideal" tissue response is minimal bubble formation and mild blanching of the trabecular meshwork. The laser is aimed at the junction of the pigmented and nonpigmented trabecular meshwork. (Reprinted with permission from Katz LJ. Argon laser trabeculoplasty.* Annual of Ophthalmic Laser Surgery *1:103–110, 1992.)*

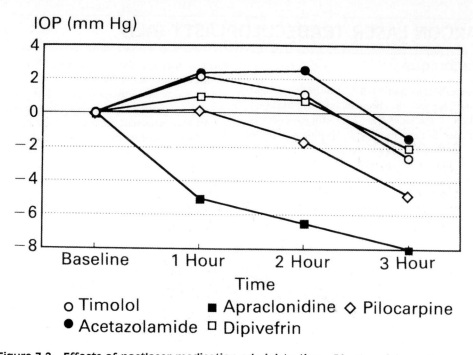

IOP (mm Hg)

o Timolol   ■ Apraclonidine   ◇ Pilocarpine
● Acetazolamide   □ Dipivefrin

Figure 7-2   Effects of postlaser medication administration   *Blunting of the postlaser intraocular pressure spike after argon laser trabeculoplasty (ALT) with apraclonidine is compared with other glaucoma medications.*

meshwork seems to be critical for the success of laser trabeculoplasty. Heavier pigmentation is a positive predictor of success. The thermal burn with the argon laser has been shown histologically to cause melting and distortion of the trabecular beams. The first theory suggested that these contraction burns over the angle mechanically helped adjacent trabecular beams open wider, thus allowing easier aqueous outflow. The second theory suggested that the laser irradiation stimulated trabecular endothelial cells to replicate (Figure 7-3). Because these cells serve a phagocytic role in the angle, it was thought that the endothelial cells keep the intratrabecular spaces free of debris that may be implicated in the increased resistance to outflow seen in glaucomatous eyes.

Efficacy

Intraocular pressure is typically reduced 20% to 30% below baseline levels with ALT. Not all eyes are responsive to laser trabeculoplasty. Positive predictors of a favorable response include heavy pigmentation of the trabecular meshwork, age (older patients), and diagnosis (pigmentary glaucoma, primary open-angle glaucoma, and exfoliation syndrome).

There is an apparent waning of the effect of ALT over time. In long-term studies of 5 to 10 years, ALT failure ranged from 65% to 90%. Re-treatment after a previous complete 360-degree application of ALT is at best a short-term benefit with failure at 1 year up to 80%. Because there is structural alteration of the outflow

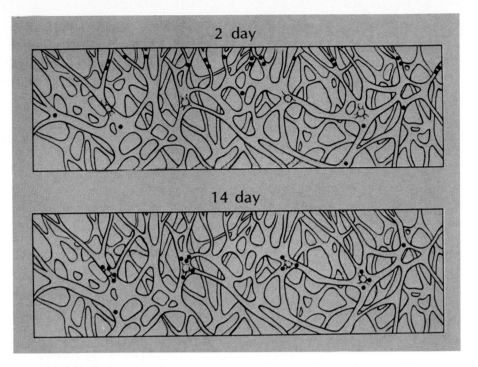

Figure 7-3 ALT: One proposed mechanism of action *Cellular theory that ALT stimulates the replication of trabecular endothelial cells that promote aqueous outflow. (Reprinted with permission from Van Buskirk EM. Pathophysiology of laser trabeculoplasty.* Surv Ophthalmol *33:264–272, 1989.)*

system with ALT, repeat treatment may lead to a paradoxical persistent elevation of intraocular pressure. Repeat argon laser application to the angle structures in animals was used by Gaasterland to create an experimental open-angle glaucoma model. If a prompt reduction in intraocular pressure is needed, or a relatively large reduction in pressure is desired (e.g., more than a 30% lowering below baseline pretreatment intraocular pressure), then ALT may not be a good choice. Medication or filtering surgery is more likely to achieve those objectives.

The current treatment paradigm for glaucoma in the United States is medication first, then ALT, and, finally, filtering surgery. This stepping regimen is only a guideline, and treatment needs to be individualized for each patient to provide optimum care. There have been studies that have reexamined the sequencing of treatments for open-angle glaucoma. In the Glaucoma Laser Trial, ALT was compared with medication as the first step in the treatment of newly diagnosed primary open-angle glaucoma. After 2 years, 44% of eyes with ALT alone were controlled as opposed to only 20% with timolol alone being adequately treated. In a subsequent paper, with a mean follow-up of 7 years, ALT alone was adequate control for 20% of eyes and timolol alone, for 15%. Although there were methodological flaws in the study design for this study, there was intriguing support to at least consider ALT as initial therapy for certain patients.

SELECTIVE LASER TRABECULOPLASTY (SLT)

Technique

A pulsed-frequency doubled neodymium (Nd):YAG laser was introduced in 1998 by Latina for trabeculoplasty. It was developed to selectively target pigmented tissue and minimize any collateral effect. In contrast with the continuous wave argon laser, the selective laser does not cause any thermal injury to the trabecular region. The fixed spot size of 400 μm dwarfs the typical 50-μm spot size used with ALT (Figure 7-4). Therefore, the spacing between laser spots with the SLT is much more

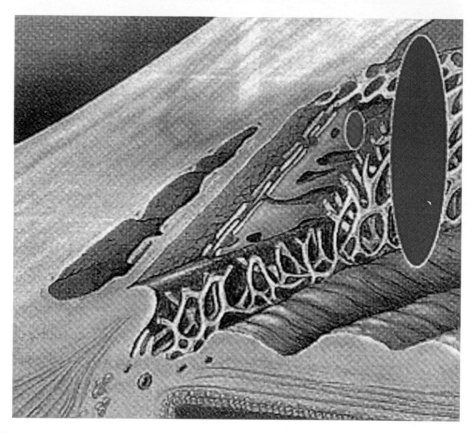

Figure 7-4 Comparison of argon and selective laser spots *Comparative size of the argon laser spot (50 μm) versus the neodymium (Nd):YAG selective laser spot (400 μm). (Courtesy of Michael S. Berlin, MD, Associate Clinical Professor, University of California–Los Angeles; Jules Stein.)*

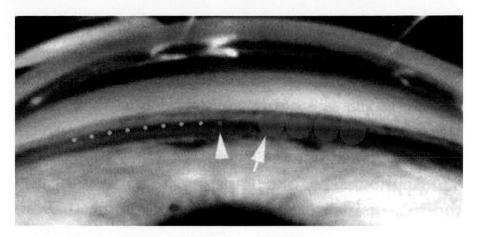

Figure 7-5 Comparison of spacing of laser spots *Spacing of the argon laser versus the close application of the selective laser. Triangle indicates approximate 50-μm spot size with ALT versus the 400-μm spot size of selective laser trabeculoplasty (SLT). (Courtesy of Michael S. Berlin, MD, Associate Clinical Professor, University of California–Los Angeles, Jules Stein.)*

compact and almost confluent (Figure 7-5). The spot size with SLT is so large that the entire angle is covered with the aiming beam. The only variables in applying the laser are the number of shots (50 to 60), extent of the angle treated (180 to 360 degrees), and the power (up to 0.8 joules).

The power endpoint is determined by the tissue reaction with the initial laser application. Blanching of the pigmented trabecular meshwork with slight bubble vaporization is ideal. If there is a great deal of bubble formation, then the power is adjusted downward. The use of low power is strongly recommended in heavily pigmented angles as seen in pigmentary glaucoma.

Mechanism of Action

Scanning electron microscopy highlights the difference between argon laser application, with the "melting" of trabecular beams, and the selective laser, with little if any observable structural alteration (Figure 7-6A,B). Therefore, the mechanical stretching theory is not applicable for the selective laser effect on the intraocular pressure. In vitro cultures of trabecular meshwork cells were irradiated by Latina with either argon or selective laser. Argon laser application damaged both pigmented and nonpigmented cells. In contrast, the selective laser targeted only the pigmented cells.

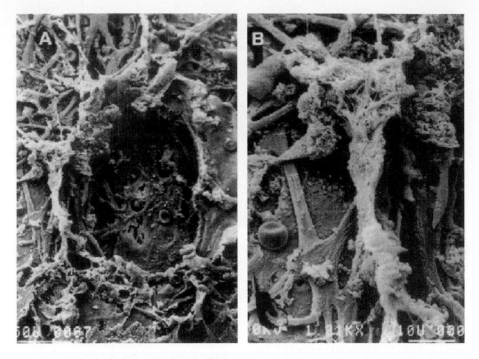

Figure 7-6A,B Scanning electron microscopy of cadaver eyes treated with argon or selective laser *A. Argon burn resulted in coagulative melting of the trabecular beam.* Left panel: *lower magnification showing the crater;* right panel: *a higher magnification view showing the curling of the collagen caused by the thermal damage. **B.** The selective laser did not cause any significant structural alteration.* Left panel: *a lower magnification view showing the absence of a crater;* right panel: *a higher magnification view showing a fracture of one of the sheets of collagen. (Reprinted with permission from Kramer TR, Noecker RJ. Comparison of the morphologic changes after selective laser trabeculoplasty and argon laser trabeculoplasty in human eye bank eyes.* Ophthalmology *108:773–779, 2001.)*

Recruitment of macrophages into the outflow system has been demonstrated in animal models and in human eyes. These macrophages may release chemical mediators that regulate the outflow rate. Elevated interleukin levels detected following laser application have been postulated to improve aqueous outflow.

Efficacy

Comparative trials have confirmed that ALT and SLT have equivalent efficacy in lowering the intraocular pressure in eyes that have failed medical therapy. Preliminary data suggest that initial therapy with SLT prior to any glaucoma medication use lowers the intraocular pressure by 24% to 30% below baseline levels. Because no structural damage is detected with SLT, repeating the laser treatment could theoretically be safely attempted and could potentially lower the intraocular pressure. In eyes that have failed previous ALT, success has been reported in using SLT to lower the intraocular pressure.

BIBLIOGRAPHY

Damji KF, Shah KC, Rock WJ, et al. Selective laser trabeculoplasty argon laser trabeculoplasty: A prospective randomised clinical trial. *Br J Ophthalmol* 83:718–722, 1999.

Feldman RM, Katz LJ, Spaeth GL, et al. Long-term efficacy of repeat argon laser trabeculoplasty. *Ophthalmology* 98:1061–1065, 1991.

Glaucoma Trial Research Group. The Glaucoma Laser Trial 2. Results of argon laser trabeculoplasty versus topical medicines. *Ophthalmology* 97:1403–1413, 1990.

Glaucoma Trial Research Group. The Glaucoma Laser Trial (GLT) and glaucoma laser trial follow-up study: 7. Results. *Am J Ophthalmol* 120:718–731, 1995.

Katz LJ. Argon laser trabeculoplasty. *Annual of Ophthalmic Laser Surgery* 1:103–110, 1992.

Kramer TR, Noecker RJ. Comparison of the morphologic changes after selective laser trabeculoplasty and argon laser trabeculoplasty in human eye bank eyes. *Ophthalmology* 108:773–779, 2001.

Latina MA, Sibayan SA, Shin DH, et al. Q-Switched 532-nm Nd:YAG laser trabeculoplasty (selective laser trabeculoplasty). *Ophthalmology* 105:2082–2090, 1998.

Spaeth GL, Baez KA. Argon laser trabeculoplasty controls one third of cases of progressive, uncontrolled, open angle glaucoma for 5 years. *Arch Ophthalmol* 110:491–494, 1992.

Van Buskirk EM. Pathophysiology of laser trabeculoplasty. *Surv Ophthalmol* 33.264–272, 1989.

Wise JB. Long-term control of adult open angle glaucoma by argon laser treatment. *Ophthalmology* 88:197–202, 1981.

Chapter 8

SURGICAL MANAGEMENT OF GLAUCOMA: TRABECULECTOMY AND GLAUCOMA DRAINAGE DEVICES

Marlene R. Moster, MD

Augusto Azuara-Blanco, MD, PhD

TRABECULECTOMY

Purpose of Procedure

Guarded filtration surgery, or trabeculectomy, is the procedure most commonly used to control the intraocular pressure in patients with glaucoma (Figure 8-1). Trabeculectomy lowers the intraocular pressure by creating a fistula between the inner compartments of the eye and the subconjunctival space (i.e., filtering bleb). Cairns reported the first series in 1968. A number of techniques are available to assist in establishing and maintaining the function of filtration blebs and avoiding complications.

Description

Any type of regional anesthesia (retrobulbar, peribulbar, and sub-Tenon's) can be used. Topical anesthesia is also possible, with topical 2% lidocaine gel, 0.1 mL of intracameral 1% nonpreserved lidocaine (Figure 8-2), and 0.5 mL of subconjunctival 1% lidocaine injected from the superior-temporal quadrant to balloon the conjunctiva over the superior rectus muscle (Figure 8-3).

Trabeculectomy should be done at the superior limbus, because inferiorly located blebs are associated with a much higher risk of bleb-associated infections. The globe can be rotated inferiorly with the use of a superior rectus traction suture (4-0 or 5-0 black silk) or a corneal traction suture (7-0 or 8-0 black silk or Vicryl on a spatulated needle); refer to Figure 8-4.

A limbus- (Figure 8-5) or fornix- (Figure 8-6) based conjunctival flap is made with Wescott scissors and nontoothed utility forceps. A fornix-based flap may be easier in cases with preexisting perilimbal scarring, and is more likely to be associated with diffuse blebs. When forming limbus-based flaps, the conjunctival incision is placed 8 to 10 mm posterior to the limbus. The conjunctival and Tenon's wound should be lengthened to approximately 8 to 12 mm cord length. The flap is then extended anteriorly to expose the corneoscleral sulcus. When making fornix-based flaps, the conjunctiva and Tenon's are disinserted. Approximately a 2-clock-hour limbal peritomy (6 to 8 mm) is sufficient. Blunt dissection is carried posteriorly.

The scleral flap should completely cover the sclerostomy to provide resistance to the aqueous

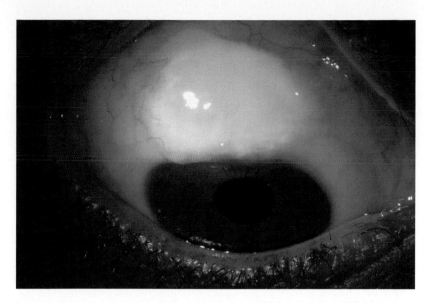

Figure 8-1 **Posttrabeculectomy eye** *Slit-lamp view of an eye that underwent trabeculectomy 3 months earlier.*

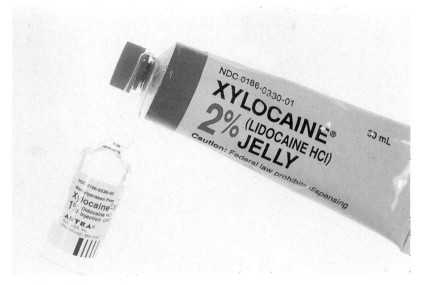

Figure 8-2 **Topical anesthetic agents** *Xylocaine 2% and lidocaine 1% nonpreserved for injection.*

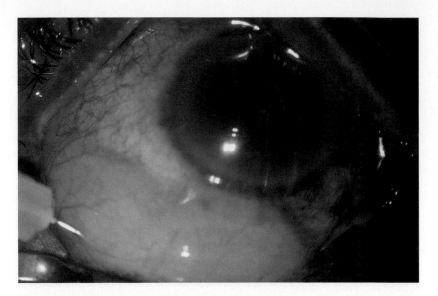

Figure 8-3   Ballooning of conjunctiva   *Ballooning of the conjunctiva with nonpreserved lidocaine 1% (0.5 mL) using a 30-gauge sharp needle in the direction of the superior rectus muscle.*

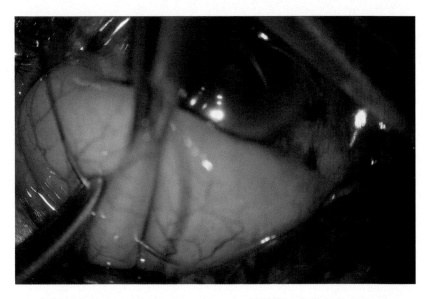

Figure 8-4   Traction suture placement   *Placement of a traction suture prior to a limbus-based trabeculectomy.*

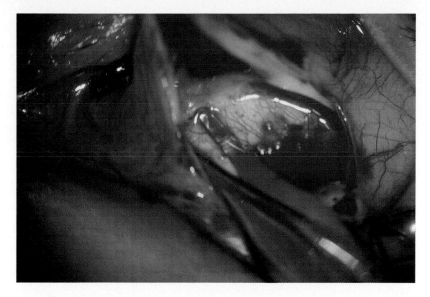

Figure 8-5 Limbus-based flap *Developing a limbus-based conjunctival-Tenon's flap.*

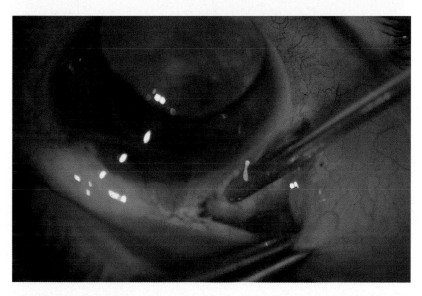

Figure 8-6 Fornix-based flap *Developing a fornix-based conjunctival-Tenon's flap.*

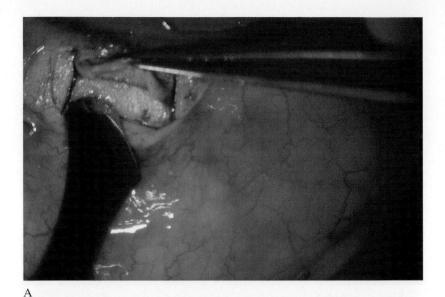

A

B

Figure 8-7   Partial-thickness flap   *Developing a one-half to two-thirds partial-thickness scleral trabeculectomy flap with a fornix-based conjunctival flap (A,B) or with a linbal-based flap (c).*

outflow. The fluid will flow around the scleral flap. Differences in the shape or size of the scleral flap probably have little effect on surgical outcome. The flap thickness should be between one half and two thirds (Figure 8-7). It is important to

dissect the flap anteriorly (approximately 1 mm into clear cornea) to ensure that the fistula is created anterior to the scleral spur and ciliary body.

A corneal paracentesis is made before opening the globe (Figure 8-8) with either a 30- or a

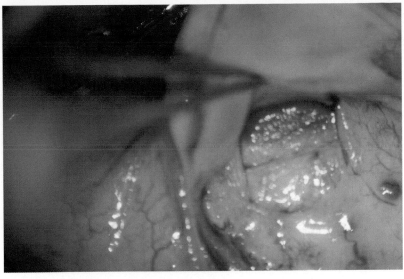

C

Figure 8-7 Partial-thickness flap *(continued)*

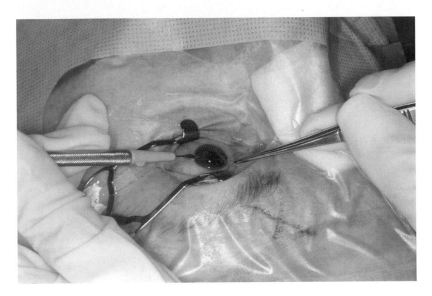

Figure 8-8 Corneal paracentesis

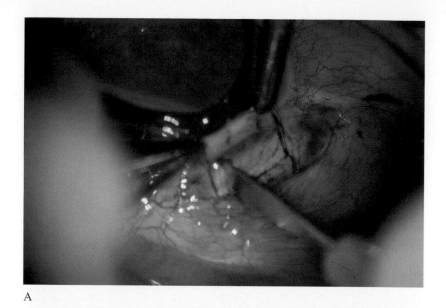

A

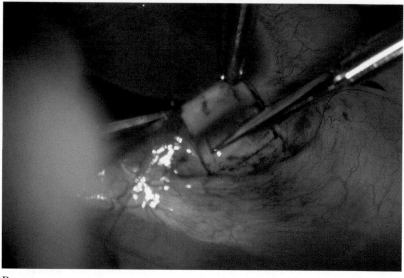

B

Figure 8-9 Removing the internal trabeculectomy block (A,B,C)

27-gauge needle or a sharp point blade. A block of tissue at the corneoscleral junction is then excised. Two radial incisions are made first with a sharp blade or knife starting in clear cornea, and extending posteriorly approximately 1 to 1.5 mm. The radial incisions are made approximately 2 mm apart. The blade or Vannas scissors are used to connect the incisions; thereby a rectangular piece of tissue is removed (Figure 8-9). Alternatively, an anterior corneal incision, parallel to the limbus and perpendicular to the eye, is made to enter into the anterior

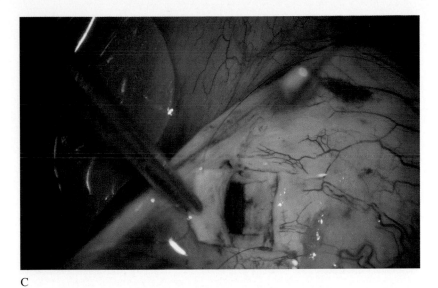

C

Figure 8-9 *(continued)*

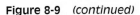

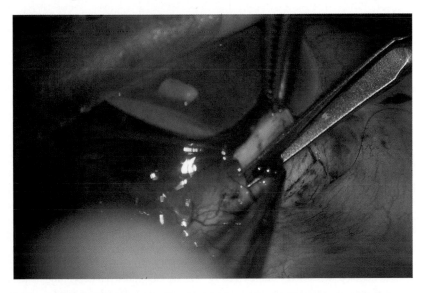

Figure 8-10   Surgical iridectomy   *Surgical iridectomy with Vannas scissors after trabeculectomy block removal.*

chamber and a Kelly or Gass punch is used to excise the tissue.

A peripheral iridectomy is then performed. The iris is grasped near its root with toothed forceps. The iris is retracted through the sclerostomy, and an iridectomy is performed with Vannas or DeWecker scissors (Figure 8-10). The iridectomy should avoid damage to the iris root and ciliary body or bleeding.

The scleral flap (Figure 8-11) is sutured initially with two interrupted 10-0 nylon sutures (in case of rectangular flap) or with one suture

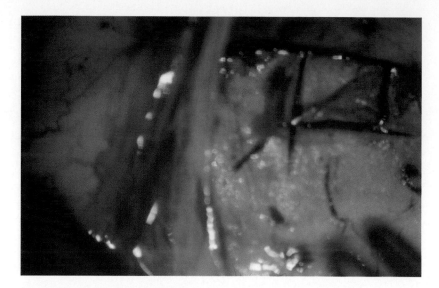

Figure 8-11   Suturing the scleral flap

(in a triangular flap). Slipknots are useful to adjust the tightness of the scleral flap and the rate of aqueous outflow. Additional sutures can be used to better control the outflow. During the suturing of the scleral flap, the anterior chamber is filled through the paracentesis, and the flow around the scleral flap is observed. If flow seems excessive, or the anterior chamber shallows, the slipknots are tightened or additional sutures are placed. If aqueous does not flow through the flap, the surgeon may loosen the slipknots, or replace tight sutures with looser ones.

Releasable sutures can be used (Figure 8-12A–C). The use of releasable sutures allows the surgeon to close the scleral flap tightly, knowing that the flow can be increased postoperatively. Externalized releasable sutures are easily removed and are effective in cases of inflamed or hemorrhagic conjunctiva or thickened Tenon's capsule.

Conjunctival closure in limbus-based flaps is done with a double or single running suture (Figure 8-13A,B), with an 8-0 or 9-0 absorbable suture, or with 10-0 nylon. Many surgeons favor a rounded-body needle. In fornix-based flaps, a tight conjunctival-corneal apposition is needed. Two 10-0 nylon sutures or a mattress suture (Figure 8-14) at the edges of the incision can be used to anchor the conjunctiva to the cornea.

After the wound is closed, a 30-gauge cannula is used to fill the anterior chamber with balanced salt solution through the paracentesis track to elevate the conjunctival bleb and test for leaks. Antibiotics and corticosteroids can be injected in the inferior fornix. Patching the eye can be individualized depending on the patient's vision and the anesthesia used.

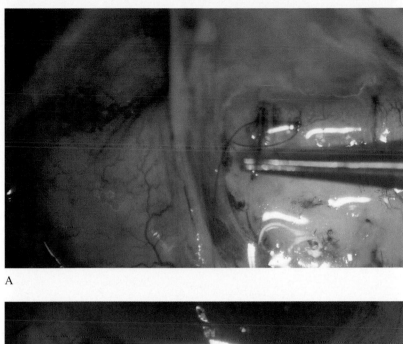

A

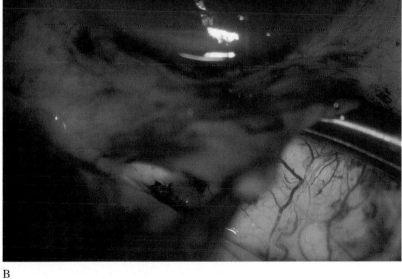

B

Figure 8-12A,B,C   Releasable sutures   *A. Placing of releasable sutures. **B.** Backhand releasable suture through clear cornea.*

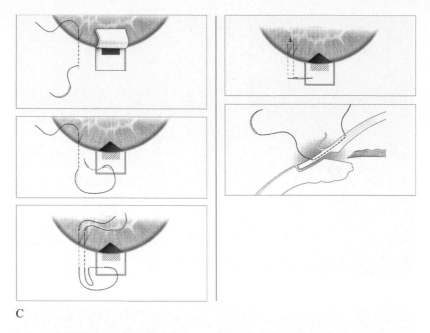

C

Figure 8-12C Releasable sutures *(continued)* *C. Releasable suture technique in a limbus-based conjuctival incision (described by Richard P. Wilson, MD). A 10-0 nylon suture is used.* ***Step 1:*** *The suture enters into the cornea 1 mm anterior to the limbus (depth: midstromal) and exits through the sclera adjacent to the flap (going underneath the corneoscleral limbus and the insertion of the conjunctiva).* ***Step 2:*** *The needle is passed through the scleral flap and sclera adjacent to the flap.* ***Step 3:*** *The needle enters the sclera and exits through the cornea (direction parallel to step 1).* ***Step 4:*** *The suture is then tied with up to seven knots.* ***Step 5:*** *Illustrates the depth of the suture. (Illustrations by Christine Gralapp). (Adapted with permission of American Academy of Ophthalmology from Moster MR, Azuara-Blanco A. Focal Points Volume XVIII, number 6. San Francisco: American Academy of Ophthalmology, 2000).*

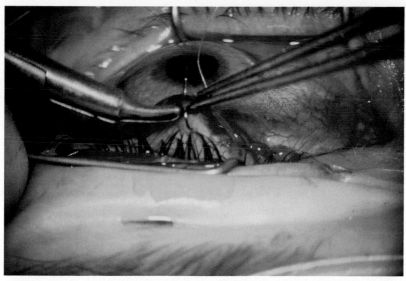

A

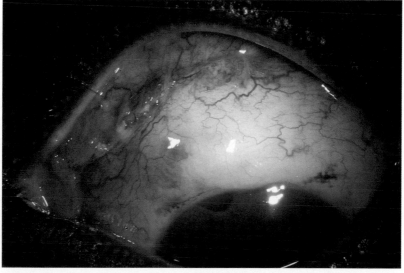

B

Figure 8-13A,B **Conjunctival closure: limbus-based flap** *A. Closed limbus-based conjunctival-Tenon's flap with running Vicryl suture.* ***B.*** *Postoperative appearance of a closed limbus-based conjunctival-Tenon's flap.*

Technique of Intraoperative Application of Antimetabolites

To reduce postoperative subconjunctival fibrosis, especially important in cases at high risk for failure, mitomycin C (Figure 8-15) and 5-fluorouracil (5-FU) are used. The use of antifibrotic agents is associated with a higher success and complication rates for primary and high-risk trabeculectomies. An individualized consideration of the risk/benefit ratio is recommended.

Mitomycin C (0.2 to 0.5 mg/mL solution) or 5-FU (50 mg/mL solution) is applied for 1 to 5 minutes using a soaked cellulose sponge (Figure 8-16) placed over the episclera or a piece that is cut to the appropriate size. Application under the scleral flap is also possible. The conjunctival-Tenon layer is draped over the sponge, avoiding contact of the mitomycin C with the wound edge. After the application, the sponge is removed and the entire area is irrigated thoroughly with balanced salt solution. The plastic devices that collect the liquid runoff (Figure 8-17) are changed and disposed of according to toxic waste regulations (Figure 8-18).

Postoperative Care

Topical steroids (e.g., prednisolone acetate 1%, four times daily) are tapered after 6 to 8 weeks. Some clinicians use topical nonsteroidal anti-inflammatory agents (e.g., 2 to 4 times a day for 1 month). Antibiotics are required for 1 to 2 weeks after surgery. Postoperative cycloplegics are utilized on an individual basis in patients with shallow anterior chambers or intense inflammation.

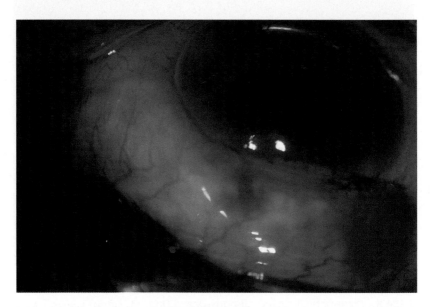

Figure 8-14 Conjunctival closure: fornix-based flap *Closure of a fornix-based conjunctival-Tenon's flap with two individual 10-0 nylon mattress sutures.*

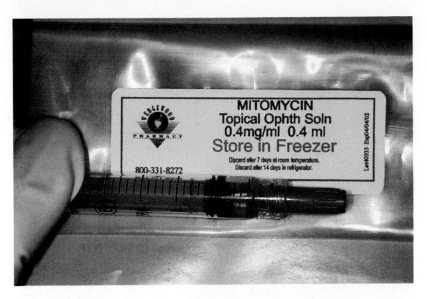

Figure 8-15 Mitomycin C *Mitomycin C as delivered to the operating room*

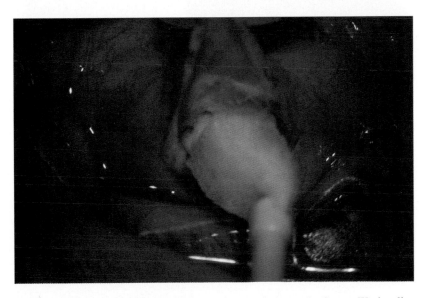

Figure 8-16 Application of mitomycin C *Delivery of mitomycin C on a Weck-cell sponge under the conjunctiva and Tenon's capsule.*

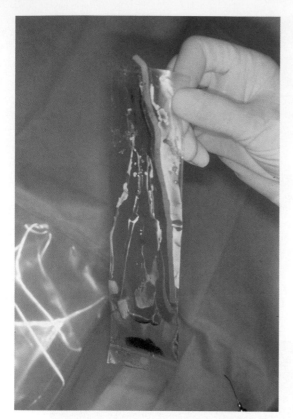

Figure 8-17 Collection of mitomycin C runoff *Collection of remnants of mitomycin C after irrigation.*

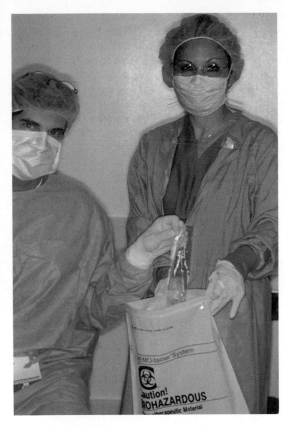

Figure 8-18   Disposal of mitomycin C runoff   *Proper disposal of mitomycin C–contaminated materials.*

In cases prone to early failure (e.g., vascularized and thickened blebs), repeated subconjunctival applications of 5-FU (5 mg in 0.1 mL solution) over the first 2 to 3 weeks are recommended.

Digital ocular compression applied to the inferior sclera or cornea through the closed inferior eyelid, and focal compression with a moistened cotton tip at the edge of the scleral flap, can be useful to elevate the bleb and reduce the intraocular pressure in the early postoperative period, especially after laser suture lysis (Figure 8-19).

Suture lysis and cutting and pulling releasable sutures are necessary when there is a high intraocular pressure, a flat filtration bleb, and a deep anterior chamber. Gonioscopy must be performed prior to the laser treatment to confirm an open sclerostomy with no tissue or clot occluding its entrance. Suture lysis and cutting and pulling releasable sutures should be done within the first 2 to 3 weeks after surgery, although it may be successful even months after surgery in patients in whom mitomycin C had been used.

Complications of Trabeculectomy

Refer to Table 8-1.

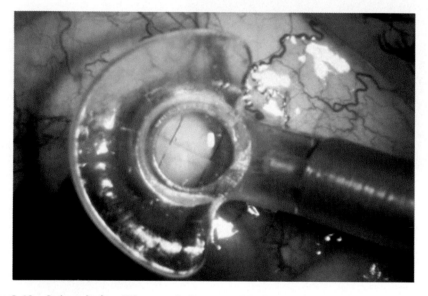

Figure 8-19 Suture lysis *(Photograph Courtesy of Richard P. Wilson, MD; Wills Eye Hospital, Philadelphia, PA).*

TABLE 8-1   COMPLICATIONS OF TRABECULECTOMY

Complication	Treatment
Conjunctival buttonholes (Figure 8-20)	Purse-string suture with 10-0 or 11-0 needle on a rounded ("vascular") needle.
Early overfiltration (Figure 8-21)	If AC is shallow or flat with no lens-cornea touch, use cycloplegics, restriction in activity, and avoidance of Valsalva maneuvers. If there is lens-corneal touch, perform urgent reformation of AC. If complication persists, resuture scleral flap.
Choroidal effusions (Figure 8-22)	Observation, cycloplegics, steroids. Drainage is considered if effusions are appositional and associated with flat anterior chamber.
Suprachoroidal hemorrhage	
Intraoperative	Prompt closure of eye and gentle reposition of prolapsed uvea. Intravenous mannitol and acetazolamide.
Postoperative	Observation; control IOP and pain. Drain (after 7–10 days) cases with persistent flat AC and intolerable pain.
Aqueous misdirection	Initial medical treatment: intensive topical cycloplegic-mydriatic regimen, topical and oral aqueous suppressants, and osmotics. In pseudophakics: Nd:YAG laser hyaloidotomy or peripheral anterior vitrectomy via AC. In phakics: phacoemulsification and anterior vitrectomy. Pars plana vitrectomy.
Bleb encapsulation (Figure 8-23)	Initial observation. Aqueous suppressants if IOP is elevated. Consider needling with 5-fluorouracil or surgical revision.
Late bleb leak (Figure 8-24)	If leak is not brisk, initial observation and topical antibiotics. If it persists, surgical revision (conjunctival advancement or autograft).
Chronic hypotony (Figure 8-25)	If there is maculopathy and visual loss: subconjunctival injection of blood or surgical revision of the scleral flap.
Blebitis (Figure 8-26), endophthalmitis	Bleb infection without intraocular involvement: intensive topical treatment with wide-spectrum fortified antibiotics. Bleb infection with mild anterior segment cellular reaction: intensive topical treatment with fortified antibiotics. Bleb infection with severe anterior segment cellular reaction or vitreous involved: vitreous sample and intravitreal antibiotics.

AC = anterior chamber; IOP = intraocular pressure.

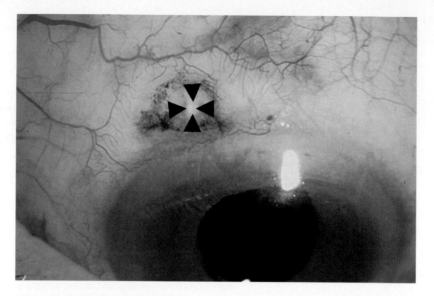

Figure 8-20   Conjunctival buttonhole   *Conjunctival buttonhole identified several weeks following trabeculectomy with mitomycin C. The* arrowheads *denote the edges of the hole.*

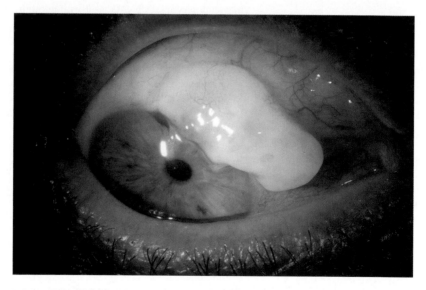

Figure 8-21   Overfiltration   *Overfiltration caused by an exuberant bleb.*

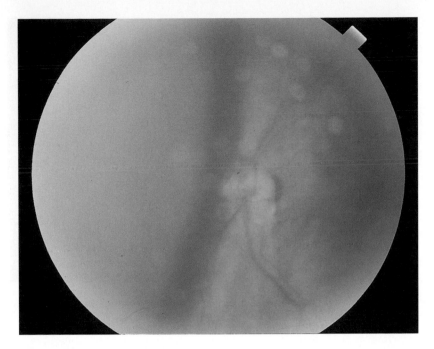

Figure 8-22 Choroidal detachment *Fundus photograph showing serous choroidal detachment obscuring the optic nerve.*

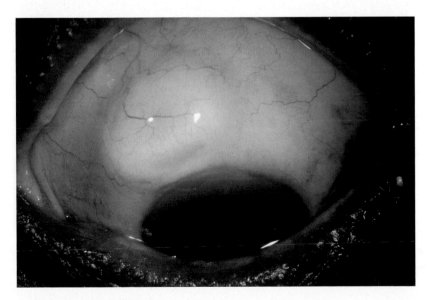

Figure 8-23 Encapsulated bleb

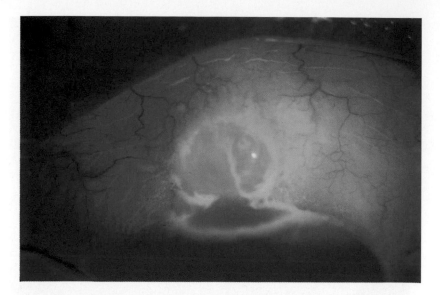

Figure 8-24 Late bleb leak *Late bleb leak 3 years following trabeculectomy surgery. Under cobalt blue light, the Seidel test shows aqueous flow from the leak.*

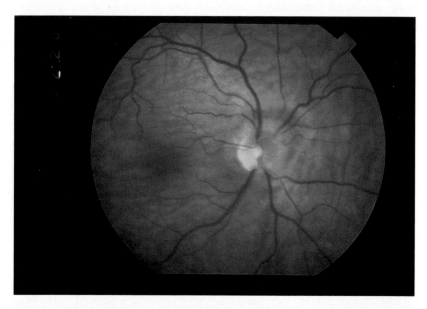

Figure 8-25 Chronic hypotony *Fundus photograph showing retinal folds through the maculopathy—so-called hypotony maculopathy.*

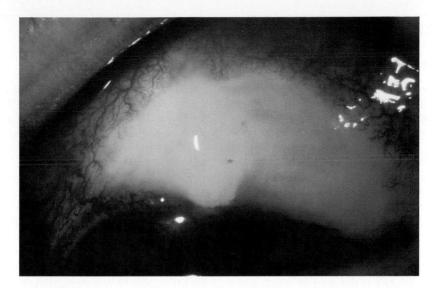

Figure 8-26   Blebitis   *Slit-lamp photograph of a case of blebitis; exudative discharge can be seen on the bleb.*

GLAUCOMA DRAINAGE DEVICES

Purpose of Procedure

Glaucoma drainage devices (GDDs), also called aqueous shunts or tube shunts, are used to reduce the intraocular pressure in patients with uncontrolled glaucoma in whom filtration surgery with antifibrotic agents has already failed or is unlikely to succeed (Figure 8-27). Aqueous shunting devices consist of a posteriorly placed, episcleral bleb-promoting explant connected to a silicone tube that is inserted into the eye, usually in the anterior chamber (occasionally through the pars plana). A posterior-filtering bleb is formed around the episcleral explant. Aqueous flow crosses passively through the wall of the capsule and is reabsorbed by venous capillaries and lymphatics.

There are now several devices available that differ regarding the presence or absence of a flow-limiting element and the design of the episcleral plate or plates. *Nonrestrictive devices* (e.g., single- or double-plate Molteno, Baerveldt; Figure 8-28) permit the free flow of fluid from the inner ostium of the tube in the anterior chamber to the episcleral explant. *Restrictive devices* (e.g., Krupin, Joseph, White, Optimed, single- or double-plate Ahmed; Figure 8-29) incorporate an element in the posterior part of the tube (i.e., valve, membrane, or resistant matrix) designed to limit fluid flow in an attempt to prevent postoperative hypotony.

Description

Implantation of GDD can usually be performed under retrobulbar, peribulbar, or sub-Tenon's anesthesia. The preferred location is the superotemporal quadrant. A superior rectus muscle or a corneal or scleral traction suture is helpful to improve exposure of the surgical site.

Either a fornix- or limbus-based conjunctival flap can be used. A 90- to 110-degree conjunctival incision is adequate for single-plate implants. The episcleral plate is placed between adjacent rectus muscles with its anterior edge at least 8 mm posterior to the limbus (Figure 8-30). Nonabsorbable sutures (6-0 to 8-0 nylon) are passed through the fixation holes of the episcleral plate and sutured to the sclera. The optimal length of tubing is estimated by laying the tube across the cornea. The tube is then trimmed bevel-up to extend 2 to 3 mm into the anterior chamber (Figure 8-31). A corneal paracentesis is done (Figure 8-32). A 23-gauge needle is used to create a limbal-scleral incision into the anterior chamber at an oblique angle, parallel to the plane of the iris, starting approximately 1 to 2 mm posterior to the corneoscleral limbus (Figure 8-33). The tube is then inserted through this entry track into the anterior chamber with smooth forceps.

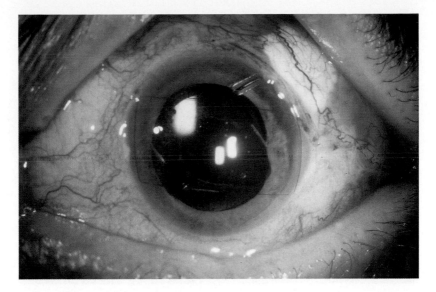

Figure 8-27   Glaucoma drainage device   *Baerveldt tube shunt in pseudophakic open-angle glaucoma with a chamber-maintaining suture in place.*

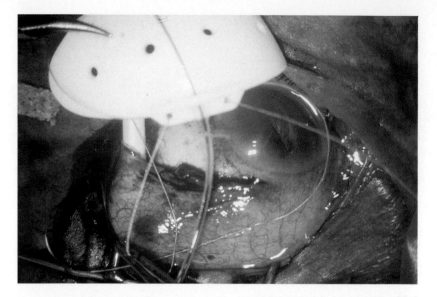

Figure 8-28   Nonrestrictive device   *Baerveldt 350 mm² tube shunt on an eye. Latina suture is in place (see text for further description).*

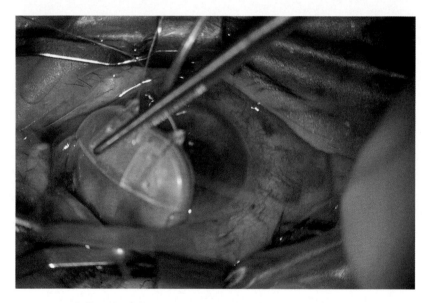

Figure 8-29   Restrictive device   *Ahmed tube shunt.*

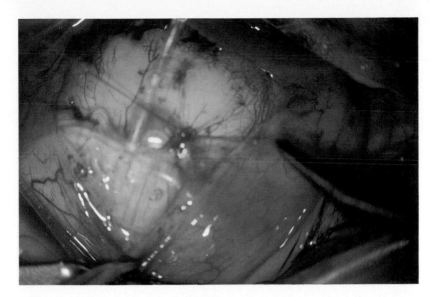

Figure 8-30 *Ahmed tube shunt sewn to sclera.*

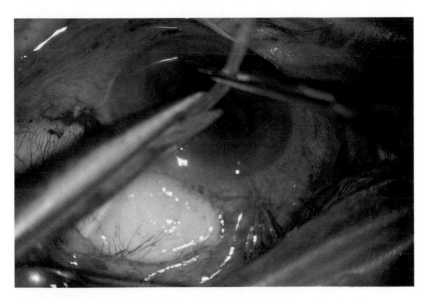

Figure 8-31 *The tube is cut to the appropriate size with Wescott scissors.*

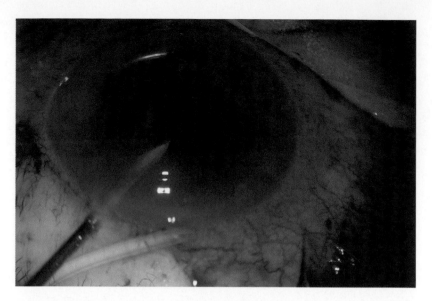

Figure 8-32 *A 23-gauge needle entering the anterior chamber prior to placement of the tube.*

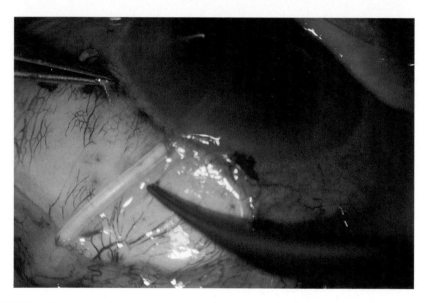

Figure 8-33 *Placement of the tube shunt into the anterior chamber.*

GLAUCOMA MANAGEMENT

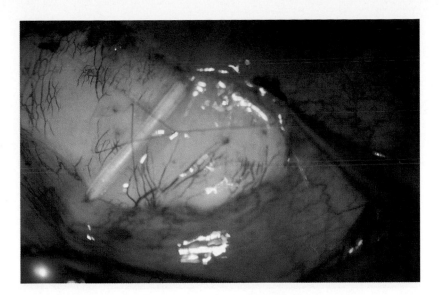

Figure 8-34 *Suturing the tube shunt to the sclera with 10-0 nylon.*

Proper positioning of the tube in the anterior chamber is essential, assuring that it does not touch the iris, lens, or cornea. The tube can be fixed to the sclera with sutures of 10-0 nylon or Prolene (Figure 8-34). This anterior suture is wrapped tightly around the tube to prevent movement into or out of the anterior chamber. To avoid postoperative conjunctival erosion of the tube, donor sclera, fascia lata, dura mater, or pericardium can be used to cover the limbal portion of the tube (Figure 8-35). The patch graft is sutured in place using interrupted 10-0 nylon, Prolene, or Vicryl sutures.

The tube can also be placed through the pars plana (Figure 8-36) in cases in which placement into the anterior chamber is difficult or undesirable (e.g., corneal graft, extensively shallow anterior chamber from iridocorneal contact, etc.). This approach requires pars plana vitrectomy with careful attention to remove the vitreous skirt in the quadrant where the tube will be inserted.

During the insertion of *nonrestrictive devices,* an additional step is needed to prevent postoperative hypotony. This step can be performed before suturing the plate to episclera. Temporary occlusion of the tube with absorbable suture can also be achieved by ligating with an absorbable 6-0 to 8-0 Vicryl suture.

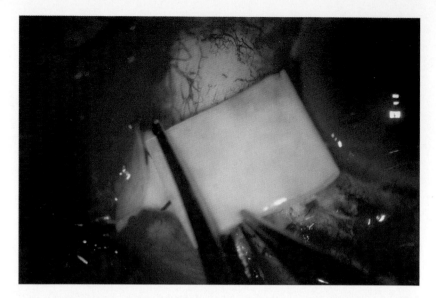

Figure 8-35 Patch graft *Tutoplast pericardium patch graft covering the tube shunt.*

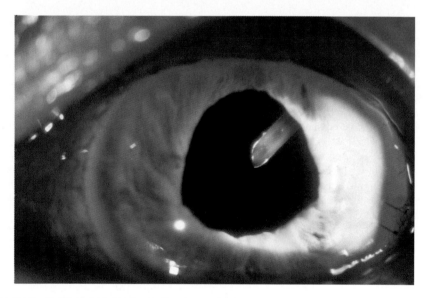

Figure 8-36 Tube shunt through the pars plana

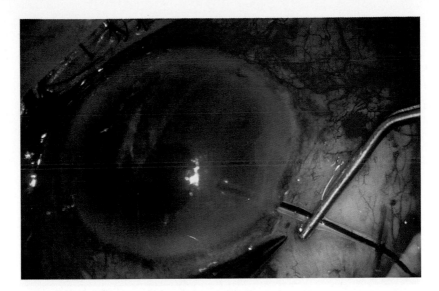

Figure 8-37   Latina suture   *Latina suture with 10-0 nylon acting as a stent through the Baerveldt tube.*

Because the tube is completely ligated, several venting slits in the anterior extrascleral portion of the tube can be made with a sharp, 15-degree blade to allow some aqueous outflow in the early postoperative period. The amount of aqueous egress can be checked with a 27-gauge cannula on a syringe with saline inserted into the end of the tube. Ligation of the tube with absorbable suture can be further modified by placing a 4-0 or 5-0 nylon suture (Latina suture; Figure 8-37) into the tube from the reservoir side with enough suture coming out of the tube to place its other end subconjunctivally in the inferior quadrant. If the pressure cannot be controlled with medication during the period before the ligature dissolves, ablating the Vicryl suture with an argon laser can open the tube. If a Latina suture had been placed, then a small cut in the inferior conjunctiva far away from the reservoirs allows the nylon suture to be pulled from the tube lumen, making the shunt functional. The Latina suture has the advantage of not requiring treatment with an argon laser if early opening of the tube is needed. A watertight conjunctival closure (see earlier discussion) completes the procedures.

Postoperative Care

The postoperative regimen includes a topical antibiotic and occasionally a cycloplegic for 2 to 4 weeks, and topical steroids for 2 to 3 months postoperatively. Nonsteroidal antiinflammatory drops can also be used concomitantly.

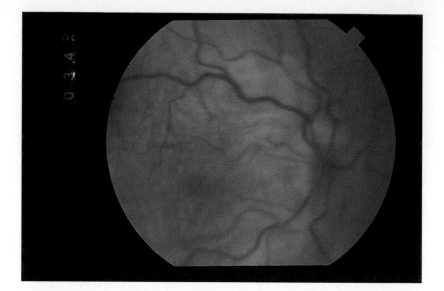

Figure 8-38 Chronic hypotony *Chronic hypotony with maculopathy and choroidal folds.*

Complications

Implantation of aqueous tube shunts is associated with a significant risk of postoperative complications. Early postoperative complications include hypotony, hypotony maculopathy (Figure 8-38), flat anterior chamber (Figure 8-39), choroidal effusions (Figures 8-20 and 8-40), suprachoroidal hemorrhage (Figure 8-41), aqueous misdirection (Figure 8-42), hyphema (Figure 8-43), and increased intraocular pressure. Hypotony, the most common complication, is usually due to excessive outflow of aqueous humor. It may result in a flat anterior chamber and choroidal detachment. Recurrent flat anterior chamber may require additional tube ligation. Restrictive or valved implants may be less commonly complicated by hypotony than nonrestrictive devices, but this has not yet been tested in a prospectively designed directly comparative study.

High intraocular pressure can be related to occlusion of the tube by fibrin, a blood clot, iris, or vitreous (Figure 8-44). Fibrin or blood may resolve spontaneously. An intracameral injection of tissue plasminogen activator may help to dissolve the clot within a few hours but can be associated with severe bleeding. When the iris tissue occludes the lumen of the tube, neodymium (Nd):YAG laser iridotomy or argon laser iridoplasty may reestablish the patency of the tube. Vitreous incarceration can be successfully treated with Nd:YAG laser, but an anterior vitrectomy may be necessary to prevent recurrence.

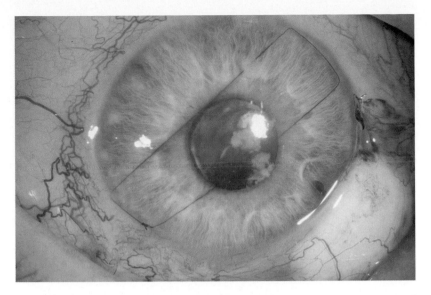

Figure 8-39 **Shallow anterior chamber** *Shallow anterior chamber following tube shunt with chamber-maintaining suture holding back the implant.*

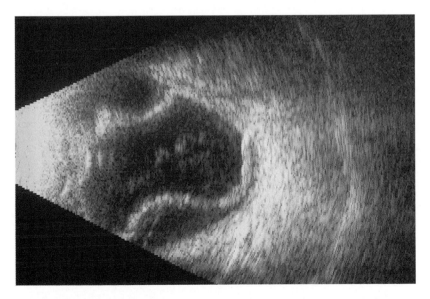

Figure 8-40 **Choroidal detachment** *B-scan ultrasound of serous choroidal detachments.*

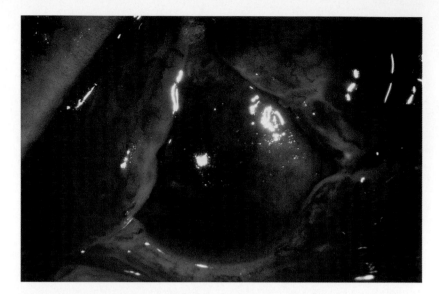

Figure 8-41 **Suprachoroidal hemorrhage** *Slit-lamp photograph of an eye with suprachoroidal hemorrhage; the retina can be seen through the pupil.*

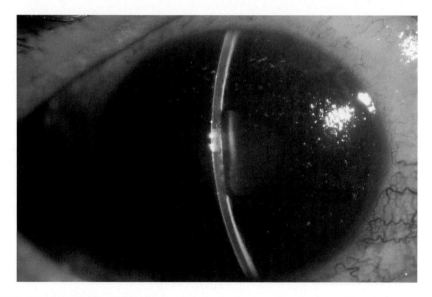

Figure 8-42 **Aqueous misdirection** *Slit-lamp photograph of an eye with aqueous misdirection in the presence of a patent iridectomy. There is a flat anterior chamber and an elevated intraocular pressure.*

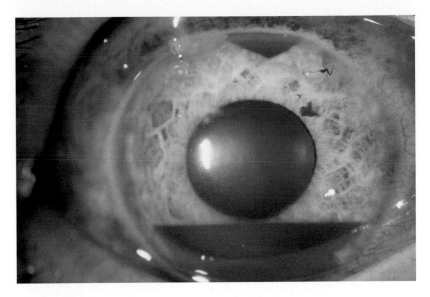

Figure 8-43   Hyphema   *Hyphema following trabeculectomy.*

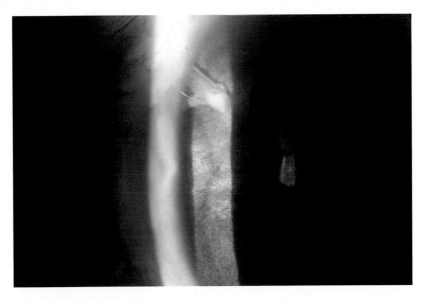

Figure 8-44   Implant occlusion   *Fibrous membrane occluding the lumen of a glaucoma drainage device.*

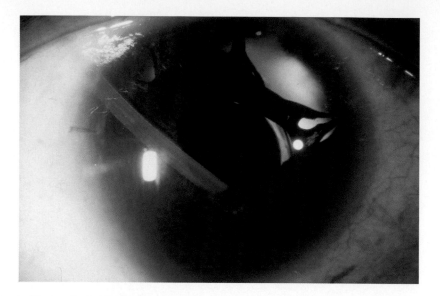

Figure 8-45   Implant migration   *Migration of the tube shunt in a 14-year-old patient with congenital cataract and glaucoma.*

Late postoperative complications of aqueous shunting procedures include increased intraocular pressure, hypotony, implant migration (Figure 8-45), conjunctival erosion (Figure 8-46), corneal edema or decompensation (Figure 8-47A,B), cataract (Figure 8-48), diplopia, and endophthalmitis (Figure 8-49). Late failure with increased intraocular pressure is usually caused by excessive fibrosis around the plate. Corneal decompensation may result from direct contact between the tube and the cornea. When the tube is touching the cornea, repositioning of the tube should be considered, especially in cases where there is the risk of endothelial failure (i.e., cases with focal corneal edema, or after penetrating keratoplasty). Diplopia can be caused by mechanical restriction of the extraocular muscles. If diplopia is persistent and not responsive to prisms, the shunt may need to be removed or relocated.

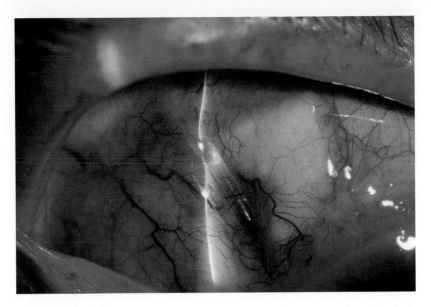

Figure 8-46 Conjunctival erosion *Erosion of the conjunctiva over a glaucoma drainage device.*

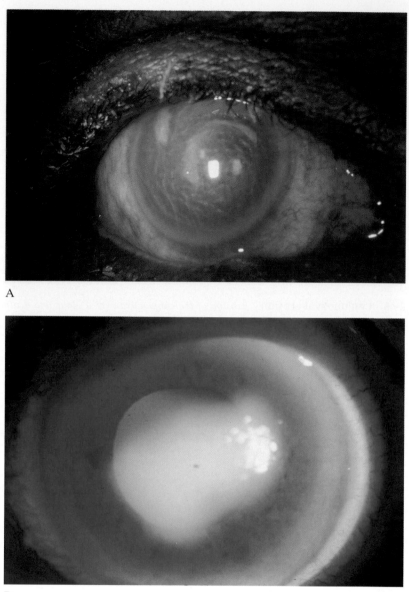

A

B

Figure 8-47A,B Corneal decompensation *A. Corneal decompensation following trabeculectomy.* ***B.*** *Breakdown of the cornea after 5-fluorouracil injection following trabeculectomy.*

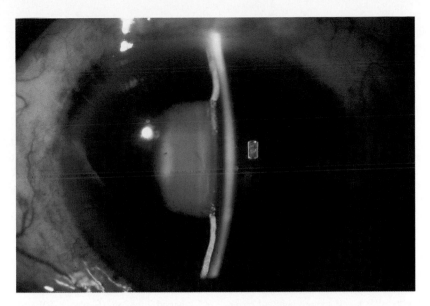

Figure 8-48 **Cataract** *Cataract development following trabeculectomy.*

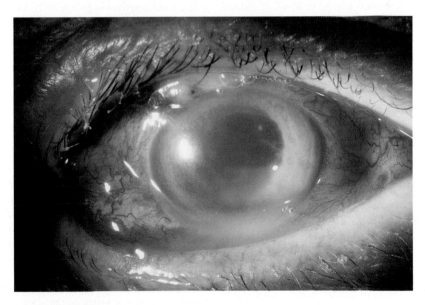

Figure 8-49 **Endophthalmitis** *Endophthalmitis 18 months following trabeculectomy.*

BEAUJON TECHNIQUE: TRABECULECTOMY WITH RELEASABLE SUTURES

Oscar V Beaujon-Balbi, MD

Oscar Beaujon-Rubin, MD

In this section, we present a technique of trabeculectomy using releasable sutures to close the scleral flap. First, we make a small, L-shaped conjunctival incision of 4 by 2 mm, situated 1 or 2 mm from the limbus, as shown in Figures 8-50A and 8-51A. *This size is intended to allow only the necessary space to perform the scleral flap.* Hemostasis can be employed if needed. Next, a scleral flap of 3 by 4 mm and two-thirds partial thickness is made (Figure 8-50B,C). Mitomycin C, 0.4 mg/dL, is applied with a Weck-cell sponge, without covering it with conjunctiva for 2 to 3 minutes. Following treatment with mitomycin C, the area is profusely washed with 60 to 80 mL of sodium chloride–balanced saline solution. Paracentesis is performed, and the scleral flap is dissected anteriorly up to Descemet's membrane to create a valve-like incision. After entering the anterior chamber, sclerectomy is performed using a Kelly Descemet punch, followed by a peripheral iridectomy made with Vannas scissors. A 10-0 nylon monofilament suture is employed to close the scleral flap in a releasable suture, as follows:

1. Entry is made in the sclera at the temporal corner, with exit on the bed of the scleral flap (Figure 8-51B).
2. A total pass is made through the flap.
3. Superficial entry is made on the surface of the flap under the conjunctiva at the limbus toward the cornea, with exit in clear cornea 1 mm from the limbus (Figures 8-50D and 8-51C).
4. With the same needle, entry is made back through clear cornea at 1 mm, with exit over the flap in a superficial manner.
5. A total pass is made on the flap.
6. Finally, entry is made on the bed of the flap, with exit on the sclera at the other corner (Figure 8-51D).

Thereafter, the surgeon places three loops of sutures, two over the scleral flap and the third over the cornea (Figure 8-51E,F). The free sides of the sutures are tied with the corresponding loop on the flap using only one lace of three loops, and then cut (Figures 8-50E and 8-51G,H). The conjunctiva is closed with a mattress suture, using the same 10-0 nylon monofilament, superficially over the flap and parallel to the limbus just under the remnant conjunctiva, closing the horizontal part of the L-shaped incision (Figure 8-50F). The other part is closed with a knot, first anchoring on episclera and then in a continuous manner just in the conjunctiva (Figure 8-50G). This creates a watertight conjunctival closure.

If it becomes necessary to release the suture, the loop can be cut on the surface of the cornea and then pulled with forceps. This is performed at the slit lamp with topical anesthesia and never with less than a 48-hour surgical evaluation or two continuous evaluation intervals.

For combined procedures (cataract and glaucoma surgery), we use a single port approach. We modified the technique by making a partial scleral flap, reducing by half the extension of the lateral incisions. This creates a 2-by-4 mm flap, 2 mm away from the limbus. After mitomycin C application, we make a scleral tunnel with a crescent knife, continuing the previously initiated groove with scleral flap dissection. Then, phacoemulsification with a foldable lens implantation is performed, followed by sclerectomy with a Kelly Descemet punch and peripheral iridectomy. Closure of the scleral flap and conjunctiva are completed as previously described.

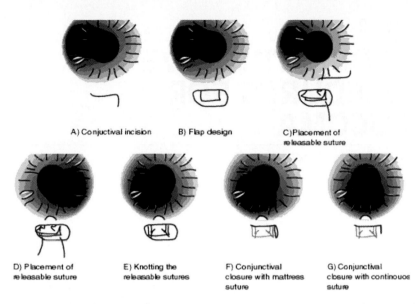

Figure 8-50A–G   Beaujon technique   *Diagram of the Beaujon technique of closure of the trabeculectomy flap with releasable sutures.*

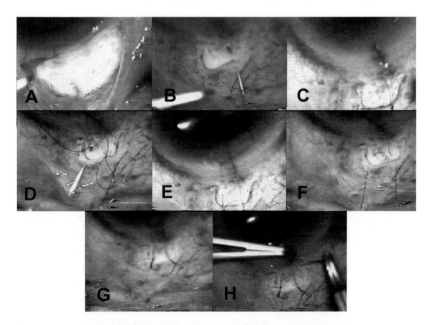

Figure 8-51A–H   Beaujon technique   *Composite photograph of surgical images of the Beaujon technique.*

Chapter 9

CYCLODESTRUCTIVE PROCEDURES FOR GLAUCOMA

Geoffrey P. Schwartz, MD

Louis W. Schwartz, MD

Intraocular pressure is the major risk factor for glaucoma that ophthalmologists are able to control. Medically, either eye drops or pills are used to decrease aqueous production or increase aqueous outflow to effectively lower intraocular pressure. Most surgical and laser procedures, trabeculotomy, filtering surgery, tube shunts, goniotomy, iridectomies, laser trabeculoplasty, and laser iridotomy decrease the intraocular pressure by increasing outflow. Cyclodestructive procedures are designed to destroy the ciliary processes, thereby decreasing aqueous production. Because of the unpredictability of these procedures in lowering intraocular pressure and the complications associated with their use, such cyclodestructive procedures are often considered a surgery of last resort.

TECHNIQUES

Several techniques are used for cyclodestruction. They include noncontact transscleral cyclophotocoagulation (CPC), contact transscleral CPC, cyclocryotherapy (CCT), transpupillary CPC, and endoscopic cyclophotocoagulation (ECP). All of the procedures may be repeated as many times as needed, with a usual interval of 1 month between re-treatments if the target pressure is not achieved.

Noncontact Transscleral Cyclophotocoagulation (CPC)

A neodymium (Nd):YAG laser is used to perform this procedure. In the past, a semiconductor diode laser, Microlase (Keeler, Inc., Broomall, PA), was also utilized.[1] Retrobulbar anesthesia is given. A lid speculum is placed if a contact lens is not used. A contact lens developed by Bruce Shields may or may not be used. The contact lens has the advantages of having markers at 1-mm intervals to better judge the distance from the limbus, blocking some of the laser light from entering the pupil, and to blanch an inflamed conjunctiva to decrease superficial charring of the conjunctiva[2] (Figure 9-1A,B). Eight to ten burns are placed 1 to 3 mm (optimal: 1.5 mm) from the limbus for 180 to 360 degrees, taking care to avoid the 3 and 9 o'clock meridians in order not to coagulate the long posterior ciliary arteries and cause anterior segment necrosis. Energy levels of 4 to 8 J are used. The laser beam is focused on the conjunctiva; however, the laser is defocused such that its effect is actually 3.6 mm beyond the conjunctival surface, with most of the

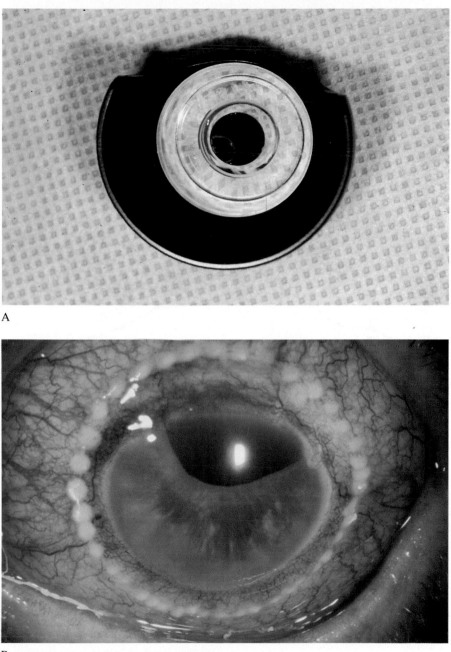

A

B

Figure 9-1A,B A. Shields lens *Shields lens for noncontact transscleral cyclophotocoagulation (CPC).* ***B.*** *Placement of laser burns 1.5 mm from the limbus. Note blanching of inflammed conjuctiva.*

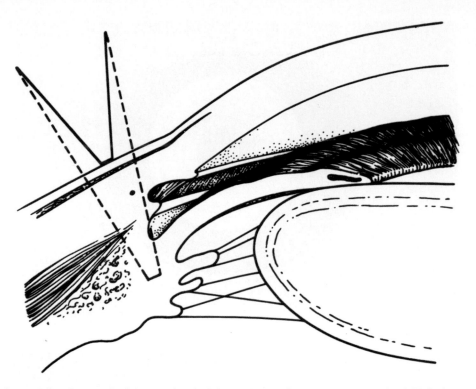

Figure 9-2   Noncontact transscleral CPC   *Diagram of noncontact transscleral CPC showing that the laser energy is actually focused within the ciliary body.*

energy being absorbed by the ciliary body (Figure 9-2). In general, the greater the energy levels used, the greater is the inflammation.[3–5]

Contact Transscleral CPC (Figure 9-3)

This technique is currently the most popular cyclodestructive procedure. It uses a contact diode laser probe that is relatively small and portable (G-Probe; IRIS Medical Instruments, Inc., Mountain View, CA). A Nd:YAG probe and a krypton laser have also been used to perform contact transscleral CPC.

In this technique, retrobulbar anesthesia is given and a lid speculum is placed. The patient is placed in the supine position. The anterior edge of the probe is placed at the limbus. Because of the design of the G-Probe, the energy is actually delivered 1.2 mm from the limbus; 30 to 40 applications of 1.5 to 2.0 watts of energy are applied for 1.5 to 2 seconds over 360 degrees, avoiding the 3 and 9 o'clock positions. The energy level is reduced by 0.25 W if an audible pop is heard, because audible pops are associated with greater inflammation and hyphema.[6]

Cyclocryotherapy (CCT) (Figure 9-4)

A nitrous oxide cryosurgical unit is used to cool the 2.5-mm probe to −80 degrees centigrade, placing it approximately 1 mm posterior to the limbus for 60 seconds. Two to three quadrants are treated with four cryolesions per quadrant, avoiding the 3 and 9 o'clock positions.[7]

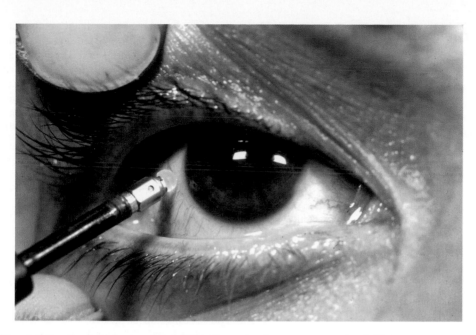

Figure 9-3 Contact transscleral CPC *Example of contact transscleral CPC.*

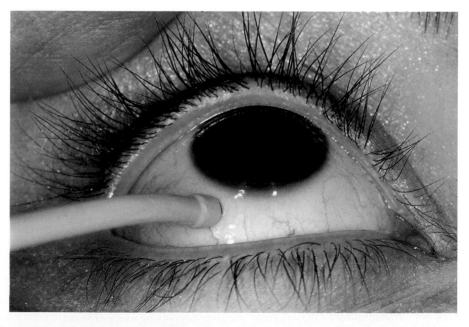

Figure 9-4 Cyclocryotherapy (CCT) *Photograph demonstrating CCT. The probe is placed approximately 1 mm posterior to the limbus.*

Transpupillary CPC (Figure 9-5)

A continuous wave argon laser is delivered by a biomicroscope. The idea behind this technique is to apply the laser energy precisely to the ciliary processes instead of having to go through other structures, such as the conjunctiva and sclera. In order to visualize the ciliary processes, a Goldmann-type gonioprism with scleral depression and large sector iridectomy are necessary. Laser settings of 50- to 100-μm spot size, 700 to 1000 mW, for 0.1 second, with the energy level being adjusted to create a whitening of the tissue, are used to treat all visible ciliary processes. The major disadvantage to this technique is visualization problems.[8]

Endoscopic Cyclophotocoagulation (ECP) (Figure 9-6A,B)

This technique is performed in the operating room under local retrobulbar anesthesia. There are two different approaches: limbal and pars plana. In the limbal approach, the pupil is maximally dilated, an incision approximately 2.5-mm in length is made with a keratome, and viscoelastic is introduced between the iris and crystalline lens or pseudophake to access the ciliary processes. A maximum of 180 degrees can be treated through the one incision, and a second incision can be made directly opposite the original one to treat the remaining 180 degrees. Viscoelastic is washed out after the procedure and the wound closed with 10-0 nylon suture. A cataract extraction may be combined with this procedure at the same time.

When performing the ECP through the pars plana incision, the patient must be aphakic or pseudophakic. A typical pars plana incision is made 3.5 to 4.0 mm from the limbus, an anterior vitrectomy is performed, and the laser endoscope is inserted. Two incisions are necessary if more than 180 degrees of ciliary processes are to be treated. The sclerotomies are closed with 7-0 Vicryl suture. The laser endoscope has an image guide, light guide, and laser guide in an 18- or 20-gauge endoprobe.

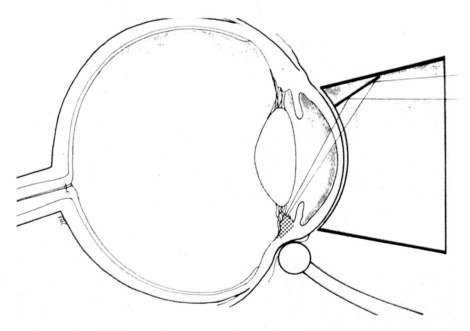

Figure 9-5   Transpupillary CPC   *Diagram showing transpupillary CPC. The laser energy is being focused by a mirrored lens onto the ciliary body, which has been moved into view by scleral depression.*

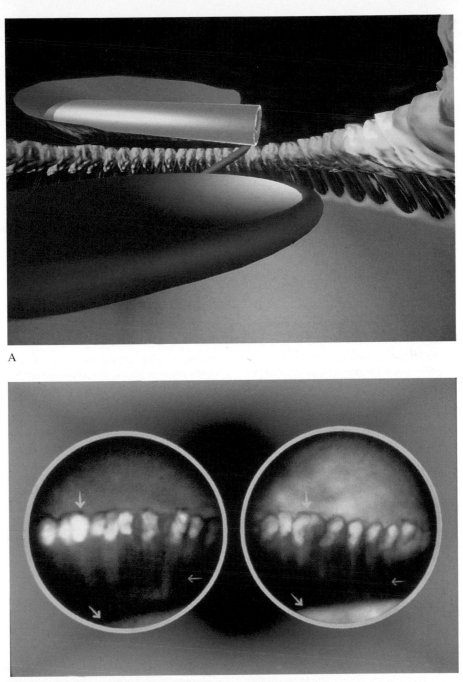

A

B

Figure 9-6A,B Endoscopic cyclophotocoagulation (ECP) *A. Diagram showing an endolaser probe delivering energy to the ciliary body. **B.** View through the endoscopic camera of the ciliary body following delivery of the laser energy. The white color of the ciliary processes indicates thermal destruction of the ciliary process* (yellow arrow). *Photos courtesy of Martin Uran, MD.*

The 20-gauge probe has a 70-degree field of view, with a depth of focus from 0.5 mm to 15 mm. The 18-gauge endoprobe has a 110-degree field of view, with a depth of focus from 1 mm to 30 mm. The probe is connected to a video camera, light source, video monitor, and video recorder. A semiconductor diode laser at 810 nM wavelength is attached to the laser guide. Laser applications from 0.5 to 2 seconds, 500 to 900 mW, are used to produce an end-point of whitening and shrinkage of each ciliary process. When popping is heard or bubbles form, laser power and duration, or both, are decreased. The surgeon performs the procedure by viewing the video monitor.[9,10]

POSTPROCEDURE CARE

In all of these treatments, topical steroids as well as sub-Tenon's steroids are given to stem the inflammation that occurs in all patients. Atropine drops may or may not be given. Analgesics and ice packs are prescribed for pain.

INDICATIONS

Cyclodestruction of the ciliary body is usually reserved for use in patients who have failed previous treatment with medicines or surgeries. The exceptions to this rule include patients who are not willing to undergo surgery, those who cannot undergo surgery owing to medical conditions, and patients in underdeveloped countries. In underdeveloped countries, where medical care is expensive and not always available, diode contact transscleral CPC, which is portable and relatively easy to use, may be the first line of treatment for glaucoma in the future.

These procedures may have benefit in controlling pain in blind, painful eyes, and may allow the patient to avoid removal of the eye as long as visualization or ultrasound reveals no intraocular tumor. Types of glaucoma that have been treated with varying degrees of success include end-stage open-angle glaucoma; neovascular glaucoma; blind, painful eye; glaucoma postpenetrating keratoplasty; advanced angle closure, both primary and secondary; traumatic glaucoma; malignant glaucoma; silicone oil glaucoma; congenital glaucoma; pseudophakic and aphakic open-angle glaucoma; and secondary open-angle glaucoma. Alternative treatments that are usually considered in this group of patients include filtering surgery with antimetabolite or tube shunts.

CONTRAINDICATIONS

There are relatively few contraindications to this procedure. A phakic patient with good vision is the primary contraindication. In this case, alternative treatments should be tried first. Marked uveitis is a relative contraindication because patients have increased inflammation following the treatment; care should be taken to try to quiet the eye as much as possible before the procedure. However, uveitic glaucoma is one of the secondary glaucomas that have been treated successfully with this procedure. For all of the procedures, except ECP, patient cooperation is required and may be a contraindication.

COMPLICATIONS

Table 9-1 lists the complications of cyclodestructive procedures. The most feared of these complications are chronic hypotony leading to phthisis, which occurs in 8% to 10% of patients, and sympathetic ophthalmia, which is extremely rare. Significant pain occurs in about 50% of patients and may last for several hours to several weeks, the usual duration being 2 to 3 days, following the procedure. One cannot predict from the type of glaucoma which patients will have this significant pain. It can be treated with analgesics and ice.

TABLE 9-1   COMPLICATIONS OF CYCLODESTRUCTIVE PROCEDURES

Uveitis-iritis (hypopyon)
Vitritis
Chronic flare
Pain
Hyphema
Vitreous hemorrhage
Corneal edema
Thinning of the sclera
Retinal detachment
Sympathetic ophthalmia
Malignant glaucoma
Anterior segment necrosis or ischemia
Decreased vision
Blindness
Chronic hypotony
Phthisis
Traumatic cataract (with ECP)

REFERENCES

1. Hennis HL, Stewart WC. Semi-conductor diode laser transscleral cyclophotocoagulation in patients with glaucoma. *Am J Ophthalmol* 113:81–85, 1992.
2. Simmons RB, Blasini M, Shields MD, et al. Comparison of transscleral neodymium:YAG cyclophotocoagulation with and without a contact lens in human autopsy eyes. *Am J Ophthalmol* 109:174–179, 1990.
3. Frankhauser F, Van der Zypen E, Kwasniewska S, et al. Transscleral cyclophotocoagulation using a neodymium YAG laser. *Ophthalmic Surg Lasers* 1:125–141, 1986.
4. Schwartz LW, Moster MR. Neodymium:YAG laser transscleral cyclodiathermy. *Ophthalmic Laser Therapy* 1:135–141, 1986.
5. Crymes BM, Gross RL. Laser placement in noncontact Nd:YAG cyclophotocoagulation. *Am J Ophthalmol* 110:670–673, 1990.
6. Allingham RR, DeKater AW, Bellows AR, et al. Probe placement and power levels in contact transscleral neodymium:YAG cyclophotocoagulation. *Arch Ophthalmol* 109:738–742, 1990.
7. Bietti G. Surgical intervention on the ciliary body: New trends for the relief of glaucoma. *JAMA* 142:889–897, 1950.
8. Shields S, Stewart WC, Shields MD. Transpupillary argon laser cyclophotocoagulation in the treatment of glaucoma. *Ophthalmic Surg Lasers* 19:171–175, 1988.
9. Uram M. Endoscopic cyclophotocoagulation in glaucoma management. *Curr Opin Ophthalmol* 6(2):19–29, 1995.
10. Mora JS, Iwach AG, Gaffney MM, et al. Endoscopic diode laser cyclophotocoagulation with a limbal approach. *Ophthalmic Surg Lasers* 28:118–123, 1997.

Section 3

DISEASE SYNDROMES

Douglas J. Rhee, MD

INTRODUCTION

The glaucoma syndromes are divided into two main categories: primary and secondary. The primary glaucomas are those for which the cause of the increased resistance to outflow and elevated intraocular pressure is unknown. The secondary glaucomas are associated with known ocular or systemic conditions responsible for the elevated intraocular pressure and resistance to outflow.

Primary open-angle glaucoma is the most common form of glaucoma in the United States. It comprises approximately two thirds of all cases of glaucoma. This particular disease syndrome is probably the final common pathway for a variety of yet undistinguished separate pathophysiologic processes. As our understanding of the genetic and pathophysiologic components continues to expand, I predict that we will eventually distinguish several other conditions with these characteristic optic nerve and visual field defects.

The chapters in this section include representative photographs and briefly describe the major glaucoma syndromes:

Congenital glaucomas
Primary open-angle glaucoma
Secondary open-angle glaucomas
Inflammatory glaucomas
Lens-associated glaucomas
Uveitic glaucomas
Primary angle-closure glaucoma
Secondary angle-closure glaucomas

Additionally, some of the delayed-onset complications from glaucoma surgery are discussed.

Chapter 10

DEVELOPMENTAL GLAUCOMAS (CONGENITAL GLAUCOMAS)

Oscar V. Beaujon-Balbi, MD

Oscar Beaujon-Rubin, MD

The developmental glaucomas are a group of conditions characterized by a developmental abnormality of the aqueous outflow system of the eye. This group includes (1) congenital glaucoma, in which the developmental abnormality of the anterior chamber angle is not associated with other ocular or systemic anomalies; (2) developmental glaucomas with associated anomalies, in which ocular or systemic anomalies are present; and (3) secondary glaucomas of childhood, in which other ocular pathologies are the cause of the impairment of the aqueous outflow.

Several different systems are used to classify developmental glaucomas. The most common are the Shaffer-Weiss and the Hoskin anatomic classifications. The former divides congenital glaucoma into three major groups: (1) primary congenital glaucoma, (2) glaucoma associated with congenital anomalies, and (3) secondary glaucomas of childhood. The latter defines the actual developmental disorder clinically evident at the time of examination and also includes three groups, as follows: (1) isolated trabeculodysgenesis with malformation of the trabecular meshwork in absence of iris or corneal anomalies, (2) iridotrabeculodysgenesis that includes angle and iris anomalies, and (3) corneotrabeculodysgenesis, usually associated with iris anomalies. The identification of anatomic defects can be useful in determining the appropriate therapy and prognostic factors.

PRIMARY CONGENITAL GLAUCOMA

Primary congenital glaucoma (PCG) is the most common form of infantile glaucoma, representing 50% of all cases of congenital glaucoma. It is characterized by a trabecular meshwork anomaly and is not associated with other ocular or systemic diseases. Seventy-five percent of PCG cases occur bilaterally. The incidence is 1 in 5000 to 10,000 live births. More than 80% of cases present before 1 year of age: 40% at birth, 70% between 1 and 6 months, and 80% before 1 year. The disorder is more common in males (70% males, 30% females), and 90% of cases are sporadic, without a family history. Although an autosomal recessive model with variable penetrance has been suggested, it is thought that most of the cases are a result of multifactorial inheritance with nongenetic factors involved (e.g., environmental factors).

Clinical Features

History Epiphora, photophobia, and blepharospasm form the classic triad. Usually, children with congenital glaucoma prefer dimly lit places and avoid exposure to intense light. The caregiver may describe an excessive amount of tearing. In unilateral cases, the mother may note an asymmetry between eyes, referring to an enlarged (affected side) or decreased (normal side) eye size (Figure 10-1).

External Examination The normal horizontal corneal diameter in a full-term newborn is 10 to 10.5 mm. This increases to the adult diameter of approximately 11.5 to 12 mm by 2 years of age. A diameter greater than 12 mm in an infant is highly suggestive of congenital glaucoma.

Measurements of the cornea are made in the horizontal meridian with calipers. Other findings include corneal cloudiness, tears in Descemet's membrane (Haab's striae), deep anterior chamber, intraocular pressure greater than 21 mm Hg, iris stroma hypoplasia, isolated trabeculodysgenesis on gonioscopy, and increased optic nerve cupping. Haab's striae may be single or multiple and are characteristically oriented horizontally or concentrically to the limbus (Figure 10-2).

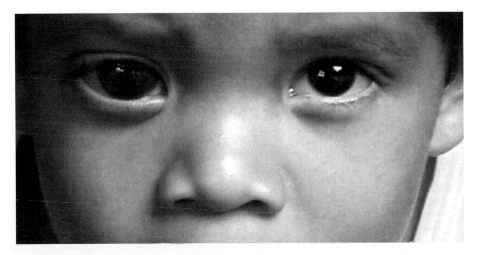

Figure 10-1   Unilateral primary congential glaucoma   *This photo demonstrates a cloudy cornea and buphthalmos.*

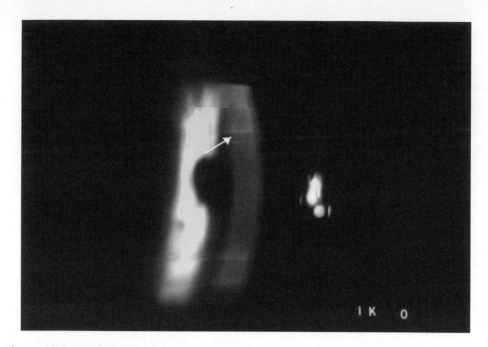

Figure 10-2　Haab's striae　Arrows *indicate breaks in Descemet's membrane.*

Optic nerve evaluation is a very important part of the glaucoma evaluation. Glaucomatous disc changes occur more rapidly in infants and at lower pressures than in older children or adults. Cup-to-disc ratios greater than 0.3 are rare in normal infants and must be considered highly suspicious for glaucoma. Asymmetry of optic nerve cupping is also suggestive of glaucoma, particularly differences of greater than 0.2 between the two eyes. The glaucomatous cupping may be oval in configuration but is more often round and central (Figure 10-3). Reversal of optic nerve cupping has been observed after normalization of intraocular pressure.

Evaluation of the anterior chamber angle is essential for an accurate diagnosis and treatment. The developmental anomalies can present in two major forms: (1) flat iris insertion, in which the iris inserts directly or anterior to the trabecular meshwork with iris processes that can overcome the scleral spur (Figure 10-4A); and (2) concave iris insertion, in which the iris is observed behind the trabecular meshwork but

is covered with a dense abnormal tissue (Figure 10-4B). For comparison, a gonioscopic photo of a normal anterior chamber angle from an infant is also presented (Figure 10-5).

Elevation of the intraocular pressure causes rapid enlargement of the globe with progressive enlargement of the cornea in children younger than 3 years of age. As the cornea enlarges, stretching leads to ruptures in Descemet's membrane, epithelial and stromal edema, and corneal clouding. The iris is stretched so that the stroma appears thinned. The scleral canal through which the optic nerve passes also enlarges with elevated intraocular pressure. This results in rapid cupping of the optic nerve, which can quickly reverse if the intraocular pressure is normalized. This dramatic reversal in cupping is not seen in adult eyes and is probably related to the greater elasticity of the optic nerve head connective tissue in the infant. If the intraocular pressure is not controlled, a buphthalmos can develop (Figure 10-6; see also Figure 10-1).

Figure 10-3 **Round cupping** *Round cupping in congenital glaucoma.*

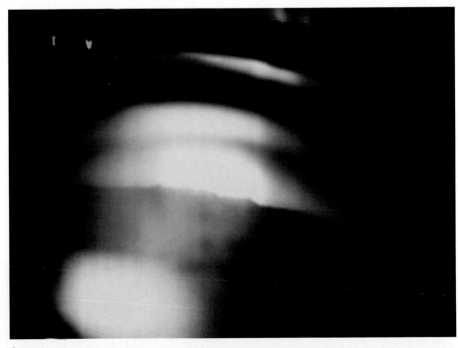

A

Figure 10-4A,B **Gonioscopy** *A. Flat iris insertion.*

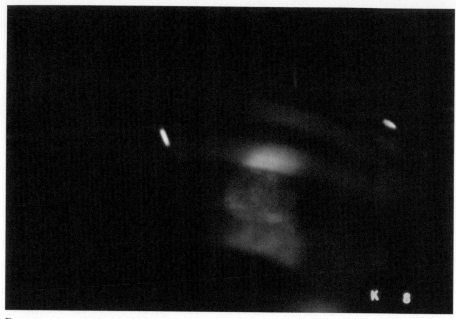

B

Figure 10-4A,B **Gonioscopy** *(continued)* ***B.*** *Concave iris insertion.*

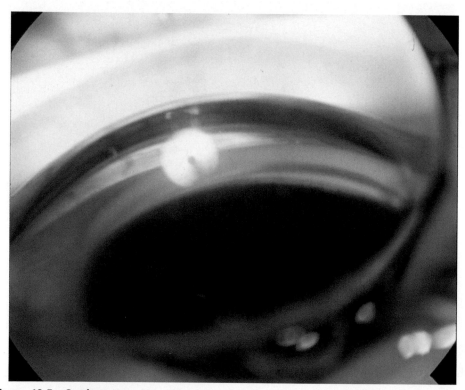

Figure 10-5 **Gonioscopy** *Note the relative paucity of anterior chamber pigment of a normal anterior chamber angle in an infant.*

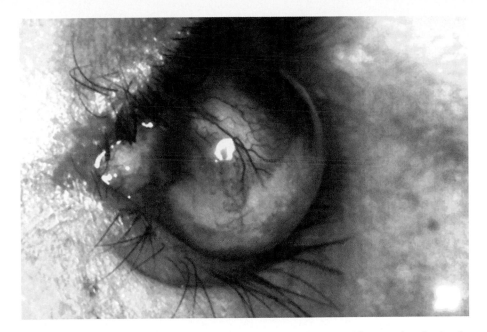

Figure 10-6 **Buphthalmos** *An extreme example of buphthalmos with corneal and scleral thinning.*

Differential Diagnosis

Other causes of corneal changes include megalocornea, metabolic diseases, corneal dystrophies, obstetric trauma, and keratitis. Epiphora or photophobia may occur in nasolacrimal duct obstruction, dacriocystitis, and iritis. Optic nerve anomalies simulating a glaucomatous nerve include optic pits, colobomas, and hypoplasia.

Management

The treatment of congenital glaucoma is always surgical. Medical treatment can be used for a limited time while the surgery is being scheduled. Procedures that involve trabecular incisions are the choice in this condition. Goniotomy requires a clear cornea for visualization of the angle. Trabeculotomy with an external approach to Schlemm's canal does not require corneal transparency. The goniotomy is performed using a goniotome and direct gonioscopy lens. We prefer the Barkan's goniolens. An incision is made in the dense abnormal tissue at the trabecular meshwork for an extension of 90 to 180 degrees using the goniotome through clear cornea (Figures 10-7 and 10-8).

In cloudy or opacified corneas, trabeculotomy is indicated. A scleral flap is made and Schlemm's canal must be found in order to perform the procedure. The trabecular meshwork is cut using a trabeculotome or by using a suture (usually propylene) through Schlemm's canal (Lynch procedure). In cases where Schlemm's canal is not found, trabeculectomy is performed. Another choice is the placement of a valved or nonvalved glaucoma-filtering device (Figure 10-9).

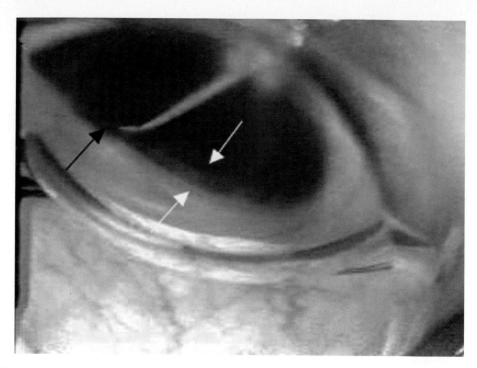

Figure 10-7 Congenital glaucoma during goniotomy *Note the difference in angle configuration between the goniotomy-treated portion of trabecular meshwork* (white arrow) *and the nontreated portion* (black arrow).

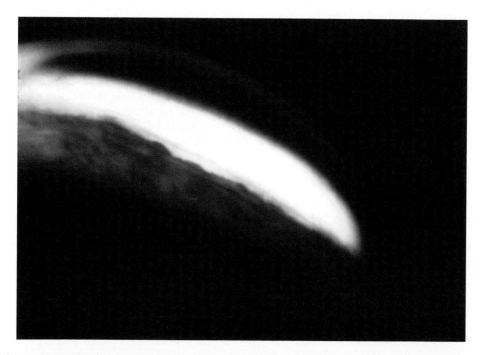

Figure 10-8 Angle visualization *Visualization of the angle after goniotomy.*

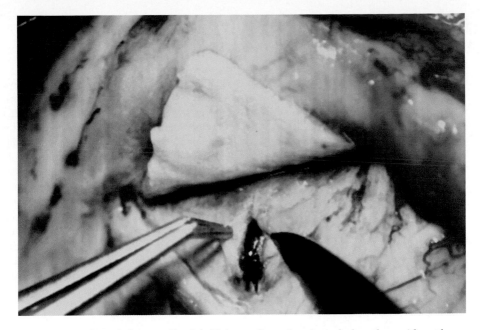

Figure 10-9 Trabeculotomy *Partial-thickness dissection through the sclera with cutdown over Schlemm's canal.*

GLAUCOMA ASSOCIATED WITH CONGENITAL ANOMALIES

Aniridia

Aniridia is a bilateral congenital anomaly in which the iris is markedly underdeveloped, but there is generally a rudimentary iris stump of variable extent visible on examination of the angle (Figure 10-10). Two thirds of cases are dominantly transmitted with a high degree penetrance. Twenty percent are associated with Wilms' tumor. A deletion of the short arm of chromosomes 11 has been associated with Wilms' tumor and sporadic aniridia. Poor visual acuity is common because of foveal and optic nerve hypoplasia. Other associated ocular conditions include keratopathy, cataract (60% to 80%), and ectopia lentis (Figure 10-11). Photophobia, nystagmus, decreased vision, and strabismus are common manifestations in aniridia. Progressive corneal opacification and pannus usually occur circumferentially in the periphery.

Glaucoma associated with aniridia does not usually develop until late childhood or early adulthood. It may be a result of trabeculodysgenesis or of progressive closure of the trabecular meshwork by the residual iris stump. If it develops during infancy, a goniotomy or trabeculotomy may be indicated. It has been suggested that early goniotomy may prevent the progressive adherence of the residual peripheral iris to the trabecular meshwork.

In older children, medical therapy to control intraocular pressure should first be attempted. Any form of surgery has the risk of injuring the unprotected lens and zonules, and filtering procedures have an increased risk of vitreous incarceration. Cyclodestructive procedures may be necessary in certain patients with uncontrolled advanced glaucoma.

Axenfeld's Anomaly

Axenfeld's anomaly is characterized by peripheral cornea, anterior chamber angle, and iris

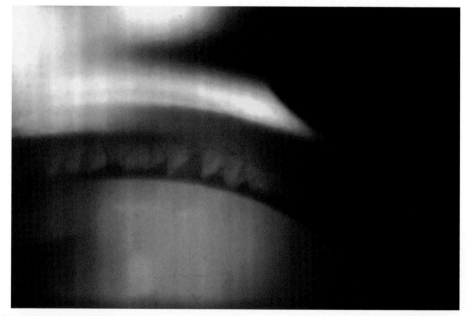

Figure 10-10 Aniridia *Gonioscopic photograph showing an iris remnant with ciliary processes below.*

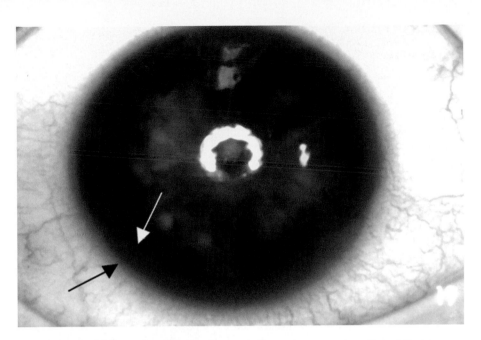

Figure 10-11   Aniridia and cataract   Arrows *indicate the remnant portion of the iris.*

anomalies. A prominent Schwalbe's line, referred to as *posterior embryotoxon,* is a peripheral cornea alteration in these patients. Iris strands attaching to the posterior embryotoxon and hypoplasia of the anterior iris stroma may be present. The disease is usually bilateral and has an autosomal-dominant inheritance (Figure 10-12).

Axenfeld's syndrome includes glaucoma and occurs in 50% of patients with the anomaly. If glaucoma occurs in infancy, goniotomy or trabeculotomy is often successful. If glaucoma occurs later, medical therapy should be tried initially, and filtering surgery should be used if needed.

Rieger's Anomaly

Rieger's anomaly represents a more advanced degree of angle dysgenesis. Besides the clinical aspect observed in Axenfeld's anomaly, a marked iris hypoplasia is observed with polycoria and corectopia. It is usually bilateral and inherited in an autosomal-dominant pattern, although the anomaly can be present sporadically. Glaucoma develops in more than half of cases, often requiring surgery.

Rieger's Syndrome

When the findings of Rieger's anomaly are associated with systemic malformations, the term *Rieger's syndrome* is preferred. The most commonly associated systemic anomalies are developmental defects of the teeth and facial bones. Dental abnormalities include a reduction of crown size (microdontia), a decreased but evenly spaced number of teeth, and a focal absence of teeth (commonly the anterior maxillary primary and permanent central incisors) (Figures 10-13A,B and 10-14).

Because of the similarity of anterior chamber angle abnormalities in these entities, it has been proposed that they represent a spectrum of developmental disorders that have been named *anterior chamber cleavage syndrome* and *mesodermal dysgenesis of cornea and iris.* They are also referred to as Axenfeld-Rieger syndrome.

Peter's Anomaly

Peter's anomaly represents a major degree of anterior chamber developmental disorder. A

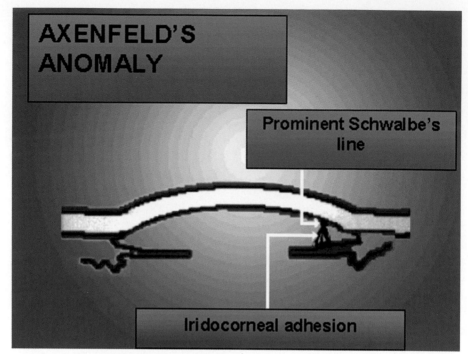

Figure 10-12   Axenfeld's anomaly diagram

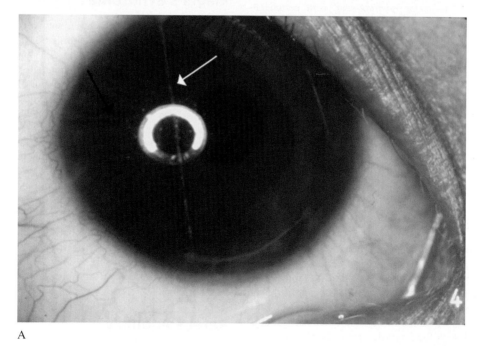

A

Figure 10-13A,B   Rieger's syndrome   *A. Notice prominent anterior embryotoxon* (white arrows) *and iris hypoplasia* (black arrow).

DISEASE SYNDROMES

corneal opacity associated with a posterior stromal defect is present, also known as Von Hippel's corneal ulcer. The iris is adherent to the cornea at the collarette. The lens can be included on these adhesions with an absent corneal endothelium. Peter's anomaly is bilateral and frequently associated with glaucoma and cataract. Corneal transplant with cataract removal to improve visual acuity has a guarded prognosis. In these cases, a trabeculectomy or glaucoma drainage implant devices are required for glaucoma control (Figure 10-15A,B).

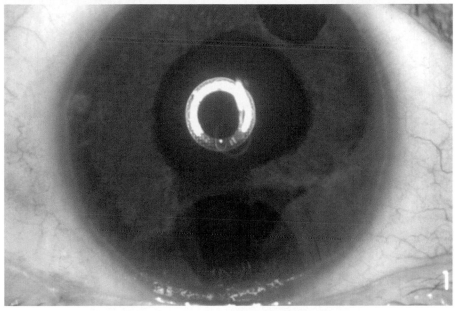

B

Figure 10-13A,B   Rieger's syndrome   (continued) B. *The mother of the patient in (A), showing prominent anterior embryotoxon, corectopia, and polycoria.*

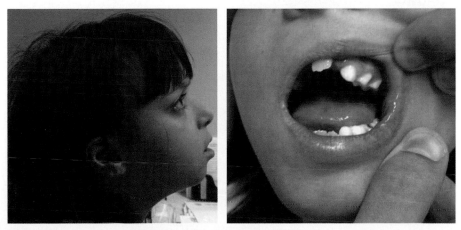

Figure 10-14   Rieger's syndrome   Left. *Facial anomalies, maxillary hypoplasia.* **Right.** *Dental anomalies, hypodontia, and anodontia. (Courtesy of Dr. Adael Soares, Escola Paulista de Medicina, UNIFESP, São Paulo, Brazil.)*

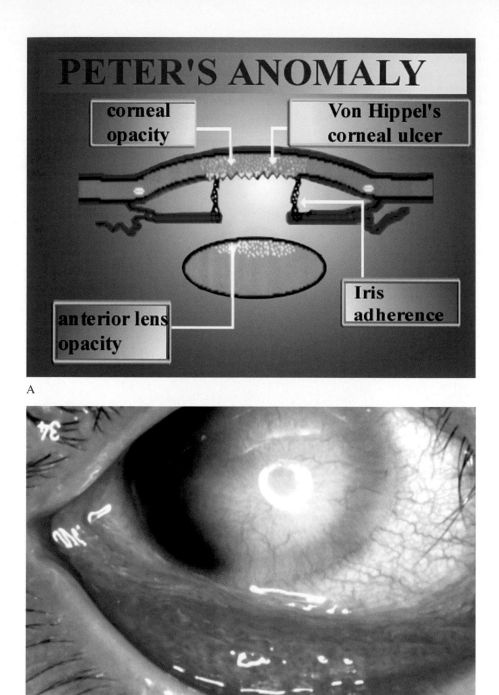

Figure 10-15A,B   Peter's anomaly   *A. Diagram of anomaly.* ***B.*** *Note the corneal opacity (leukoma), along with corneal pannus.*

DISEASE SYNDROMES

MARFAN SYNDROME

Marfan syndrome is characterized by musculoskeletal abnormalities, such as arachnodactyly, excessive height, long extremities, hyperextensive joints, and scoliosis; cardiovascular disease; and ocular abnormalities. Transmission is autosomal dominant with high penetrance, although approximately 15% of cases are sporadic (Figure 10-16A,B).

Ocular features include ectopia lentis, microphakia, megalocornea, myopia, keratoconus, iris

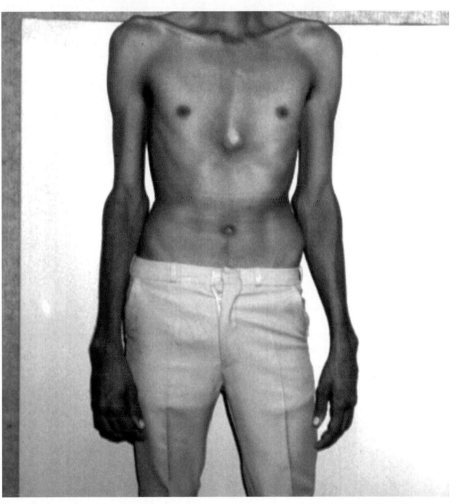

A

Figure 10-16A,B Marfan syndrome *A. Note the tall and thin body habitus; this patient also has pectus excavatum.*

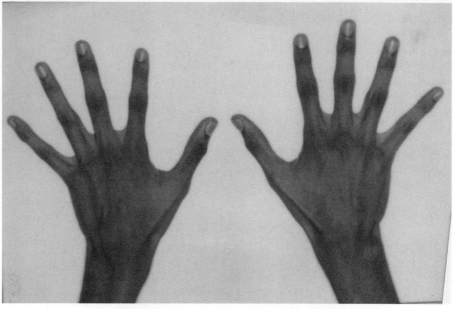

B

Figure 10-16A,B Marfan syndrome *(continued)* ***B.*** *Arachnodactyly.*

hypoplasia, retinal detachment, and glaucoma (Figure 10-17). The zonules are often attenuated and broken, leading to upward subluxation of the lens (The lens may also become dislocated into the pupil or anterior chamber, leading to lens-induced glaucoma).

Open-angle glaucoma may also develop, frequently in childhood or adolescence, and is associated with congenital abnormalities of the anterior chamber angle. Dense iris processes bridge the angle recess, inserting anterior to the scleral spur. Iris tissue sweeping across the recess may have a concave configuration. Usually the glaucoma occurs in older childhood, and the medical therapy should first be attempted.

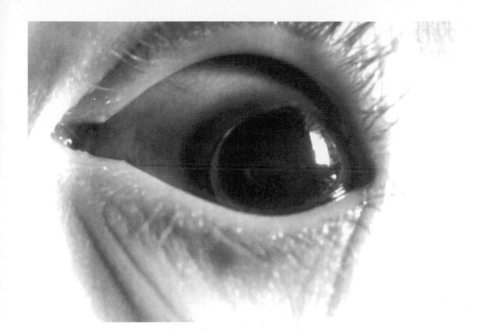

Figure 10-17   Marfan syndrome   *Anterior ectopia lentis. In this eye, the crystalline lens has dislocated anteriorly.*

MICROSPHEROPHAKIA

Microspherophakia may occur as an isolated disorder that is inherited as an autosomal-recessive or -dominant trait or it may be associated with Weill-Marchesani syndrome. That syndrome is characterized by short stature, brachydactyly, brachycephaly, and microspherophakia.

The lens is small and spherical and may move anteriorly, resulting in pupillary-block glaucoma (Figure 10-18). Angle-closure glaucoma can be treated using mydriatics, iridectomy, or lens extraction. Glaucoma usually occurs in late childhood or early adulthood.

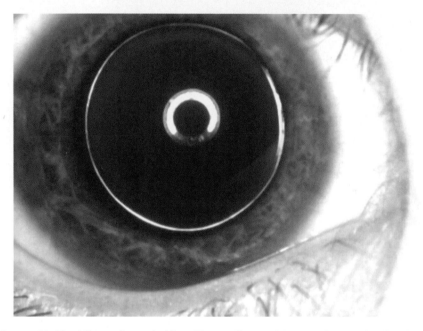

Figure 10-18 Microspherophakia *The small, round lens can be visualized within the aperture of the dilated pupil.*

STURGE-WEBER SYNDROME (ENCEPHALOTRIGEMINAL ANGIOMATOSIS)

Patients with Sturge-Weber syndrome have a facial hemangioma following the distribution of the trigeminal nerve. The facial hemangioma is usually unilateral but may be bilateral. Conjunctival, episcleral, and choroidal hemangiomas are also common abnormalities. Diffuse uveal involvement has been termed the "tomato-catsup" fundus. No clear hereditary pattern has been established.

Glaucoma more often occurs when the ipsilateral facial hemangioma involves the lids and conjunctiva. Glaucoma may occur in infancy, late childhood, or young adulthood. The glaucoma that occurs in infancy looks and behaves like glaucoma associated with isolated trabeculodysgenesis and responds well to goniotomy.

The glaucoma that appears later in life is probably related to elevated episcleral venous pressure from arteriovenous fistulas. In older children medical therapy should be attempted first. However, if this is not successful, trabeculectomy should be considered. Filtering surgery has an increased the risk of choroidal hemorrhage, resulting in shallowing or flattening of the anterior chamber related to the diminution of the intraocular pressure at the moment of surgery. This probably occurs when the intraocular pressure level falls below that of arterial blood pressure and results in effusion of choroidal fluid into surrounding tissues (Figures 10-19 and 10-20A–D).

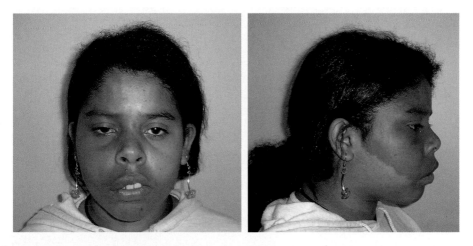

Figure 10-19　Sturge-Weber syndrome　*Note unilateral frontal and maxillary distribution. (Courtesy of Dr. Claudia Pabon Bejarano, Escola Paulista de Medicina, UNIFESP, São Paulo, Brazil.)*

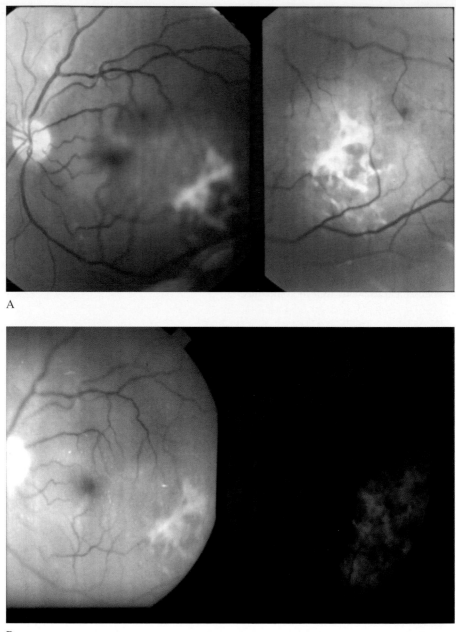

A

B

Figure 10-20A–C   Sturge-Weber syndrome   *Choroid hemangioma. (Courtesy of Dr. Dario Fuenmayor, Caracas, Venezuela.)*

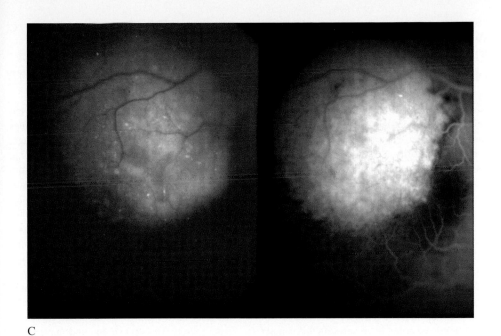

C

Figure 10-20A–C   Sturge-Weber syndrome   *(continued)*

NEUROFIBROMATOSIS (VON RECKLINGHAUSEN'S DISEASE AND BILATERAL ACOUSTIC NEUROFIBROMATOSIS)

Neurofibromatosis is an inherited disorder of the neuroectodermal system that results in hamartomas of the skin, eyes, and nervous system. The syndrome primarily affects tissue derived from the neural crest, particularly the sensitive nerves, Schwann's cells, and melanocytes.

Neurofibromatosis has two forms: NF-1, or classic Von Recklinghausen's neurofibromatosis; and NF-2, or bilateral acoustic neurofibromatosis. NF-1 is the most common form and includes involvement of skin with café-au-lait spots and cutaneous neurofibromas, iris hamartomas called Lisch nodules, and optic nerve gliomas (Figure 10-21). NF-1 occurs in an estimated 0.05% of population and has a prevalence of 1 in 30,000. It is inherited in an autosomal-dominant pattern with complete penetrance. NF-2 is less common, with an estimated prevalence of 1 in 50,000.

Cutaneous involvement includes café-au-lait spots, which appear as hyperpigmented macules on any part of body and tend to increase in age; and multiple neurofibromas, which are benign tumors of nerve connective tissue and vary from tiny, isolated nodules to huge pedunculous soft tissue masses. Ophthalmic involvement includes (1) iris hamartomas, clinically observed as bilateral, raised, smooth-surfaced, dome-shaped lesions: (2) plexiform neurofibromas of the upper lid, which appear clinically as an area of thickening of the lid margin with ptosis and an S-shaped deformity; (3) retinal tumors, most commonly astrocytic hamartomas; and (4) optic nerve gliomas, which manifest as unilateral decreased visual acuity or strabismus and have been observed in 25% of cases. Ipsilateral glaucoma is also occasionally seen and is usually associated with plexiform neurofibroma of the upper lid.

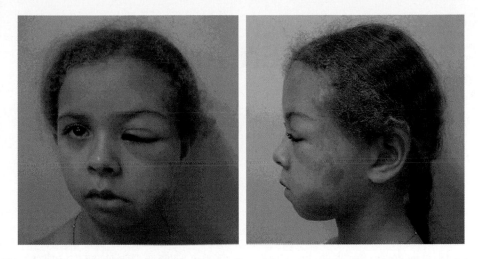

Figure 10-21   Neurofibromatosis   *Note café-au-lait spots and plexiform neurofibroma of the upper lid. (Courtesy of Dr. Claudia Pabon Bejarano, Escola Paulista de Medicina, UNIFESP, São Paulo, Brazil.)*

Chapter 11

PRIMARY OPEN-ANGLE GLAUCOMA

George L. Spaeth, MD

Worldwide, glaucoma, in its many forms, is the leading cause of irreversible blindness. The glaucomas can be classified roughly into the primary glaucomas, in which the process affects both eyes and is not the result of any recognized trauma occurring during a person's lifetime, and the secondary glaucomas, which often affect only one eye (though with certain types of secondary glaucomas, may be bilateral) and are a consequence of a recognized trauma such as infection, mechanical injury, or neovascularization.

The primary glaucomas are further divided on the basis of the anterior chamber angle. The angle-closure glaucomas are those in which the pressure becomes elevated as a consequence of

interference with aqueous outflow due to adhesions developing between the iris and the trabecular meshwork, and the open-angle glaucomas those in which aqueous humor has a clear access to the trabecular meshwork. The primary glaucomas are further divided according to the age of onset of the condition. Those occurring at or shortly after birth are termed *congenital*; those occurring after infancy and prior to age 40 years are termed juvenile glaucomas; and those first becoming apparent after the age of 40 are termed adult-onset open-angle glaucoma (Figure 11-1). The glaucomas occurring in infants represent a separate group and are discussed elsewhere in this text (see Chapter 10).

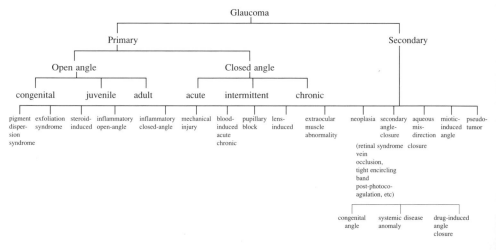

Figure 11-1   Classification of glaucoma

DEFINITION OF GLAUCOMA

The definition of glaucoma has changed so dramatically since it was first used in ancient Greece that the word has come to mean different things to different people. The definition is still evolving, as a consequence of which there are unfortunate and disturbing confusions regarding communication. Figure 11-2 illustrates a rough timeline of these changes.

Until the late 19th century, the definition of glaucoma was based largely on the presence of symptoms, blindness, or, later, pain. The development of statistical theory, the availability of the tonometer, and the concept of disease as a deviation from normal led to glaucoma being defined solely in terms of elevated intraocular pressure (IOP) above 21 mm Hg (that is, greater

than two standard deviations above the mean) or IOP above 24 mm Hg (greater than three standard deviations above the mean).

Studies conducted largely in the 1960s that showed that only around 5% of individuals with an IOP above 21 mm Hg ever develop actual optic nerve damage and visual field loss forced a total rethinking of the definition of glaucoma, as did studies showing that somewhere around one third of the patients who had the optic nerve and visual field changes characteristic of glaucoma had IOPs in the range of normal. Many authors began using the terms "low-tension glaucoma" or "normal-pressure glaucoma" or "high-tension glaucoma." As more and more attention became concentrated on the optic

How the Definition of Glaucoma Has Changed Over the Years

~500 BC   noninflammatory blindness
                            ↓

~1850   elevated intraocular pressure
                            congestive
                            noncongestive
                            ↓

~1900   intraocular pressure over 21 mm Hg
                            closed angle
                            open angle
                            ↓

~1970   intraocular pressure over 21 mm Hg
                            with visual field loss
                            ↓

~1980   intraocular pressure-mediated optic nerve damage
                            low-tension glaucoma
                            high-tension glaucoma
                            ↓

~1990   characteristic optic neuropathy
                            ↓

~2000   process leading to characteristic ocular tissue
                            damage at least partially related to
                            intraocular pressure
                            ↓

~2005   ?

Figure 11-2 How the definition of glaucoma has changed over the years

nerve, many leading contributors to the field ignored the classic changes caused by the angle-closure glaucomas—specifically, pain along with corneal, iris, and lens damage—and concentrated solely on the optic nerve. This led to a definition of glaucoma as a characteristic optic neuropathy. Recently, some authors have subdivided glaucoma into pressure-dependent and pressure-independent types.

My preference is shown in Figure 11-2, in which glaucoma is defined as the process lead-ing to characteristic ocular tissue damage at least partially caused by IOP, regardless of the level of IOP. Because almost all findings and symptoms of glaucoma in its early and moderate stages are found in people who do not have glaucoma, identification of characteristics that occur only (or almost only) in glaucoma is important (Figure 11-3).

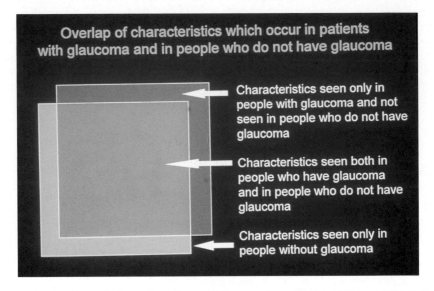

Figure 11-3   Overlap of characteristics which occur in patients with and without glaucoma

EPIDEMIOLOGY

Glaucoma affects individuals of all ages and in all geographic areas. It is not surprising that estimates of the presence of glaucoma vary widely (Figure 11-4). This variation is related to the differing definitions of glaucoma, differing methods of examination, and different expression of the constellation of loosely related conditions called primary open-angle glaucoma. Congenital glaucoma represents a distinct entity that is extremely rare. Most juvenile glaucoma is genetically determined, and while much more common than the congenital types of open-angle glaucoma, it is still relatively uncommon. The majority of patients with glaucoma are older than

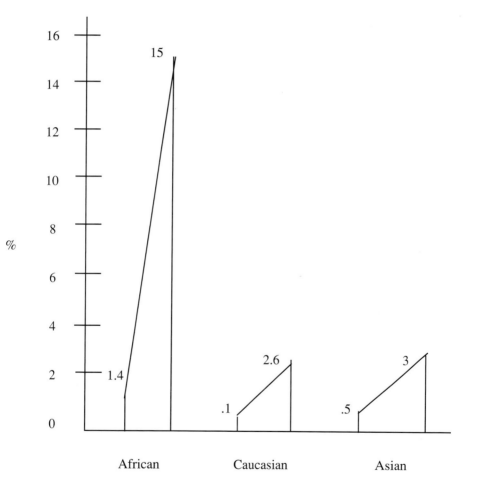

Figure 11-4 Prevalence of open-angle glaucoma in different populations

60 years of age. The relationship between the prevalence of glaucoma and age is illustrated in Figure 11-5. The prevalence of glaucoma in African Americans over the age of 80 may be more than 20%.

It is difficult to generalize regarding the amount of blindness caused by glaucoma. Again, glaucoma is a variable condition, with variable definitions. However, the incidence clearly increases markedly with age and especially in African Americans (Figure 11-6).

Worldwide, the incidence of glaucoma is estimated at around 2.5 million per year. The prevalence of blindness due to primary open-angle glaucoma is probably around 3 million. In the United States around 100,000 individuals are blind in both eyes as a result of glaucoma.

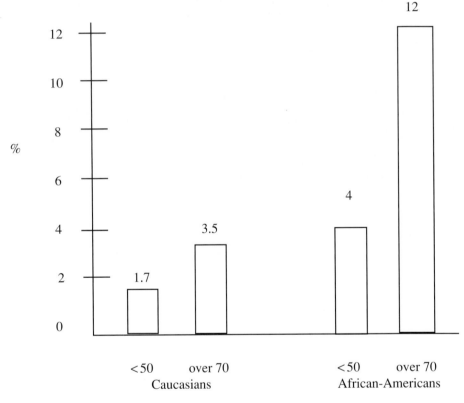

Figure 11-5   Relation between prevalence of glaucoma and aging

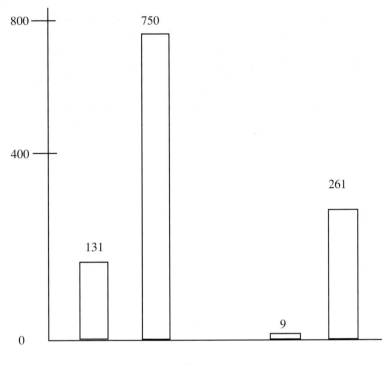

Cases of blindness
per 100,000 people

800

750

400

261

131

9

0

45-64   over 85   45-64   over 85
African-Americans   Caucasians

Years

Figure 11-6   Blindness caused by glaucoma

PATHOPHYSIOLOGY

The hallmark of glaucoma is ocular tissue damage, especially to the optic nerve. Figure 11-7 illustrates two of many possible ways in which the tissue damage can develop. In Figure 11-7A, the initiating factor is IOP within the normal or the elevated range, causing mechanical deformation and leading to subsequent damage. In Figure 11-7B, factors that are presumably less directly related to the structural deformation caused by IOP play a predominant role. Toxic agents or autoimmune mechanisms cause damage and eventual death of the retinal ganglion cells, leading to loss of tissue and structural damage, which itself may facilitate the IOP-related damage similar to that listed in Figure 11-7A.

The final common pathway in all the primary open-angle glaucomas is the death, sometimes by necrosis, but usually by apoptosis, of the retinal ganglion cell. This may lead to further damage, in the retina, optic nerve, and brain. Feedback loops make this oversimplified schema far more complex. For example, the last change noted under B in Figure 11-7, "structural change," itself predisposes to cell damage as listed under both A and B. Some of the factors that may be involved in this cascade of events are shown in Table 11-1.

Pathogenesis of Ocular Tissue Damage in Glaucoma

A.

Intraocular Pressure (any level)
↓

mechanical deformation of tissue (cornea, lamina, neuron, blood vessels)
↓

cell damage - vascular damage
↓

cell death by necrosis, but usually by apoptosis
↓

tissue loss (nerve fiber layer thinning, etc)

B.

Excitotoxicity, deficient growth factors, autoimmune mechanisms
↓

cell damage
↓

cell death (especially retinal ganglion cell)
↓

tissue loss
↓

structural change

Figure 11-7A,B   Pathogenesis of ocular tissue damage in glaucoma   *A. Intraocular pressure causes mechanical deformation and subsequent damage. **B.** Factors less directly related to damage caused by intraocular pressure are involved.*

Mechanical Injury
    Stretching of lamina cribrosa, blood vessels, corneal endothelial cells, etc.
Abnormal Glial, Neural, or Connective Tissue
Metabolic Deprivation
    Direct compression of neurons, connective tissue, and vasculature by intraocular pressure
    Lack of neurotrophins
        secondary to mechanical blockade of axons
        genetically determined
        deficient nerve growth factors
    Ischemia and hypoxia
        abnormal autoregulation of retinal and choroidal vessels
        decreased perfusion
            acute/chronic
            primary/secondary
        abnormal oxygen transfer
Autoimmune Mechanisms
Defective Protective Measures
    Deficient or inhibited nitric oxide synthase
    Abnormal heat-shock protein
Toxicity to retinal ganglion cells and other tissues
    Glutamate
Genetic Predisposition
    Abnormal optic nerve structure
        large laminar pores
        large scleral canal
        abnormal connective tissue
        abnormal vasculature
    Abnormal trabecular meshwork
        decreased permeability of extracellular matrix
        abnormal endothelial cells
        abnormal molecular biology

HISTORY

A thorough history is the most important single part of the examination of a patient with primary open-angle glaucoma. Even though the disease is relatively free of symptoms in its early stages, the history is the part of the examination that develops the relationship between the patient and the physician that is essential to successful diagnosis and management of glaucoma. Additionally, a meticulous history will frequently uncover symptoms of the disease, even in the moderate stages; for example, difficulty seeing in the dark, mild eye ache, a sense that vision simply is not as good as it was. Furthermore, history leads to eliciting the risk factors for glaucoma, and even more importantly, the risk factors for becoming blind from glaucoma (Tables 11-2 and 11-3).

The essential question in history-taking is, "How are you?" The physician must stress that the most important part of that question is the word "you." Glaucoma is a frightening condition that frequently decreases the patient's quality of life simply as a result of the patient knowing he or she has glaucoma. Additionally, there is such a long history of associating glaucoma with IOP that the physician at every appropriate opportunity must indicate to the patient that both the patient's and physician's concern relates to the patient's health, not primarily to the patient's IOP. An evaluation of health requires taking a competent, compassionate history.

TABLE 11-2   RISK FACTORS FOR THE DEVELOPMENT OF GLAUCOMA

1. Genetic Make-up
   Positive family history of glaucomatous visual loss
   Identification of glaucoma-related gene

2. Intraocular Pressure Considerations

mm Hg	likelihood of eventually developing glaucoma
>21	5%
>24	10%
>27	50%
>39	90%

3. Age

age in years*	prevalence of glaucoma
<40	rare
40–60	1%
60–80	2%
>80	4%

4. Vascular Factors
   Migraine
   Vasospastic disease
   Raynaud's disease
   Hypotension
   Hypertension

5. Myopia

6. Obesity

*These figures are for Caucasians and Asians; the prevalence in Africans is approximately four times higher.

TABLE 11-3 RISK FACTORS FOR BECOMING BLIND FROM GLAUCOMA

1. Disease process capable of causing blindness*
2. Lack of access to care
   geographic
   economic
   care unavailable
3. Lack of self-care competence
   intellectual limitation
   emotional limitation
   socioeconomic deprivation

*There is a great variation of disease severity with primary open-angle glaucoma; some patients do not get worse even in the absence of any treatment, whereas others go rapidly blind even with treatment.

CLINICAL EXAMINATION

The clinical examination of the patient suspected of having primary open-angle glaucoma differs only from the standard examination in emphasis. An essential part of the examination is a meticulous search for the presence or absence of a relative afferent pupillary defect (APD). An APD can be present prior to detectable field loss. Additionally, the presence of APD indicates that there is definite optic nerve damage, which triggers a necessary search for the cause of that damage. Checking the patient for an APD is a part of every complete examination of the patient with glaucoma.

External and Biomicroscopic Examination

Biomicroscopic examinations of the patient with glaucoma differ only from the standard biomicroscopic examination in that the physician searches for the topical side effects of the medications that the patient may be using (Figure 11-8A–C), and findings that may be associated with glaucoma such as a Krukenberg spindle.

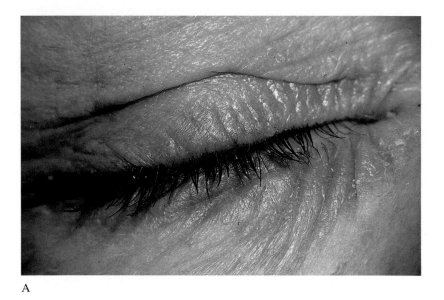

A

Figure 11-8 *A. External exam showing erythema and edema from an allergic reaction to timolol. B. Contact dermatitis involving the periorbital area of the left eye. There is also some conjuctival infection. C. Corneal epithelial pseudoendrites as a result of latanoprost (photo courtesy of Christopher Rapuano, M.D.; Wills Eye Hospital, Philadelphia, PA).*

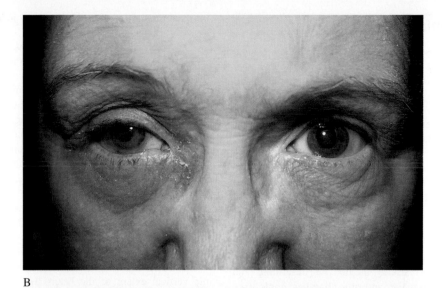

B

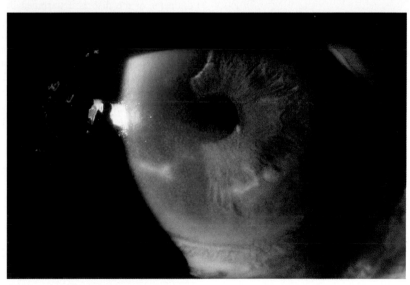

C

Figure 11-8 *(continued)*

Gonioscopy

Gonioscopy is an essential part of the evaluation of a patient with glaucoma. The examiner needs to search for the signs of pigment dispersion syndrome, exfoliation syndrome, and angle recession. Gonioscopy needs to be repeated at about yearly intervals, because anterior chamber angles that are initially deep may become increasingly narrow with age, leading eventually to chronic or, in rare cases, acute angle closure. Because miotics can cause marked shallowing of the anterior chamber angle, gonioscopy should be performed after any miotic is started or after a concentration of a miotic is changed. The Spaeth Gonioscopic Grading System provides a rapid, quantitative, clinically useful method of describing and recording the anterior chamber angle (see Chapter 3).

Posterior Pole

Primary open-angle glaucoma is primarily a disease of the optic disc. Consequently, knowledgeable, extensive evaluation of the optic nerve is a mandatory part of the evaluation of the patient suspected of having glaucoma and of the continuing evaluation of the patient. In the *diagnosis* of primary open-angle glaucoma, evaluation of the optic nerve is the single most important aspect of the assessment. In the *management* of glaucoma, the nature of the optic disc is the second most important aspect of the examination, a meticulous history being the first.

The optic disc is best examined with the pupil in a dilated state. After dilation the optic nerve is examined stereoscopically at the biomicroscope using a strong plus lens such as a 60- or 66-diopter lens. This is best done with the beam narrowed to a thin slit and the magnification on high (1.6 or 16X) using a Haag-Streit 900 series slit-lamp biomicroscope. The examiner gains an idea of the disc topography by this method. Also, the size of the disc is measured. To measure the vertical height of the disc the beam is widened so that the horizontal extent of the beam is the same width as the width of the optic nerve (Figure 11-9). The beam is then narrowed vertically until the vertical diameter of the optic disc exactly matches the vertical extent of the beam. The vertical diameter of the disc is determined by reading the reticule on the slit lamp and applying the appropriate correction factor. Though these factors vary slightly with the Volk and the Nikon lenses, a rough approximation is that for the 60-diopter lens one multiplies the reading on the reticule by 0.9; for the 66-diopter, no correction factor is needed; and for the 90-diopter, the measurement on the reticule is multiplied by 1.3. The normal disc has a diameter between 1.5 and 1.9 mm vertically.

The next step employs the direct ophthalmoscope. The beam of the ophthalmoscope should be narrowed so that it projects a beam on the retina approximately 1.3 mm in

1. Size

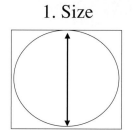

2. Read reticule

3. Use correction factor

Figure 11-9 Method of measuring vertical diameter of the disc

diameter. This is the size of the middle-sized beam on some Welch-Allyn ophthalmoscopes and of the smallest beam on some other Welch-Allyn ophthalmoscopes. The examiner should learn the size of the beam for the ophthalmoscope he or she is using. This can be readily done by projecting the beam on the retina next to the optic nerve, noting the height of that beam relative to the optic nerve, and then using the strong plus lens to get an exact measurement of the height of the projected beam. Once this has been determined, the size of the optic nerve can be determined relatively accurately with the direct ophthalmoscope itself. In eyes with more than 5 D of hyperopia or 5 D of myopia, the disc size will be abnormally large or abnormally small, respectively, when viewed with the strong plus lens due to magnification or minification.

The optic nerve can be best examined using a direct ophthalmoscope with both the patient and the examiner in the seated position. The examiner's head must be in a position to avoid obstructing the patient's gaze with the other eye, because that other eye must fixate firmly to allow careful evaluation of the eye being examined. The examiner directs primary attention to the 6 and 12 o'clock positions of the nerve: What is the rim width? Is an acquired pit or a disc hemorrhage present? Is there peripapillary atrophy? Are the vessels displaced, bent, engorged, narrowed, or "bayonetted"? The examiner also estimates the width of the neuroretinal rim at the 1, 3, 5, 7, 9, and 11 o'clock positions. This is done in terms of a rim-to-disc ratio; that is, the relative width of the rim in comparison to the diameter of the optic nerve in that axis. Thus, the maximum rim-to-disc ratio is 0.5.

In Figure 11-10, the rim-disc ratio at 1 o'clock is 0.2; at 3 o'clock, 0.15; at 5 o'clock, 0.0; at 7 o'clock, 0.25; at 9 o'clock, 0.20, and at 11 o'clock, 0.25. Figure 11-11A illustrates a disc with a narrow rim that respects Jonas's ISNT rule, which states that the rim should be widest *i*nferiorly, next widest *s*uperiorly, next widest *n*asally, and narrowest *t*emporally. Despite the large cup, there is no visual field loss (Figure 11-11B). Figure 11-12 shows a disc

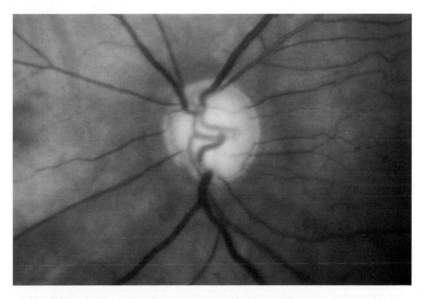

Figure 11-10 Optic nerve photograph of a left eye showing an acquired pit at approximately 5 o'clock

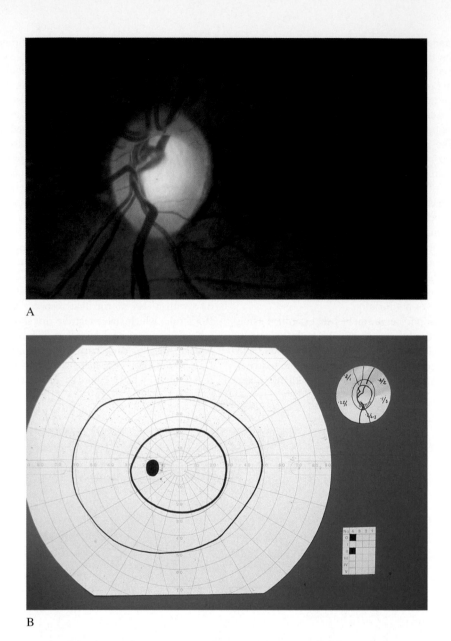

Figure 11-11 *A. A disc with a narrow rim that respects Jonas's ISNT rule. **B.** Corresponding Goldmann Visual Field showing no abnormality*

DISEASE SYNDROMES

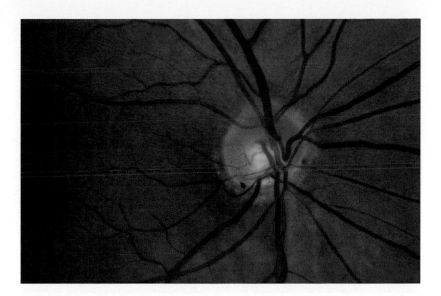

Figure 11-12 Small cup-to-disc ratio *A disc with a relatively small cup-disc ratio, but a rim-disc ratio of 0 at the inferior pole.*

with a relatively small "cup-disc ratio," but a rim-disc ratio of 0 at the inferior pole. Cup-to-disc ratios are misleading and should not be used. Figure 11-13 shows two discs of different sizes. Figure 11-13A is a small disc with a disc diameter of approximately 1.2 mm. Figure 11-13B is a large disc with a disc diameter of approximately 2.2 mm. The examiner may be misled by the relative size of the cup in these two discs and incorrectly conclude that the disc in Figure 11-13B is less healthy than that in Figure 11-13A. In actuality, it is the other way around.

The rim area is relatively constant in all healthy discs. Thus, in large discs, the rim area is spread over a much greater area (recall that area involves the square of the radius). The consequence of this is that the normal rim of the large, *healthy* disc is narrower than the normal rim of the small, *healthy* disc. The rim area in Figure 11-13B is actually greater than the rim area in Figure 11-13A.

The relative health of the optic nerve can be estimated by staging the disc according to the system illustrated in Figure 11-14.

In younger patients, or patients whose optic nerves are in the relatively early stages of glaucomatous damage, specifically stages 0 to 3, evaluation of the nerve fiber layer can be helpful. The examiner focuses meticulously on the retinal surface, preferably with a red-free light in the direct ophthalmoscope, and looks for lines that would follow the course of the nerve fiber layers. A trough can indicate the presence of such a defect illustrated in Figure 11-15. In most cases, however, the topography of the optic nerve provides more valuable clues than does the nature of the nerve fiber layer.

The optic nerves of the two eyes should be symmetric. Where asymmetry is present, one of the nerves is almost always abnormal, unless the optic nerves are of different sizes, as indicated in Figure 11-13. Figure 11-16 shows the right and left eyes of a patient with unilateral optic nerve damage resulting from glaucoma.

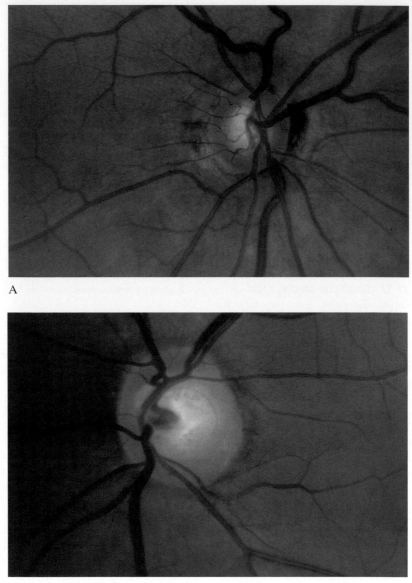

Figure 11-13A,B Two discs of different sizes *A. Small disc with a disc diameter of approximately 1.2 mm. **B.** Large disc with a disc diameter of approximately 2.2.*

THE DISC DAMAGE LIKELIHOOD SCALE – DDLS

DDLS	Thinnest width of rim (rim/disc ratio)			DDLS Stage	EXAMPLES		
	For Small Disc < 1.50 mm	For Average Size Disc 1.50 – 2.00 mm	For Large Disc > 2.00 mm		Small Optic Nerve	Average Optic Nerve	Large Optic Nerve
0a	.5	.4 or more	.3 or more	0a			
0b	.4 up to .5	.3 to .4	.2 to .3	0b			
1	.3 up to .4	.2 to .3	.1 to .15	1			
2	.2 up to .3	.1 to .2	.05 to .1	2			
3	.1 up to .2	less than .1	.01 to .05	3			
4	less than .1	$0 < 45^0$	0 for 45^0	4			
5	no rim for < 45^0	0 for 45^0 to 90^0	0 for 45^0 to 90^0	5			
6	no rim for 45^0 to 90^0	0 for 90^0 to 180^0	0 for 90^0 to 180^0	6			
7	no rim for more than 90^0	0 for more than 180^0	0 for more than 180^0	7			

The DDLS is based on the radial width of the neuroretinal rim measured at its thinnest point. The unit of measurement is the rim/disc ratio, that is, the radial width of the rim compared to the diameter of the disc in the same axis. When there is no rim remaining the rim/disc ratio is 0. The circumferential extent of rim absence (0 rim/disc ratio) is measured in degrees. Caution must be taken to differentiate the actual absence of rim from sloping of the rim as, for example, can occur temporally in some patients with myopia. A sloping rim is not an absent rim. Because rim width is a function of disc size, disc size must be evaluated prior to attributing a DDLS stage. This is done with a 60D to 90D lens with appropriate corrective factors. The Volk 60D lens minimally underestimates the disc size. Corrective factors for other lenses are: Volk 60D × .88, 78D × 1.2, 90D × 1.33. Nikon 60D × 1.03, 90D × 1.63.

Figure 11-14. The Disc Damage Likelihood Scale: *A method of grading the amount of disc damage that takes into account the size of the optic disc*

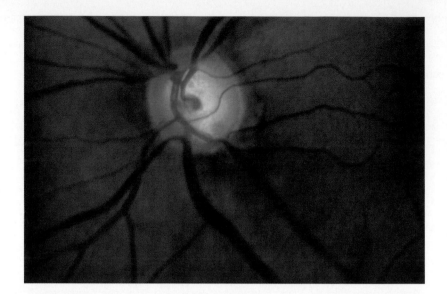

Figure 11-15   A disc with an inferotemporal notch and a nerve fiber layer defect inferotemporally

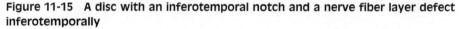

The examiner should search out the presence of an acquired pit of the optic nerve. These localized defects immediately adjacent to the outer edge of the rim, just temporal to the inferior or superior pole of the disc, are pathognomonic for glaucomatous damage. The observer also specifically looks for the presence of a disc hemorrhage on the retina crossing the rim. Such hemorrhages are usually signs that the glaucomatous process is out of control. Further information about the optic disc is found in Chapter 4.

presence or absence of defects. The evaluation of the visual field with the Esterman test on a Humphrey field analyzer correlates well with the level of functional loss caused by the glaucoma. The standard monocular visual field examination, preferably with an automated perimeter such as the Octopus or Humphrey field analyzer, is a standard part of assessing the amount of monocular damage, and whether or not change is occurring. Visual fields are addressed in detail in Chapter 5.

Special Tests

The evaluation of the visual field by confrontation with a red object gives a good idea of the

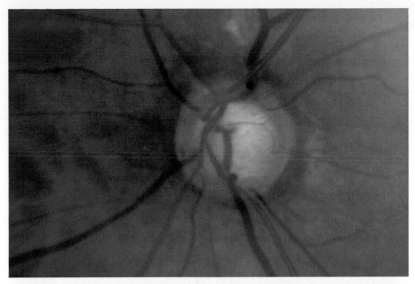

A

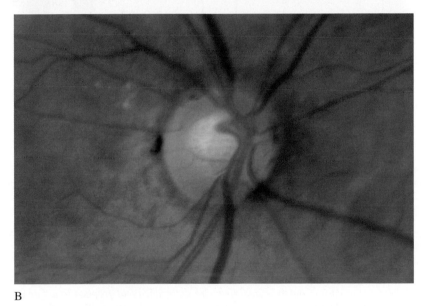

B

Figure 11-16   Unilateral optic nerve damage from glaucoma   *Right and left eyes of a patient with unilateral optic nerve damage caused by glaucoma.*

MANAGEMENT

The goal of management of a patient with primary open-angle glaucoma is the maintenance or enhancement of the patient's health. Both the physician and the patient wish to ensure that the patient does not develop functional loss prior to his or her death. Estimating the need to start treatment or the need to change the vigor of treatment requires that the physician have a good idea of the likelihood or lack of likelihood that the patient's glaucoma will ultimately cause visual functional problems. To make this determination, the physician must know three things: (1) the stage of the glaucoma, (2) the rate of change of that stage of glaucoma, and (3) the duration that the glaucoma will continue to exist. The use of the glaucoma graph can be of great help in this regard (Figure 11-17).

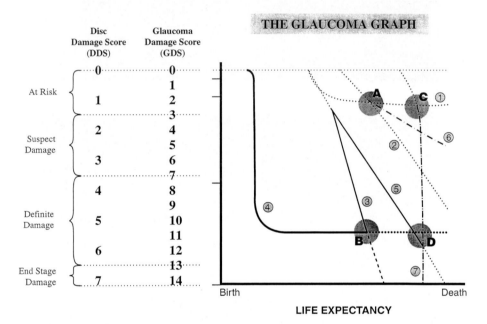

Figure 11-17   Glaucoma graph and explanation The Glaucoma Graph George Spaeth, MD   *The glaucoma graph is a way of determining and understanding the clinical course of glaucoma in an individual patient.*

On the y axis of the graph is the stage of the glaucoma, and on the x axis is the life expectancy. The slope and the curve of each of the individual lines are determined and graphed in different ways:

- *dotted lines indicate that the slope and the curve have been determined by plotting the results of serial studies, such as repeated disc photographs taken yearly or repeated visual field examinations.*
- *solid lines depict the clinical course as described in the patient's history.*
- *dashed lines are extrapolations that are presumed to represent what will happen in the future. These hypothetical, extrapolated future courses are based on the nature of the previous courses and on knowledge of what has happened since a known point in time.*

This illustration shows the courses of seven different patients with different manifestations of glaucoma:

- *A patient at point "A" has minimal glaucoma, and about one third of his or her life still to live.*

Figure 11-17 *(continued)*

- *A patient at point "B" has advanced glaucoma and has about one third of his or her life still to live.*
- *A patient at point "C" has very early glaucoma and only a few years to live*
- *A patient at point "D" has advanced glaucoma and only a few years to live.*
- *Patient no. 1, considered at point "A" has one third of his or her life to live and is in an early stage of glaucoma. About one third of his or her life earlier, this patient was noted to have elevated pressure and followed without treatment. The patient continued to be followed without treatment and no damage to the optic nerve or visual field was ever noted. It is reasonable to assume that, if the patient continues to have intraocular pressures around the same level as those noted initially, he or she will probably follow the course described by **line 1**, and will die without any evidence of glaucoma damage.*
- *Patient no. 2, also considered at **point "A"**, ie, having minimal damage with one third of his or her life left to live. In this case, however, the patient's intraocular pressure rose continuously, and the patient was noted to develop early disc and field damage, which then continued at the rate depicted by the **dashed line 2**. This patient, if untreated, would develop definite asymptomatic damage. However, the patient would have no functional loss at the time of his or her death.*
- *Patients nos. 3 and 4, at point "B": both have advanced glaucoma and one third of their lives left to live. However, **patient no. 3** is deteriorating rapidly and will be blind long before he or she dies, whereas **patient no. 4**, who has a blow to the eye as a child and lost vision to a steroid-induced glaucoma at that time, has had stable vision for most of his or her life, and it is reasonable to expect that it will continue to be stable.*
- *Patients **at points "C" and "D"** both have only a few years to live, but those at **point "C"** (like **patients nos. 1 and 2** at **point "A"**) have minimal damage, and those at **point "D"** (like **patient no. 4** at **point "B"**) have marked damage.*
- *Patient no. 5 started with a clinical course similar to that of **patient no. 3** (advanced glaucoma and deteriorating rapidly), but around the midpoint of his or her life, the glaucoma became less severe. Nevertheless, this patient will be blind at the time of his or her death unless there is effective intervention. Compare **patient no. 4**, who at **point "D"** has the same life expectancy and the same amount of damage as **patient no. 5** (only a few years to live and advanced glaucoma). **Patient no. 4**, however, has a stable clinical course and does not appear to need a change in therapy. In contrast, **patient no. 5** needs lowering intraocular pressure urgently.*
- *Patient no. 6, at around **point "C"** also has only a few years of life remaining, but has a glaucoma that is getting worse a little bit more slowly than that affecting **patients nos. 2 and 5**. However, since **patient no. 6** has so little damage to start with, no treatment is necessary, even though he or she is getting worse. Even without treatment, he or she will not have enough damage or visual loss due to glaucoma at the time of death that he or she will have any awareness of being sick, and will have no limitation in function.*
- *Patient no. 7 at point "C" has only a few years left to live, but has a type of glaucoma which is deteriorating so rapidly that even though he or she has only a short period of time to live, he or she will be blind well before the time of death.*

Using the glaucoma graph to define and characterize the nature of the clinical course helps the physician and patient to understand that:

- *Patients nos. 1, 4, and 6 do not need any treatment at all; **patient no. 1** will never develop damage, **patient no. 4** has marked damage but it is not getting worse, and **patient no. 6** is getting worse so slowly that it will not interfere with his or her life.*
- *Patients nos. 3, 5, and 7 can be seen to need treatment urgently in order to prevent them from becoming totally blind prior to the time of their deaths.*
- *Patient no. 2: The need for treatment is controversial. Since this patient would never develop glaucoma, perhaps he or she should not be treated at all. But since he or she would develop **some** damage, those would want to prevent any damage at all would advise therapy.*

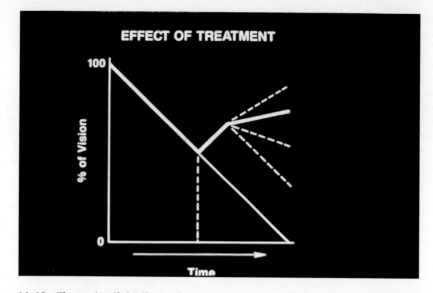

Figure 11-18   The potential effect of treatment on the course of visual field decline: *Continuing deterioration, worsening, or actual benefit*

The *stage* of the glaucoma is determined by utilizing the disc-staging nomogram in Figure 11-14. The *rate of change* is determined by serial evaluations of the history, visual field, and the optic nerve. The *duration* the glaucoma will continue to cause damage with primary open-angle glaucoma is determined by a reasonable estimate of the patient's life expectancy (Figure 11-17).

Appropriate management of primary open-angle glaucoma requires thoughtful balance of (1) the *risks* of pain or functional loss in the face of no intervention, (2) the potential *benefit* of an intervention (in terms of retardation or stabilization of deterioration of visual function or actual improvement), and (3) the potential risks introduced by the intervention itself (Tables 11-4 and 11-5).

The only proven beneficial treatment for primary open-angle glaucoma is lowering IOP. The amount that the IOP should be lowered in each individual in order to prevent deterioration, stabilize the condition, or result in improvement (Figure 11-18) also varies from individual to individual, but guidelines have been developed (Tables 11-6 and 11-7).

TABLE 11-4 RISKS AND BENEFITS OF TREATMENT

Risks Attendant to No Intervention	Risks Attendant to Intervention	Benefits of Intervention
pain	local side effects pain redness cataract infection bleeding allergy abnormal flashes increased pigmentation etc.	improvement of visual function
visual loss minimal moderate total	systemic side effects fatigue malaise cardiovascular changes neurologic changes psychologic changes pulmonary changes etc.	stabilization of deterioration of function
		retardation of rate of deterioration of function

TABLE 11-5 RISK OF LOSING FUNCTION IF NO INTERVENTION

Low
1. healthy optic nerve
2. negative family history of visual loss due to glaucoma
3. good self-care skills
4. good access to good care
5. life expectancy less than 10 years
6. intraocular pressure below 15 mm Hg
7. no exfoliation or pigment dispersion syndrome changes
8. normal cardiovascular status

High
1. damaged optic nerve
2. positive family history of visual loss due to glaucoma or presence of recognized "gene" for glaucoma
3. poor self-care skills
4. poor access to good care
5. life expectancy over 10 years
6. intraocular pressure over 30 mm Hg
7. exfoliation syndrome
8. poor cardiovascular status

TABLE 11-6 EXPECTED BENEFIT OF TREATMENT*

Expected benefit great if intraocular pressure-lowering greater than 30%
Expected benefit possible to probable if intraocular pressure-lowering is 15–30%
No benefit expected if intraocular pressure-lowering is less than 15%

*In some cases stabilization of intraocular pressure appears to be beneficial in itself.

TABLE 11-7

Usual decrease in intraocular pressure	
in response to medications	approx 15% (range 0–50%)
in response to argon laser trabeculoplasty	approx 20% (range 0–50%)
in response to filtering surgery	approx 40% (range 0–80%)
Likelihood of side effects as a result of treatment	
from medications	~30%
from argon laser trabeculoplasty	almost none
from filtering surgery	~60%*

*The lower the final intraocular pressure the greater the likelihood of side effects from the surgery.

Some physicians recommend setting a target pressure; that is, an IOP level believed likely to be low enough to prevent further damage. Two methods of arriving at a target pressure are shown in Figure 11-19. It is important to remember, however, that the target IOP is but a rough guide to treatment. The only valid method of establishing the state of control in a patient with primary open-angle glaucoma is by establishing stability of the optic nerve or visual field, or both. Thus, if the optic nerve and visual field are stable despite an IOP higher than the calculated target pressure, it is not wise to attempt to lower the pressure more vigorously in order to achieve the target IOP. Conversely, if the target pressure is achieved, but the optic nerve or visual field continue to deteriorate, then the target pressure is too high, there is another cause for the continuing deterioration other than glaucoma, or the neurons are so badly damaged that deterioration will progress no matter what level IOP is achieved.

In conclusion, primary open-angle glaucoma is an important cause of irreversible blindness around the world. Its diagnosis rests primarily on establishing the presence of optic nerve damage. The goal of treatment is maintenance of the health of the individual by using the minimum therapy necessary to retard the rate of deterioration of visual function, in order to assure that the affected person still has good visual function at the time of his or her death. To make a conclusion in this regard, the treating physician must know the stage of the glaucoma, the rate of change of the glaucoma, and the life expectancy of the patient.

Two Methods of Estimating the Target Intraocular Pressure

1. $D - (D \times D) - FF = $ target IOP
   $(\overline{100})$

2. $D - (D \times .30) - FF = $ target IOP

$D = $ IOP in mm Hg at which optic nerve damage occurs

$FF = $ 1 mm Hg for moderate optic nerve damage
   2 mm Hg for severe optic nerve damage
   1 mm Hg when D is below 20 mm Hg
   2 mm Hg when D is below 16 mm Hg

Figure 11-19   Two methods of estimating the target intraocular pressure (IOP)

Chapter 12

SECONDARY OPEN-ANGLE GLAUCOMA

Jonathan S. Myers, MD

PIGMENT DISPERSION SYNDROME (FIGURES 12-1 TO 12-7)

Definition

Pigment dispersion syndrome (PDS) is a condition in which pigment is dislodged from the pigmented epithelium on the posterior surface of the iris, and is then deposited on various structures throughout the anterior segment. Obstruction of the trabecular meshwork by pigment, and subsequent damage to the meshwork, can lead to elevated intraocular pressure and secondary open-angle glaucoma.

Epidemiology

Pigment dispersion syndrome occurs most frequently in young (aged 20 to 45 years), myopic, Caucasian men. Approximately one third of PDS patients may go on to develop pigmentary glaucoma.

Pathophysiology

Currently, it is believed that contact between the iris pigment epithelium and the lens zonular fibers leads to release of the pigment into the anterior chamber and the characteristic peripheral iris transillumination defects. The liberated pigment may then be deposited throughout the anterior segment. Obstruction of the trabecular meshwork by pigment and subsequent damage may reduce aqueous outflow, increasing intraocular pressure, and leading to subsequent nerve damage if untreated.

History

Patients often relate a history of myopia and a family history of glaucoma. Most patients are asymptomatic, but some may experience pigment storms during or after strenuous physical activity. Jarring exercise (or dilation) may lead to dramatically increased pigment dispersion, a so-called pigment storm, leading to sudden elevations of intraocular pressure. Patients may then experience blurred vision and headaches.

Clinical Examination

Slit Lamp   Characteristic findings include the Krukenberg spindle, a vertical deposition of pigment on the corneal endothelium, pigment deposition on the anterior surface of the iris, peripheral iris transillumination defects (best seen on retroillumination with a small beam through the pupil), and pigment deposition on the zonular fiber attachments near the equator of the lens.

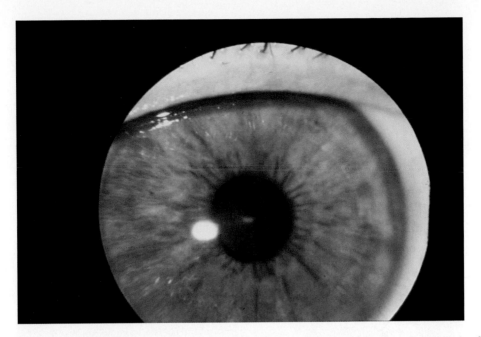

Figure 12-1 Krukenberg spindle *A vertical endothelial deposition of pigment characteristic of PDS. May slowly resolve when pigment shedding stops, but may persist for many years or forever. Pattern of deposition is thought to be related to convection currents of aqueous within the eye.*

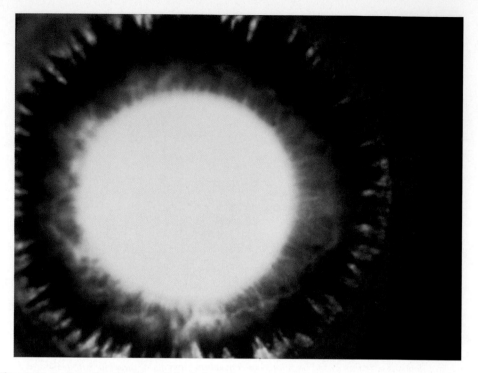

Figure 12-2 Transillumination defects in PDS *Marked peripheral and mid-peripheral transillumination defects in PDS. Many patients may present with only several mild radial spoke-like defects.*

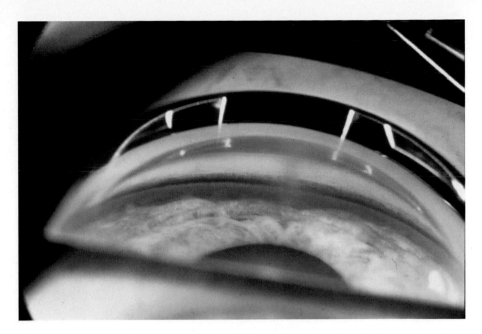

Figure 12-3   PDS, dense pigmentation and Krukenberg spindle   *Krukenberg spindle (foreground), heavily pigmented deep angle (background). Characteristic homogeneous dense pigmentation of trabecular meshwork.*

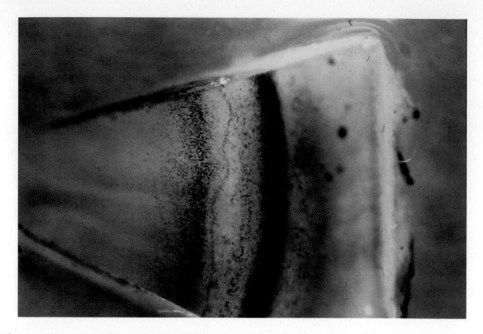

Figure 12-4   PDS, pigment deposition   *Pathology specimen showing pigment deposition on trabecular meshwork and anterior to meshwork.*

DISEASE SYNDROMES

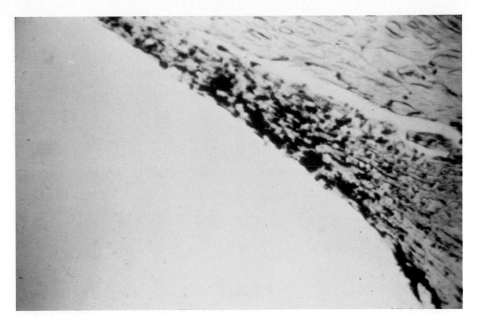

Figure 12-5   PDS, pigment deposition   *Pathology specimen showing pigment deposition within beams of trabecular meshwork.*

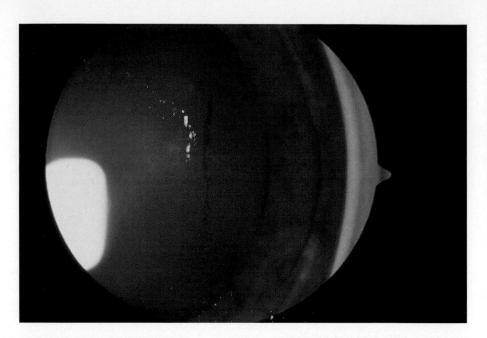

Figure 12-6 PDS, Zentmeyer's line *Deposition of pigment near equator of lens, at insertion of lens zonular fibers. Variously referred to as Zentmeyer's line or Scheie's stripe.*

DISEASE SYNDROMES

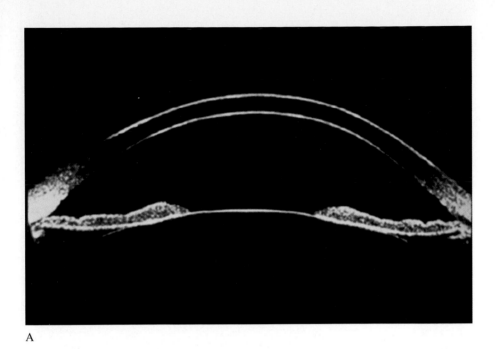

A

Figure 12-7A,B   PDS, bowing of peripheral iris   *A. UBM of patient with PDS, showing backward bowing peripheral iris in contact with lens surface.*

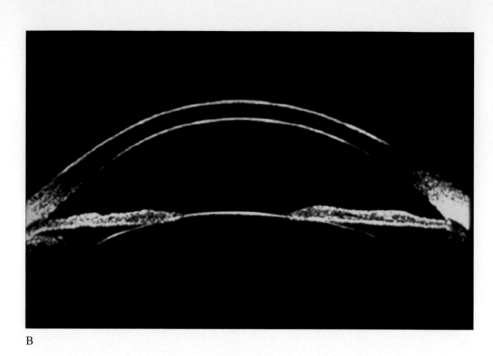

B

Figure 12-7A,B   PDS, bowing of peripheral iris   *(continued)*   *B. UBM, same patient, following iridotomy, showing anterior relaxation of iris with reduced contact with lens.*

Gonioscopy Patients may have backward bowing of the peripheral iris, increasing lens-iris contact. The angle is typically very widely open, with moderate to heavy pigmentation, which is relatively homogeneously spread over the entire circumference of the angle.

Posterior Pole Characteristic glaucomatous optic atrophy is seen with prolonged elevation of intraocular pressure or intermittent pressure spikes. Myopic patients, and possibly especially those with pigment dispersion syndrome, are prone to peripheral retinal tears, necessitating close examination.

Management

The goal of therapy is to control intraocular pressure in patients with significantly elevated pressure or glaucomatous nerve changes, usually through aqueous suppressants. Miotics reduce pigment shedding and reduce intraocular pressure, but are often poorly tolerated in this young population and may increase the risk of retinal detachment while making monitoring of the retina periphery more difficult. Laser peripheral iridotomy also may reduce pigment shedding, because it allows the posteriorly bowed iris to move anteriorly as any built-up fluid pressure in the anterior chamber is then normalized with the posterior chamber (relief of so-called reverse pupillary block). This may help prevent glaucoma in individuals at higher risk. Argon laser trabeculoplasty and filtering surgery are also effective in individuals who are uncontrolled medically.

EXFOLIATION SYNDROME (FIGURES 12-8 TO 12-12)

Definition

Exfoliation syndrome (XFS) is a systemic condition that can lead to a secondary open-angle glaucoma. The characteristic flaky white material, seen throughout the anterior segment, can obstruct the trabecular meshwork and has also been isolated in tissues throughout the body.

Epidemiology

Exfoliation syndrome ranges in prevalence from near zero in Eskimos to near 30% in people in Scandinavian countries. Its incidence increases with age and time, as does binocular versus monocular involvement. XFS-associated glaucoma may account for varying proportions of patients with glaucoma, from very small to the majority, depending on the population studied. Although patients with XFS are at an increased risk for the development of glaucoma (estimated in the Blue Mountains Eye Study at fivefold greater), the majority of these patients do not develop glaucoma.

Pathophysiology

The exact nature of the exfoliation material is not well understood, but the material has been isolated from the iris, lens, ciliary body, trabecular meshwork, corneal endothelium, and endothelial cells in blood vessels throughout the eye and orbit, as well as the skin, myocardium, lung, liver, gallbladder, kidney, and cerebral meninges. The material leads to blockage of the trabecular meshwork and thereby a secondary open-angle glaucoma. It also leads to iris peripupillary ischemia and posterior synechiae. This results in pigment release, increasing the burden on the trabecular meshwork, and increased pupillary block, predisposing to angle closure.

History

Although patients will rarely have symptomatic elevations of intraocular pressure, most patients have no contributory history. Some patients report a family history, but no clear hereditary pattern is known. A history of complicated cataract surgery is potentially suggestive.

Clinical Examination

Slit Lamp   The hallmark of XFS is the flaky white material seen most often at the edge of the pupil and in concentric rings on the anterior surface of the lens capsule after dilation. This material may also be seen deposited on the iris, angle structures, endothelium, lens implant, and vitreous face in aphakic patients. Peripupillary transillumination defects and atrophy of the pigmented ruff are often seen. Peripupillary pigment shedding is also frequent. Affected eyes are often more miotic and dilate poorly secondary to synechiae and iris ischemia. Pigment liberation with dilation may cause significant pressure spikes. Cataract formation is more frequent.

Gonioscopy   The anterior chamber angle is often more narrow in XFS, especially inferiorly relative to superiorly. Acute angle-closure glaucoma is a risk, and therefore continued monitoring of the angle is necessary. There is irregular pigmentation of the meshwork, with large, dark pigment particles. The deposition of pigment anterior to Schwalbe's line results in the characteristic, wavy Sampaolesi line.

Posterior Pole   Characteristic glaucomatous optic atrophy is seen with prolonged elevation of intraocular pressure or intermittent pressure spikes.

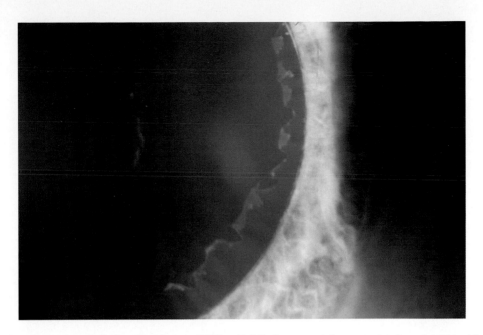

Figure 12-8 Exfoliation syndrome (XFS) *Exfoliation material on anterior lens capsule with clear zone in region between undilated pupil zone and more peripheral lens. Presumably, the movement of the iris clears exfoliative material from this area.*

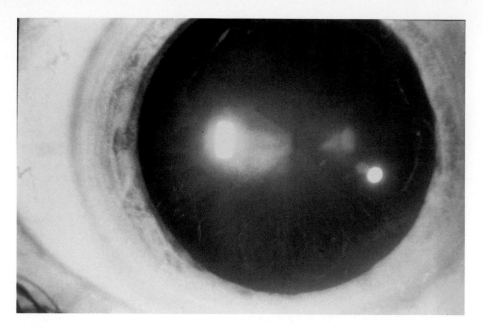

Figure 12-9   XFS, exfoliation material   *Exfoliation material on lens surface. Note typical scrolled edges.*

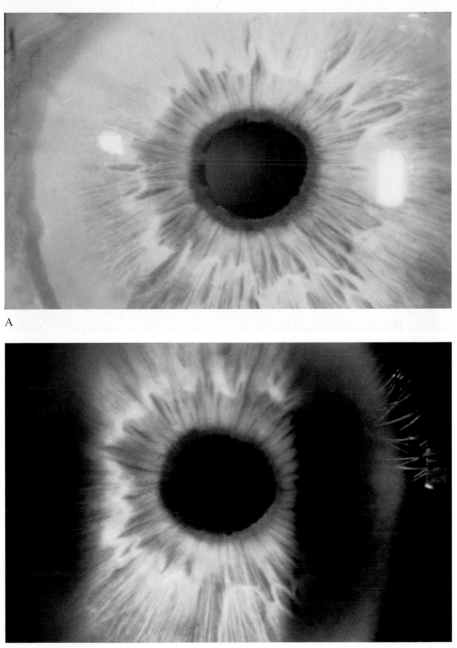

A

B

Figure 12-10A,B,C   Comparison of XFS and normal eyes   *Slit-lamp photos of (A) affected, and (B) clinically unaffected eyes. In (A), there is atrophy of the pigmented ruffs, seen in XFS; whereas it is preserved in (B).*

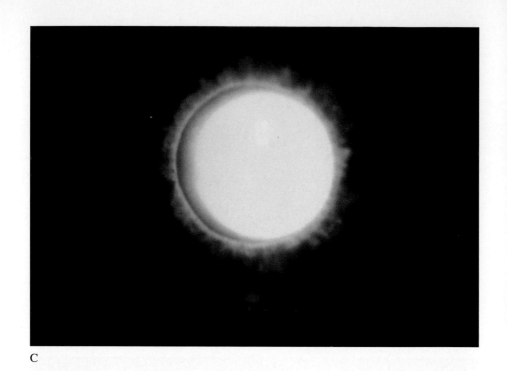

C

Figure 12-10A,B,C Comparison of XFS and normal eyes *(continued)* *C. Peripupillary transillumination corresponding to iris pigment epithelial atrophy in (A).*

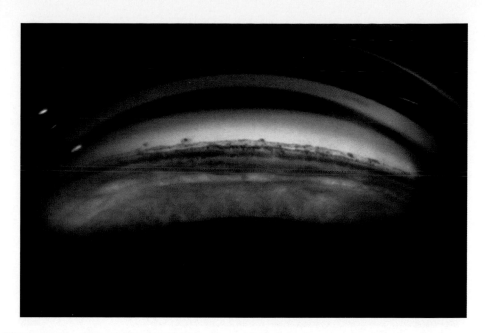

Figure 12-11   XFS, angle structures   *Heavy, dark, irregular pigmentation of angle structures in XFS.*

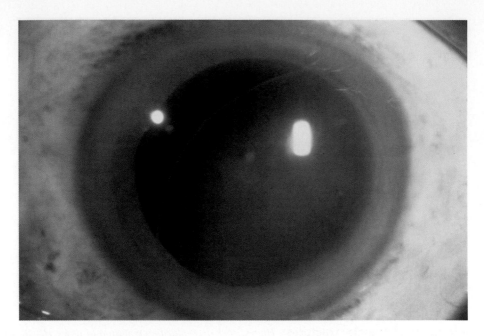

Figure 12-12   XFS, dislocated lens   *Spontaneously dislocated lens in a patient with XFS highlights fragility of zonular support.*

Management

XFS-related glaucoma often leads to higher pressures with greater diurnal fluctuation. Topical medications are appropriate but have been reported to be less effective. Argon laser trabeculoplasty is effective, although there are reports of increased postoperative elevations in intraocular pressure. Typically, the heavily pigmented meshwork will respond to lower laser energies, which may reduce postoperative pressure spikes. The results of filtration surgery are similar to those seen in primary open-angle glaucoma. Cataract surgery should be performed with extra caution, given the known fragility of the capsule and zonular fibers in these patients.

STEROID-RESPONSIVE GLAUCOMA (FIGURES 12-13 AND 12-14)

Definition

A secondary open-angle glaucoma may result from nearly any route of steroid administration. Elevations in intraocular pressure may be severe and prolonged.

Epidemiology

The incidence of steroid-induced glaucoma in the general population is unknown. Significant elevations in intraocular pressure in response to topical steroids have been reported in 50% to over 90% of glaucoma patients and 5% to 10% of patients with normal pressure. The incidence of the steroid response is related to the type, dose, and route of steroid administration. Elevated intraocular pressure has been observed with topical, intraocular, periocular, inhaled, oral, intravenous, and dermatologic administrations of steroids, as well as with endogenous elevations of steroids in Cushing's syndrome.

Pathophysiology

Increased glycosaminoglycans in the trabecular meshwork in response to steroids impede aqueous outflow and lead to elevated intraocular pressures. Steroids may reduce the membrane permeability of the trabecular meshwork, as well as reduce local phagocytic activity by cells and the breakdown of extracellular and intracellular structural proteins, further contributing to reduced meshwork permeability. The myocillin/TIGR (trabecular meshwork–inducible glucocorticoid response) gene has been shown to be upregulated in trabecular meshwork endothelial cells in response to steroid application. The link this gene may have to glaucoma and steroid-responsive intraocular pressure has not yet been fully elucidated.

History

Steroid use of any type is a crucial aspect of the history. Prior use of steroids in the distant past with subsequent normalization of intraocular pressure may present as an apparent normal-tension glaucoma. A history of asthma, skin disorders, allergies, autoimmune disorders, or the like may thus suggest possible past or current steroid use. Occasionally, patients note changes in vision related to advanced visual field loss.

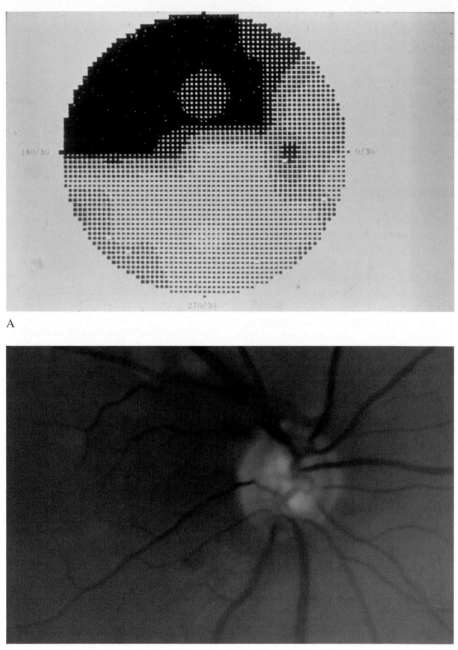

A

B

Figure 12-13A–C Steroid-responsive glaucoma *(A). Visual field defect seen in a 28 year old internal medicine resident self-medicating atopic blepharoconjunctivitis with topical steroids. Intraocular pressures were greater than 40 mm Hg, with advanced (**B** and **C**) optic nerve cupping and associated visual field loss. The patient later underwent a trabeculectomy.*

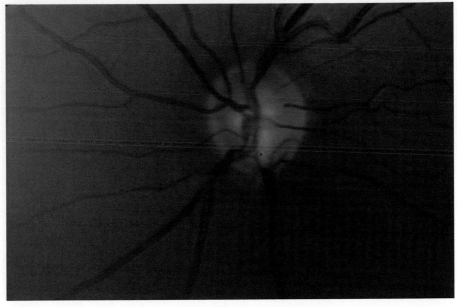

C

Figure 12-13A–C Steroid-responsive glaucoma *(continued)*

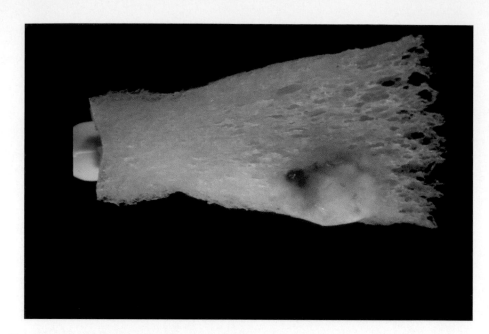

Figure 12-14 Steroid-responsive glaucoma *Excised steroid depot 5 months following vitrectomy for Eales disease on a Weck-cell sponge.*

Postop Day	IOP (mm Hg)	Course and Medications
Surgery #1: Vitrectomy/Membranectomy with Subconjunctival Depot Steroid		
1	25	Prednisolone, hyoscine, erythromycin
6	45	Add timolol, iopidine, acetazolamide
16	20	Stop acetazolamide
30	29	Add dorzolamide, taper prednisolone
48	19	Take off prednisolone
72	27	Continue timolol, apraclonidine, dorzolamide
118	44	Add latanoprost; consult glaucoma
154	31	Arrange steroid depot excision
Surgery #2 Excise Depot Steroid		
1	32	Add timolol, dorzolamide
4	28	Continue same
23	24	Continue same
38	14	Stop dorzolamide

Note: Patient later discontinued timolol; IOP has been 10–14 mm Hg since discontinuation of drug.

IOP = intraocular pressure.

Clinical Examination

Slit Lamp Usually unremarkable. Even in cases with extreme elevations of intraocular pressure, the chronicity usually prevents corneal edema.

Gonioscopy Usually unremarkable.

Posterior Pole Typical glaucomatous optic nerve changes are noted if elevation of intraocular pressure is sufficiently high and prolonged.

Special Tests Discontinuation of the steroids, if possible, may lead to a steady reduction of intraocular pressure. The time course is variable and may be prolonged in cases of prolonged steroid use. In cases in which there is concern regarding halting an ocular steroid (e.g., a corneal graft at high risk of rejection), contralateral steroid challenge may demonstrate intraocular pressure elevation and confirm the diagnosis.

Management

Discontinuation of the steroids, if possible, may yield complete resolution. If ocular steroids are used, weaker or less-pressure–inducing steroids may help (e.g., loteprednol, rimexolone, fluorometholone). Patients with significant uveitis present a special challenge because they may require steroids to control the uveitis. Additionally, the uveitis may itself lead to various forms of glaucoma, or may mask glaucoma with aqueous hyposecretion. Topical antiglaucoma medications of all types are often helpful for steroid-induced elevations of intraocular pressure. In general, laser trabeculoplasty is less effective for these patients than for those with other types of glaucomas. Filtering surgery has similar results to those in primary open-angle glaucoma.

BIBLIOGRAPHY

Campbell DG. Pigmentary dispersion and glaucoma: A new theory. *Arch Ophthalmol* 97:1667, 1997.

Gandolfi SA, Vecchi M. Effect of a YAG laser iridotomy on intraocular pressure in pigment dispersion syndrome. *Ophthalmology* 103:1693–1695, 1996.

Johnson DH, Bradley JM, Acott TS. The effect of dexamethasone on glycosaminoglycans of human trabecular meshwork in perfusion organ culture. *Invest Ophthalmol Vis Sci* 31:2568–2571, 1990.

Johnson D, Gottanka J, Flugel C, Hoffmann F, Futa R, Lutjen-Drecoll E. Ultrastructural changes in the trabecular meshwork of human eyes treated with corticosteroids. *Arch Ophthalmol* 115:375–383, 1997.

Mitchell P, Cumming RG, Mackey DA. Inhaled corticosteroids, family history, and risk of glaucoma. *Ophthalmology* 106:2301–2306, 1999.

Mitchell P, Wang JJ, Hourihan F. The relationship between glaucoma and pseudoexfoliation: The Blue Mountains Eye Study. *Arch Ophthalmol* 117:1319–1324, 1999.

Ritch R, Schlotzer-Schrehardt U. Exfoliation syndrome. *Surv Ophthalmol* 45:265–315, 2001.

Chapter 13

UVEITIC GLAUCOMAS

Ronald Buggage, MD

The development of increased intraocular pressure and glaucoma in patients with uveitis is a multifactorial process that can be viewed as a complication of the intraocular inflammation. Both directly and by the induction of structural changes, inflammation in the eye can alter the aqueous humor dynamics resulting in high, normal, or low intraocular pressures. The glaucomatous optic nerve damage and visual field defects that occur in patients with uveitis are primarily an effect of the uncontrolled intraocular pressure. The primary treatment objective for patients with uveitis-induced ocular hypertension and glaucoma is the control of the inflammatory disease and the prevention of permanent structural alterations to aqueous outflow by the use of appropriate antiinflammatory therapy. Management of the intraocular pressure, either medically or surgically, is a secondary objective.

This chapter defines and discusses the pathophysiologic mechanisms, diagnosis, and treatment strategies for patients with uveitis and elevated intraocular pressure or secondary glaucoma. The chapter concludes with a description of specific uveitic entities in which increased intraocular pressure and glaucoma most commonly occur.

In common usage the term *uveitis* is used to encompass all causes of intraocular inflammation. Uveitis can cause acute, transient, or chronic elevations in the intraocular pressure. The terms *inflammatory glaucoma* and *uveitic glaucoma* are commonly used to refer to any patient with uveitis and increased intraocular pressure. In patients with uveitis and no demonstrable

"glaucomatous" optic nerve damage or "glaucomatous" visual field defects, it is more correct, however, to use terms such as *uveitis-induced ocular hypertension, ocular hypertension secondary to uveitis,* or *secondary ocular hypertension* to refer to those with uveitis and only elevated intraocular pressure. With resolution or appropriate management of the intraocular inflammation, the increased intraocular pressure need not progress to secondary glaucoma.

The terms *inflammatory glaucoma, uveitic glaucoma* or *glaucoma secondary to uveitis* should be reserved for those patients with uveitis, increased intraocular pressure, and "glaucomatous" optic nerve or "glaucomatous" visual field defects. In most cases of uveitic glaucoma, the glaucomatous optic nerve injury is primarily a sequela of the elevated intraocular pressure; therefore, the diagnosis of uveitic glaucoma should be questioned in a patient with no known history of increased intraocular pressure. Additionally, the diagnosis of glaucoma secondary to uveitis should be questioned in any patient with visual field defects atypical for glaucoma and a normal-appearing optic nerve head. This is because many types of uveitis, particularly those affecting the posterior segment, are characterized by chorioretinal and optic nerve lesions that can produce visual field defects that do not represent glaucoma. This distinction is important, because the visual field defects in patients with active inflammatory disease may resolve or improve with appropriate therapy, whereas true glaucomatous visual field defects in patients with uveitis are irreversible.

Epidemiology

Uveitis ranks as the fourth most common cause of blindness in developing countries, behind macular degeneration, diabetic retinopathy, and glaucoma. The prevalence of uveitis from all causes is estimated at 40 cases per 100,000 persons, with an annual incidence of about 15 cases per 100,000.[1] Found in patients of all ages, uveitis is most frequently diagnosed in patients 20 to 40 years of age. Children constitute 5% to 10% of patients with uveitis.[2] Common causes of visual loss in patients with uveitis include secondary glaucoma, cystoid macular edema, cataract, hypotony, retinal detachment, subretinal neovascularization or fibrosis, and optic nerve atrophy.

About 25% of all patients with uveitis will develop increased intraocular pressure at some time during the course of their inflammatory disease.[3] In general, uveitis-induced ocular hypertension and uveitic glaucoma are more commonly complications of anterior uveitis and panuveitis because the inflammation in the anterior segment can interfere directly with the aqueous outflow route (Table 13-1). Uveitic glaucoma is also more common in cases of granulomatous than nongranulomatous uveitis. When all causes of uveitis are considered, the prevalence of glaucoma secondary to uveitis in adults varies from 5.2% to 19%.[4] The overall prevalence of glaucoma in children with uveitis is similar to adults, ranging from 5% to 13.5%; however, the reported visual prognosis for children with uveitic glaucoma is worse.[4,5]

TABLE 13-1   **UVEITIC CONDITIONS COMMONLY ASSOCIATED WITH SECONDARY GLAUCOMA**

Anterior Uveitis
   Juvenile rheumatoid arthritis
   Fuchs's heterochromic uveitis
   Glaucomatocyclitic crisis (Posner-Schlossman syndrome)
   HLA-B27–associated uveitidies (ankylosing spondylitis, Reiter's syndrome, psoriatic arthritis)
   Herpetic uveitis
   Lens-induced uveitis (phacoantigenic uveitis, phacolytic glaucoma, lens particle, phacomorphic glaucoma)

Panuveitis
   Sarcoidosis
   Vogt-Koyanagi-Harada syndrome
   Behçet's syndrome
   Sympathetic ophthalmia
   Syphilitic uveitis

Intermediate Uveitis
   Intermediate uveitis of the pars planitis subtype

Posterior Uveitis
   Acute retinal necrosis
   Toxoplasmosis

Etiology

The intraocular pressure depends on the balance of aqueous secretion and aqueous outflow. In most cases of uveitis, no single mechanism can account for the development of elevated intraocular pressure; rather, it is the result of a combination of several pathologic factors. The final common pathway of all mechanisms contributing to increased intraocular pressure in uveitis, however, is the impairment of aqueous outflow through the trabecular meshwork. Intraocular inflammation can impair aqueous outflow by causing derangements in aqueous secretion, producing changes in aqueous content, infiltrating ocular tissues, and inducing irreversible alterations in the anterior segment anatomy such as peripheral anterior synechiae and posterior synechiae that can lead to angle closure. These changes can produce a glaucoma that is not only severe but also resistant to all medical therapy. Paradoxically, the treatment of the uveitis with corticosteroids can also contribute to the development of elevated intraocular pressure.

The pathophysiologic mechanisms resulting in the development of elevated intraocular pressure in patients with uveitis can be simply classified as either open angle or closed angle. This classification is clinically useful because the initial treatment approach differs between these two groups.

Open-Angle Mechanisms

Abnormal Aqueous Secretion Inflammation of the ciliary body usually results in decreased aqueous production. Decreased aqueous secretion in eyes with normal outflow facility results in the decreased intraocular pressure or hypotony that is frequently encountered in eyes with acute uveitis. If, however, there is concomitant or greater impairment of the aqueous outflow in eyes with decreased aqueous production, the intraocular pressure may be normal or possibly increased. There is disagreement as to whether or not aqueous hypersecretion can result from the breakdown of the blood-aqueous barrier in uveitic eyes. If this were possible, increased aqueous production could contribute to the development of high intraocular pressure in uveitic eyes. Relative to ciliary body function, the most likely explanation for the elevated intraocular pressure in eye with intraocular inflammation, however, is that the aqueous production remains normal while the aqueous outflow is reduced.

Aqueous Humor Proteins Alteration in the aqueous humor content was one of the first hypotheses offered to explain the onset of elevated intraocular pressure associated with uveitis. The influx of proteins into the eye resulting from the breakdown of the blood-aqueous barrier is the earliest change in uveitic eyes that can affect the balance of aqueous flow and increase the intraocular pressure. In normal eyes, the protein content of the aqueous humor is approximately 100 times less than that in normal serum.[6] However, when the blood-aqueous barrier is disrupted, the aqueous protein concentration can resemble that of undiluted serum. An increased aqueous protein concentration can impair aqueous outflow by decreasing the flow rate of aqueous into the anterior chamber angle, mechanically obstructing the trabecular meshwork, and causing dysfunction of the endothelial cells lining the trabecular meshwork beams. Additionally, the proteins promote the development of posterior or peripheral anterior synechiae. If the integrity of the blood-aqueous barrier is restored, the effect of the aqueous protein concentration on the aqueous outflow and intraocular ocular pressure can be reversed. However, if the permeability of the blood-aqueous barrier is permanently damaged, leakage of serum proteins into the anterior chamber may persist even after the intraocular inflammation has resolved.

Inflammatory Cells An influx of inflammatory cells that secrete inflammatory mediators such as prostaglandins and cytokines occurs shortly after the protein influx in eyes with uveitis. Inflammatory cells in the anterior segment are believed to have a more direct effect on the intraocular pressure than aqueous proteins. Inflammatory cells can increase the intraocular pressure by infiltrating the trabecular meshwork and Schlemm's canal, creating a mechanical obstruction to aqueous outflow. The risk for increased intraocular pressure is higher in granulomatous uveitis because of the greater infiltration of macrophages and lymphocytes compared with nongranulomatous uveitis entities in which the cellular infiltrate may contain higher proportions of polymorphonuclear cells. Chronic, severe, or recurrent episodes of uveitis can cause permanent damage to the trabecular meshwork from injury to the trabecular endothelial cells, scarring in the trabecular meshwork and Schlemm's canal, or from the formation of a hyaline membrane overlying the trabeculum. Inflammatory cells and cellular debris in the anterior chamber angle can also contribute to the formation of peripheral anterior and posterior synechiae.

Prostaglandins   Prostaglandins are known to produce many of the signs of ocular inflammation, including vasodilatation, miosis, and increased vascular permeability, and have complex interactions on the intraocular pressure.[7,8] Whether or not prostaglandins are directly responsible for increased intraocular pressure in uveitic eyes is unclear. Through their action on the blood-aqueous barrier, they may indirectly contribute to increased intraocular pressure by enhancing the influx of aqueous protein, cytokines, and inflammatory cells. Alternatively, they can also decrease the intraocular pressure by the enhancement of uveoscleral outflow.

Trabeculitis   Trabeculitis is diagnosed when the intraocular inflammatory response is localized to the trabecular meshwork. Clinically, trabeculitis is characterized by the presence of inflammatory precipitates on the trabecular meshwork in the absence of other signs of active intraocular inflammation such as keratic precipitates, aqueous cells, or flare. The aqueous outflow in trabeculitis is decreased by mechanical obstruction of the trabecular meshwork resulting from the accumulation of inflammatory cells, swelling of the trabecular beams, and decreased phagocytosis of the trabecular endothelial cells. Because aqueous production in the ciliary body function is usually unaffected, the intraocular pressure in eyes with trabeculitis can be significantly elevated from the reduced aqueous outflow.

Steroid-Induced Ocular Hypertension   Corticosteroids are considered first-line drug therapy for patients with uveitis. Whether given topically, systemically, or by periocular or sub-Tenon's injection, corticosteroids are known to accelerate the formation of cataracts and cause increased intraocular pressure. By inhibiting the catalytic enzymes and the phagocytic activity of the trabecular endothelial cells, corticosteroids cause the accumulation of glycosaminoglycans and inflammatory material in the trabecular meshwork, resulting in decreased aqueous outflow through the trabecular meshwork.[4] Inhibition of prostaglandin synthesis is another mechanism by which corticosteroids may impair outflow facility.

The terms *steroid-induced ocular hypertension* and *steroid responder* are used to refer to patients who develop elevated intraocular pressures related to corticosteroid therapy. About 5% of the population is estimated to be steroid responders, and a steroid response can be anticipated in approximately 20% to 30% of patients after prolonged corticosteroid use.[9] The risk of a steroid response is related to the duration and the dose of corticosteroid therapy. Patients with glaucoma, diabetes, high myopia, and children younger than 10 years of age are at greatest risk for a steroid response.[4] Although steroid-induced ocular hypertension may occur at any time after the induction of corticosteroid therapy, it is most frequently detected within 2 to 8 weeks after the treatment is started. Compared with the other routes of administration, topical steroids are most frequently associated with a steroid response. Periocular steroid injections can cause an acute pressure rise in susceptible patients and, therefore, should be avoided in patients with known ocular hypertension. In most cases, the intraocular pressure returns to normal after discontinuation of the corticosteroid; however, in some cases, particularly following a steroid depot injection, the intraocular pressure can remain elevated for 18 months or longer. In these cases, surgical removal of the depot steroid or filtration surgery may be required if the intraocular pressure cannot be controlled medically (Figure 13-1).

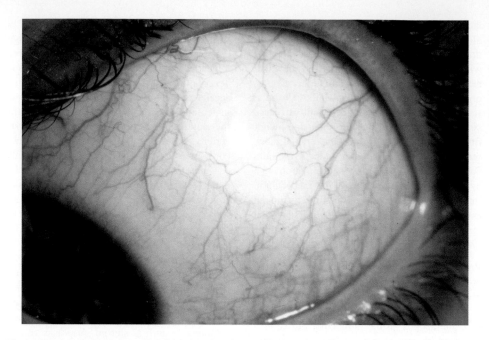

Figure 13-1 Periocular steroid injection in a steroid responder *Periocular steroid injections, useful in treating both anterior and posterior uveitis, can sometimes induce a severe elevation in the intraocular pressure in patients with ocular hypertension and known steroid responders. The anteriorly placed steroid depot in this 16-year-old patient with presumed sarcoidosis was removed when medical therapy failed to control his elevated intraocular pressure. Subsequently, his pressures normalized.*

When a patient with uveitis who is being treated with corticosteroids develops an increased intraocular pressure, it is often difficult to know if the pressure rise is a result of the restored aqueous secretion, of impaired aqueous outflow caused by the intraocular inflammation, a steroid response, or a combination of all three. Although a fall in the intraocular pressure as the steroid is tapered may be evidence of steroid-induced ocular hypertension, the decline in pressure could also be secondary to improved outflow through the trabecular meshwork or a recurrence of inflammation with aqueous hyposecretion. If a steroid response is suspected in a patient who maintains active intraocular inflammation requiring systemic corticosteroids, this may be an indication for the initiation of a steroid-sparing agent. If steroid-induced ocular hypertension is suspected in a patient with controlled or quiescent uveitis, a reduction in the concentration, dose, or frequency of the corticosteroid used should be attempted.

Closed-Angle Mechanisms

Morphologic changes in the anterior chamber structures as a result of uveitis are often irreversible and lead to significant elevations in the intraocular pressure by altering or preventing the flow of aqueous from the posterior chamber to the trabecular meshwork. The structural changes that typically lead to secondary angle closure include peripheral anterior synechiae, posterior synechiae, and pupillary membranes that can cause pupillary block and, less commonly, forward rotation of the ciliary body.

Peripheral Anterior Synechiae Peripheral anterior synechiae are adhesions between the iris and the trabecular meshwork or cornea that can completely block or impair access of the aqueous to the trabecular meshwork. Best detected by gonioscopy, peripheral anterior synechiae are a common complication of anterior uveitis and occur more commonly in granulomatous than nongranulomatous causes of uveitis. Peripheral anterior synechiae result from the organization of inflammatory material that pulls the iris surface into the angle. They develop more frequently in eyes with preexisting narrow angles or those narrowed by iris bombé. The iris attachments are usually broad, covering large segments of the angle, but can also be patchy or peaked, affecting only small portions of the trabecular meshwork or cornea (Figure 13-2). In cases of peripheral anterior synechiae related to uveitis, even though large portions of the angle may remain open the patient may still have increased intraocular pressure because the remaining angle

is functionally compromised because of prior inflammatory damage that may not be detectable by gonioscopy.

In cases of recurrent or chronic uveitis, continued peripheral anterior synechiae formation can result in complete angle closure. Neovascularization of the iris and the angle should be sought in all cases of uveitis presenting with angle closure or extensive peripheral anterior synechiae. Contraction of the fibrovascular tissue in the angle or anterior iris surface may rapidly induce a complete and severe angle closure. Neovascular glaucoma secondary to uveitis is typically resistant to medical and surgical therapy and has a poor prognosis (Figure 13-3A,B).

Posterior Synechiae Inflammatory cells, protein, and fibrin in the aqueous humor can stimulate posterior synechiae formation. Posterior synechiae are adhesions between the posterior iris surface and the anterior lens capsule, the

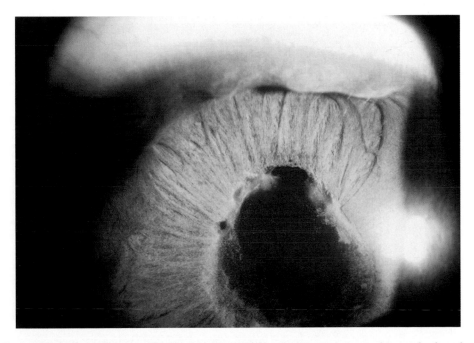

Figure 13-2   HLA-B27–associated anterior uveitis *Both posterior synechiae and a broad area of peripheral anterior synechiae obliterating the anterior chamber angle and extending onto the cornea (superior) are seen in this patient with HLA-B27–associated anterior uveitis following a severe exacerbation of intraocular inflammation.*

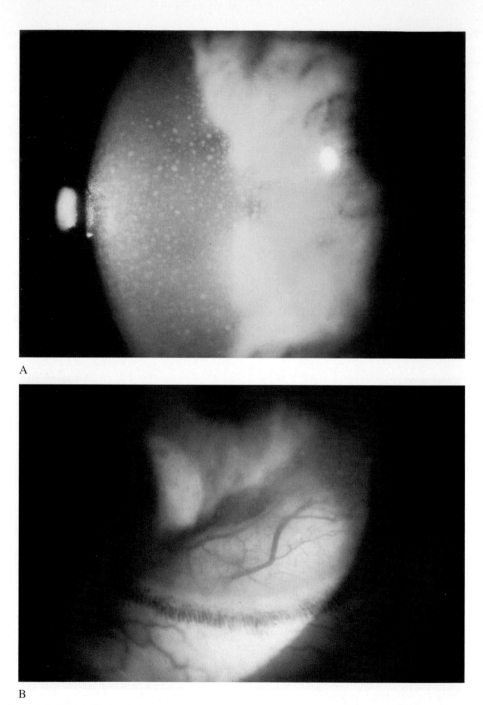

Figure 13-3A,B Neovascular glaucoma *This patient with granulomatous panuveitis developed intractable neovascular glaucoma, one of the most severe complications of uveitis. Note the diffuse, mutton fat keratic precipitates and iris bombé (**A**) and the neovascularization in the broad peripheral anterior synechiae (**B**).*

DISEASE SYNDROMES

vitreous face in aphakic patients, or the intraocular lens in pseudophakic individuals. The likelihood of developing posterior synechiae is related to the type, duration, and severity of the uveitis. Posterior synechiae are more common in granulomatous than nongranulomatous uveitis. The greater the extent of the posterior synechiae, the less the pupil is able to dilate and the greater the risk for further synechiae formation in subsequent uveitic recurrences.

The term *pupillary block* is used to denote impaired aqueous flow between the posterior and anterior chamber through the pupillary aperture as a result of posterior synechiae. Seclusio pupillae, posterior synechiae that extend for 360 degrees around the pupil and pupillary membranes, can cause complete pupillary block. In this condition, there is no flow of aqueous from the posterior to the anterior chamber. The buildup of aqueous in the posterior chamber may produce a severe elevation of the intraocular pressure that causes forward bowing of the iris into the anterior chamber, or iris bombé (Figure 13-4). Iris bombé in an eye with ongoing inflammation may result in the rapid development of angle closure caused by the formation of peripheral anterior synechiae, even in an eye that may have previously had an open angle. In some cases of uveitis with pupillary block, if the iridolenticular adhesions are sufficiently broad only the peripheral iris may bulge forward and the iris bombé may be difficult to diagnose without the use of gonioscopy.

Forward Rotation of the Ciliary Body Acute intraocular inflammation can cause ciliary body swelling and supraciliary or suprachoroidal effusions that may result in the forward rotation of the ciliary body, causing angle closure not associated with pupillary block. Elevated intraocular pressure due to this type of angle closure occurs most often in patients with iridocyclitis, annular choroidal detachments, and posterior scleritis, and can be seen in the acute stage of Vogt-Koyanagi-Harada syndrome.

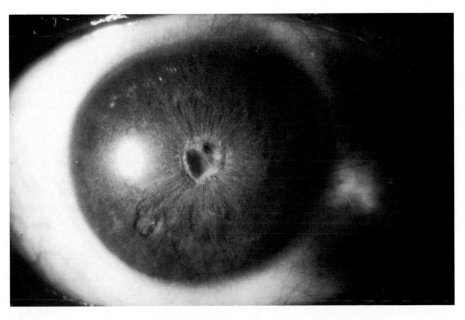

Figure 13-4   Posterior synechiae causing pupillary block and iris bombé *This patient with Vogt-Koyanagi-Harada syndrome presented with anterior segment inflammation and increased intraocular pressure as a result of posterior synechiae causing pupillary block with iris bombé. The uveitis was managed with topical and systemic corticosteroids, and the elevated intraocular pressure normalized following a laser iridotomy.*

Diagnosis

The accurate diagnosis and management of glaucoma in patients with uveitis relies on a thorough ophthalmic examination and the appropriate use of ancillary tests. Slit-lamp examination is required to establish the classification of the uveitis, the degree of inflammatory activity, and the type of inflammatory reaction. Uveitis can be classified anatomically as anterior, intermediate, posterior, or panuveitis according to the primary site of the inflammation in the eye.

The likelihood of uveitic glaucoma is greater in cases of anterior uveitis and panuveitis in which the structures involved in the aqueous outflow are more likely to be damaged by intraocular inflammation. The severity of the intraocular inflammation can be determined by assessing the aqueous cells and flare in the anterior chamber and the vitreous cells and haze. Additionally, the structural changes in the ocular architecture induced by the inflammatory disease, such as peripheral anterior and posterior synechiae, should be noted.

The inflammatory response in eyes with uveitis can be either granulomatous or nongranulomatous. Signs of granulomatous uveitis in the anterior segment include mutton fat keratic precipitates and iris nodules (Figures 13-3A,B and 13-5A,B). Granulomatous uveitis is associated with a higher incidence of uveitic glaucoma than nongranulomatous uveitis.

Gonioscopy is the most critical part of ophthalmic examination in patients with uveitis and increased intraocular pressure and should be performed using a lens that indents the central cornea and pushes the aqueous into the angle. Gonioscopic examination reveals the presence of inflammatory material, peripheral anterior synechiae, and neovascularization in the angle, allowing differentiation between open-angle and closed-angle glaucoma.

On fundus examination, particular attention should be directed to the optic nerves, which should be assessed for excavation, hemorrhage, edema, or hyperemia. The retinal nerve fiber layer should also be evaluated. The diagnosis of uveitic glaucoma should not be made without documented glaucomatous disk damage and or visual field loss. Although retinal or chorioretinal lesions in the posterior pole do not contribute to the development of uveitic glaucoma, the presence and location of such lesions that may manifest as a visual field defect and result in an incorrect diagnosis of uveitic glaucoma should be noted (Figure 13-6A,B).

Applanation tonometry is required during every clinical assessment, and reliable personnel should routinely perform visual field testing. Other ancillary tests that may be useful for the diagnosis and follow-up of patients with uveitis and increased intraocular pressure include laser flare photometry and ocular ultrasonography. Laser flare photometry is able to detect slight changes in the aqueous humor flare or protein content that cannot be assessed by the slit-lamp examination. The changes detected by the photometer have been shown to be useful in determining the activity of the uveitis.[3] B-scan ultrasonography and ultrasound biomicroscopy are useful in the assessment of uveitic glaucoma by demonstrating the morphology of the ciliary body and iridocorneal angle, which is helpful in determining the cause of both elevated and abnormally low intraocular pressures in patients with uveitis.

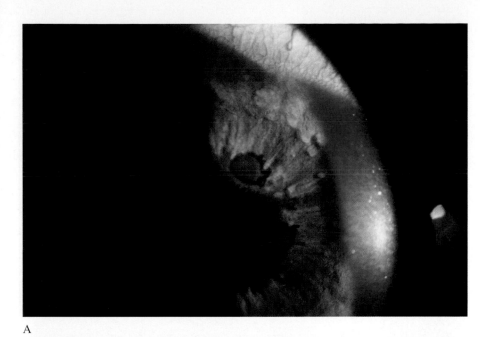

A

B

Figure 13-5A,B   Sarcoidosis and active granulomatous panuveitis   *This patient with sarcoidosis presented with an active granulomatous panuveitis, including Busacca nodules (seen here in the iris stroma) and secondary glaucoma resulting from posterior synechiae with pupillary block (**A**). Despite management with topical and systemic corticosteroids and topical antiglaucoma medications, his intraocular pressures were uncontrolled. Examination of the optic nerve head and visual field testing were consistent with glaucoma. Two months following tube shunt placement for uveitic glaucoma, the intraocular pressures were controlled and the iris nodules were resolved (**B**).*

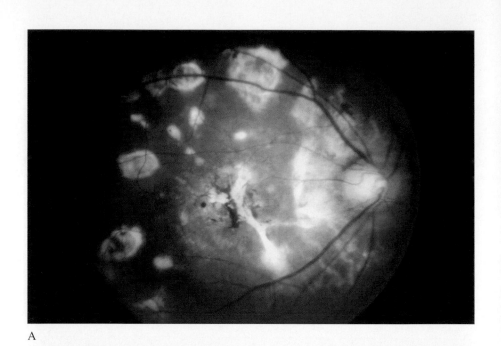

A

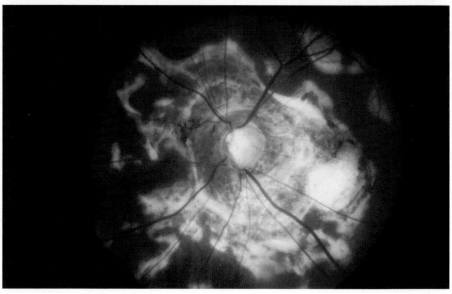

B

Figure 13-6A,B   Multifocal choroiditis   *This patient with multifocal choroiditis demonstrates the need for careful examination of the optic nerve for evidence of glaucoma in patients with uveitis. Because of the extensive posterior pole lesions, visual field testing did not reliably demonstrate the development of glaucoma in the left eye, evidenced by the progressive cupping off the optic disc. **A.** Right eye. **B.** Left eye.*

Management

The first goal in the treatment of patients with uveitis-induced ocular hypertension or uveitic glaucoma is the control of the intraocular inflammation and prevention of permanent structural changes in the eyes. In some patients, resolution of the intraocular inflammation with appropriate therapy alone may normalize the intraocular pressure. Additionally, irreversible consequences of uveitis such as peripheral ante rior and posterior synechiae can be prevented with early antiinflammatory therapy combined with mydriatics and cycloplegics.

The first-line treatment in most cases of uveitis requires the use of corticosteroids topically, locally via periocular or sub-Tenon's injection, or systemically. Topical corticosteroids are useful for anterior segment inflammation but alone are inadequate therapy for a phakic patient with active posterior segment inflammation. The frequency of administration of the topical corticosteroids depends on the severity of the inflammation in the anterior segment. Prednisolone acetate (pred-forte) is superior to other topical corticosteroid formulations for the control of anterior segment inflammation. Likewise, it is also the topical steroid formulation that is most likely to cause steroid-induced intraocular hypertension and posterior subcapsular cataracts. Less-potent topical steroid formulations such as rimexolone, fluorometholone, medrysone, and loteprednol etabonate (Lotemax) are less likely to cause a steroid response but are also less effective in controlling the intraocular inflammation. In our experience, topical nonsteroidal antiinflammatory agents play no significant role in the treatment of uveitis or its complications.

Periocular steroid injections of triamcinolone (Kenalog, 40 mg/mL) into sub-Tenon's space or transseptally through the lower lid can be effective for the control of both anterior and posterior segment intraocular inflammation. The main drawback of periocular steroids is their greater potential to cause elevated intraocular pressure and cataract in susceptible patients. Consequently, it is not advisable to administer periocular injections of depot steroid in patients with uveitis and intraocular hypertension because of their long-lasting effect, which cannot be readily discontinued.

Oral corticosteroids are the mainstay of uveitis therapy, with starting doses as high as 1 mg/kg per day, depending on the severity of the disease. Systemic steroids should be tapered once the intraocular inflammation is controlled. If sustained control of the intraocular inflammation using corticosteroids alone is not possible because of their side effects or because of persistent disease activity, a second-line immunosuppressant or a steroid-sparing medication may be needed. Steroid-sparing agents commonly used for the treatment of uveitis include cyclosporine, methotrexate, azathioprine, and, most recently, mycophenolate mofetil.[10,11] Of these, cyclosporine is considered the most effective for most causes of uveitis and should be instituted first if not contraindicated. The remaining agents are to be considered if the patient is intolerant or poorly controlled with steroids or cyclosporine used alone or in combination. Alkylating agents, cyclophosphamide, and chlorambucil are generally reserved for severe cases of uveitis.[10]

Mydriatic and cycloplegic agents are used in the treatment of patients with anterior segment intraocular inflammation to relieve the pain and discomfort associated with ciliary muscle and iris sphincter spasm. Because these agents also dilate the pupil, they are also useful in preventing and breaking synechiae, which can alter aqueous flow and contribute to elevated intraocular pressure. Commonly prescribed agents for this purpose are atropine, 1%; scopolamine, 0.25%; homatropine, 2% or 5%; phenylephrine, 2.5% or 10%; and tropicamide, 0.5% or 1%.

Medical Therapy

Once the intraocular inflammation has been adequately addressed, specific therapy should also be administered to control the intraocular pressure. In general, the medical therapy for uveitis-induced ocular hypertension and uveitic glaucoma relies primarily on aqueous suppressants for pressure control. Antiglaucoma medications used in the treatment of uveitic glaucoma include beta-blockers, carbonic anhydrase inhibitors, adrenergic agents, and hyperosmotic agents for emergent control of acute pressure elevations. As a group, miotic agents and prostaglandin-like agents are generally avoided in patients with uveitis because they can exacerbate the intraocular inflammation. Topical adrenergic antagonists are the drugs of choice for the treatment of increased intraocular pressure in patients with uveitic glaucoma because they decrease aqueous humor production without affecting the pupil size. Beta-blockers commonly used in patients with uveitis include timolol, 0.25% to 0.5%; betaxolol, 0.25% to 0.5%; carteolol, 1% to 2%; and levobunolol. Betaxolol, which has fewer pulmonary side effects, may be safer to use in patients with sarcoid uveitis and known pulmonary disease. Metipranolol has been reported to cause a granulomatous iridocyclitis in some patients and should probably be avoided in patients with uveitis.[12]

Carbonic anhydrase inhibitors that reduce intraocular pressure by inhibiting aqueous humor production can be given topically, orally, or intravenously. The oral carbonic anhydrase inhibitor acetazolamide (Diamox) has been reported to reduce cystoid macular edema, which is a common cause of visual loss in patients with uveitis.[13] It is likely that a topical carbonic anhydrase would not have a similar effect on macular edema because sufficient concentrations probably do not reach the retina.

Adrenergic agents that are used in the treatment of uveitic glaucoma include apraclonidine, particularly to control acute intraocular pressure elevations that can occur after a neodymium (Nd):YAG capsulotomy, and brimonidine, 0.2% (Alphagan), which is an alpha-2 agonist that lowers intraocular pressure by decreasing aqueous humor production and increasing uveoscleral outflow. Although they are now used infrequently, epinephrine, 1%, and dipivefrin, 0.1%, which both lower intraocular pressure primarily by increasing aqueous outflow, also cause mydriasis, which could be helpful in the prevention of synechiae in uveitic eyes.

Prostaglandin analogues are thought to reduce intraocular pressure by increasing uveoscleral outflow.[3] Although effective at lowering intraocular pressure, the benefit of this class of agents in the treatment of uveitis is questioned because latanoprost (Xalatan) has been reported to induce intraocular inflammation and cytoid macular edema.[14]

Hyperosmotic agents rapidly lower intraocular pressure, primarily by a reduction in the vitreous volume, and are helpful in the management of uveitic patients with acute angle closure. Glycerin and isosorbide can be administered orally, whereas mannitol is given intravenously.

Cholinergic agents such as pilocarpine, echothiophate iodide, eserine, and carbachol are generally avoided in patients with uveitis. This is because the induced miosis caused by these agents may potentiate formation of posterior synechiae, aggravate ciliary body muscle spasm, and contribute to a prolongation of the ocular inflammatory response by enhancing the breakdown of the blood-aqueous barrier.

Management of Angle-Closure Glaucoma

Iris bombé and angle closure caused by pupillary block are frequently the cause of severe intraocular pressure elevations and secondary glaucoma in patients with uveitis. When pupillary block is responsible for the obstruction of aqueous outflow, a communication between the posterior and anterior chambers can be reestablished using an argon or Nd:YAG laser iridotomy or a surgical iridectomy. Laser iridotomy may worsen or reactivate anterior chamber inflammation. To lessen the likelihood of this complication prior to and after the procedure, the patient should be treated aggressively with topical corticosteroids. Compared with the argon laser, the Nd:YAG laser requires the delivery of less energy and induces less postoperative inflammation. Because laser iridotomies are prone to closure, particularly in eyes with active inflammation, several iridotomies should be performed to ensure adequate aqueous flow (Figure 13-7). Repeat procedures are needed in approximately 40% of uveitic eyes.[4] Laser iridectomy should not be performed in eyes with severe active uveitis or corneal edema, or in the areas of peripheral anterior synechiae to reduce the risk of endothelial damage.

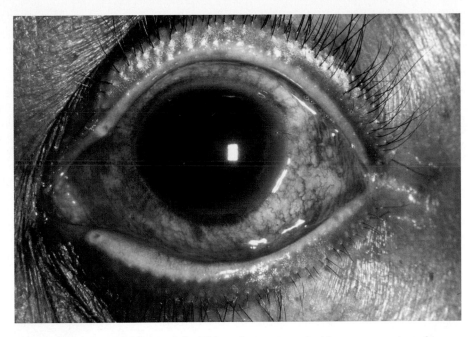

Figure 13-7   Recurrent iris bombé   *This patient presented with acute eye pain and increased intraocular pressure from recurrent iris bombé when the previous laser iridotomy site closed during a uveitic flare associated with the tapering of her systemic immunosuppression.*

Surgical iridectomy is indicated when laser iridotomies are unsuccessful or the use of laser is contraindicated. Surgical iridectomy is reported to be successful in uveitic eyes with peripheral anterior synechiae that involves less than 75% of the angle.[4] Although generally more effective than laser iridotomy, the procedure can lead to severe surgically induced postoperative inflammation that may be blunted by the use of aggressive preoperative and postoperative antiinflammatory therapy. Compared with a laser iridotomy, a large-sector surgical iridectomy may delay cataract progression.

In uveitic eyes in which the angle closure is caused by forward rotation of the ciliary body without evidence of pupillary block, laser iridotomy and surgical iridectomy are of no use. The angle closure and elevated intraocular pressure in this rare group of patients are best treated with immunosuppressive therapy and aqueous suppressants. A surgical filtration procedure may be required in these cases if the intraocular pressure cannot be controlled medically and the angle closure cannot be reversed because of the formation of peripheral anterior synechiae.

Goniosynechiolysis has been reported to be successful in lowering the intraocular pressure and establishing a normal anterior chamber angle in cases of acute angle closure resulting from extensive and recent formation of peripheral anterior synechiae. Trabeculodialysis, the disinsertion of the trabeculum from the scleral spur using a goniotomy knife, allows the aqueous direct access into Schlemm's canal and has been used in children and young adults with uncontrolled uveitic glaucoma.[4]

Argon laser trabeculoplasty is not recommended for the treatment of uveitis-induced ocular hypertension or the treatment of uveitic glaucoma because the thermal energy and additional laser-induced inflammation may further damage the previously injured trabecular meshwork.

In secondary uveitic glaucoma, the damaging mechanism is nearly always intraocular hypertension. Because there is usually no primary disc pathology and because patients with uveitis are relatively young, there is a tendency to tolerate hypertension for longer periods and to tolerate higher levels of intraocular pressure before using surgical intervention. However, when the intraocular pressure remains uncontrolled in patients receiving maximal medical therapy or there is evidence of optic nerve injury or visual field defects, surgical intervention to control the intraocular pressure is required.

Surgical procedures performed in patients with uveitic glaucoma include trabeculectomy with and without the use of antimetabolites and tube shunt procedures such as the Ahmed, Baerveldt, and Molteno implants[3,4,15] (Figure 13-8A,B). The best surgical procedure for patients with uveitic glaucoma has not been established.

All surgical procedures performed on patients with uveitis carry the risk of a postoperative flare, which typically occurs in the first postoperative week. Postoperative inflammation or reactivation of uveitis has been reported to occur in 5.2% to 31.1% cases of uveitic glaucoma treated surgically.[16] The risk of a postoperative flare is decreased in eyes that are quiescent prior to the surgical procedure. For elective surgeries, we require that the eyes remain quiet for at least 3 months prior to the operative procedure. To help to decrease the risk of a postoperative flare, approximately 1 week prior to the planned

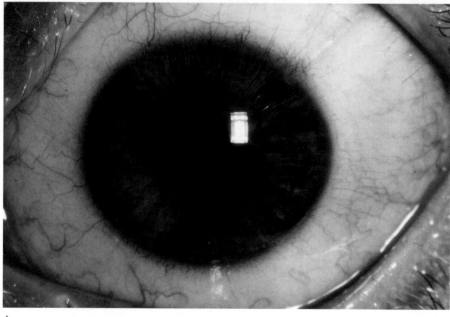

A

Figure 13-8A,B   Bilateral Baerveldt implants in patient with JRA   *This 16-year-old female patient developed bilateral anterior uveitis at the age of 3 years that has been well managed with a combination of topical and systemic antiinflammatory therapy. Because of uncontrolled intraocular pressure, she underwent bilateral Baerveldt implants as a primary glaucoma procedure with excellent results. A. Right eye showing the implant tube in the anterior chamber.*

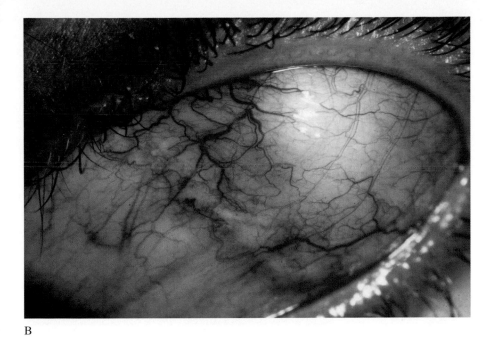

B

Figure 13-8A,B   Bilateral Baerveldt implants in patient with JRA *(continued)* **B.** *Right eye looking down and nasally, revealing the conjunctival bleb over the implant.*

surgery day, the patient's topical or systemic immunosuppressive regimen, or both, is increased and tapered postoperatively according to inflammatory response. Intraoperatively, periocular steroids are routinely given. For emergent glaucoma procedures in patients with active disease, an exacerbation of the existing inflammation should be expected; therefore, aggressive topical therapy and the use of high-dose oral (0.5 to 1.5 mg/kg per day) or even intravenous corticosteroids may be required in the perioperative period.

Reported success rates for trabeculectomy in patients with uveitis glaucoma range from 73% to 81%.[17] However, the true significance of such findings is not entirely clear. In trabeculectomy cases performed in patients with uveitis, the postoperative inflammatory response is believed to accelerate the wound healing process and cause failure of the filtering procedure.[18] The outcome for trabeculectomies in patients with uveitis may be improved by the use of aggressive

perioperative antiinflammatory therapy and antimetabolites such as mitomycin C, which is favored over 5-fluorouracil.[4] The higher success rates of filtering surgery with the use of wound-modulating agents, however, is associated with an elevated risk for hypotony, bleb leaks, and endophthalmitis, which has been reported in up to 9.4% of eyes following trabeculectomy.[19] Cataract progression is also very common after filtration surgery for uveitic glaucoma.

Implant drainage procedures have also been used for the treatment of uveitic glaucoma, most commonly in patients who have failed previous filtering procedures.[4,15] They have been reported to be more successful than a repeat trabeculectomy in patients with uveitis.[17] Postoperative complications such as choroidal effusion, choroidal hemorrhage, and shallow anterior chambers may be greater in eyes with uveitic glaucoma as compared with eyes with primary open-angle glaucoma (Figure 13-9A,B).

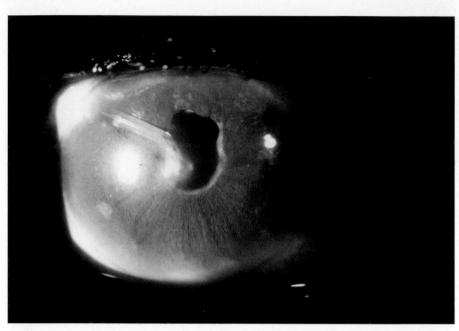

A

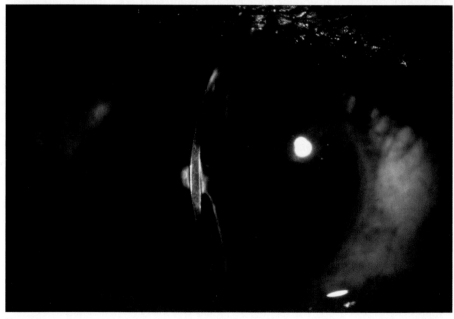

B

Figure 13-9A,B   Complications of glaucoma surgery in uveitis patient   *Hypotony with choroidal effusion and a shallow anterior chamber (**A**, diffuse illumination; **B**, slit beam) is a common complication of implant drainage procedures in patients with uveitis.*

DISEASE SYNDROMES

Ciliary body destructive procedures should be considered as a last resort for the treatment of uveitic glaucoma in which intraocular pressure is not amenable to any other medical or surgical glaucoma treatment. Cyclocryotherapy and contact and noncontact laser cycloablation procedures are generally similar in their ability to successfully lower the intraocular pressures. The primary disadvantage of cycloablative treatments is the induction of a severe intraocular inflammatory response and the development of phthisis bulbi in about 10% of treated eyes.[20]

SPECIFIC ENTITIES

Fuchs's Heterochromic Iridocyclitis

Fuchs's heterochromic iridocyclitis is typically a unilateral, chronic, low-grade, nongranulomatous anterior uveitis that is associated with secondary posterior subcapsular cataract and glaucoma in 13% to 59% of cases.[21] The heterochromia that characterizes the condition is a result of the intraocular inflammation that causes iris atrophy in the affected eye.

Epidemiology Fuchs's heterochromic iridocyclitis is thought to be a relatively uncommon cause of anterior uveitis, accounting for 1.2% to 3.2% of all uveitis cases.[22] The condition is unilateral in 90% of cases and appears to affect men and women equally. The disease is most commonly diagnosed in the third to fourth decades of life. Uveitic glaucoma has been reported in 15% of patients at the time of diagnosis with the onset of glaucoma in another 44% during the course of follow-up.[23] Estimates of the overall incidence range from 13% to 59% and may be higher in patients with bilateral disease and in African-American patients.[4]

Etiology The increased intraocular pressure in Fuchs's heterochromic iridocyclitis is thought to be the result of decreased aqueous outflow caused by inflammatory cells or a hyaline membrane obstructing the trabecular meshwork.

History Patients with this condition are typically asymptomatic, although some patients may have mild ocular discomfort and blurred vision. Patients are not known to have associated systemic disease. They frequently come to medical attention because of decreased vision associated with cataract progression.

Ophthalmic Examination External examination typically reveals a white, quiet eye. The anterior segment generally shows a unilateral, low-grade, nongranulomatous anterior uveitis. The cornea shows stellate keratic precipitates scattered over the entire endothelium, which are an important clue to the diagnosis (Figure 13-10A). In patients with dark irides, the stromal atrophy that results from the intraocular inflammation will cause the iris in the affected eye to appear lighter in color (Figure 13-10B). In patients with light irides, however, the stomal atrophy will cause the affected eye to appear darker in color because of the exposure of the iris pigment epithelium. Another important diagnostic finding in patients with Fuchs's heterochromic iridocyclitis is the identification of iris neovascularization or neovascularization of the angle by gonioscopy. Despite the chronicity of the intraocular inflammation in these patients, peripheral anterior synechiae and posterior synechiae almost never form. However, posterior subcapsular cataract is a common complication. Although the posterior segment examination is usually normal, chorioretinal lesions have been reported in patients with Fuchs's heterochromic iridocyclitis.

Differential Diagnosis The differential diagnosis for Fuchs's heterochromic iridocyclitis includes the Posner-Schlossman syndrome, sarcoidosis, syphilis, herpetic uveitis, and, in those cases with posterior pole lesions, toxoplasmosis.

Laboratory Studies There are no laboratory studies that allow for the diagnosis of Fuchs's heterochromic iridocyclitis. Lymphocytes and plasma cells have been identified in aqueous humor from affected patients. The diagnosis is made clinically based on the distribution of the keratic precipitates, the low-grade anterior uveitis, heterochromia, absence of synechiae, and the lack of ocular symptoms.

Course The anterior uveitis in Fuchs's heterochromic iridocyclitis is insidious and slowly progressive. The neovascularization of the iris and angle may cause mild intraocular hemorrhage with minor trauma but does not cause peripheral anterior synechiae or neovascular glaucoma. Cataract and glaucoma are the most common complications. Cataract formation has been reported in more than 50% of patients with the condition. Cataract extraction, when required, is generally uncomplicated and is less likely to be complicated by the postoperative

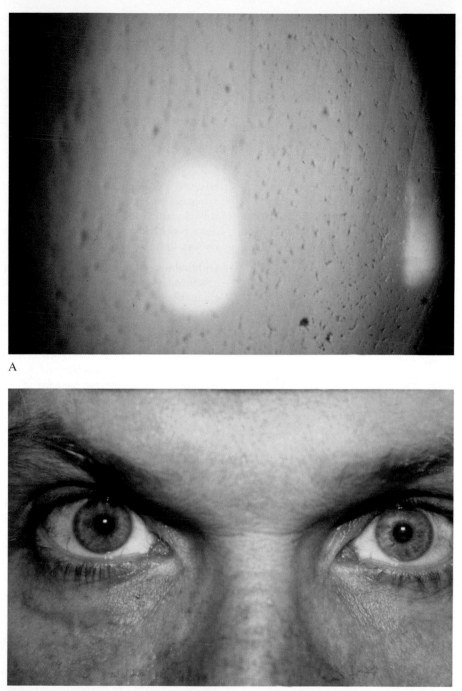

A

B

Figure 13-10A,B   Fuchs's heterochromic iridocyclitis *Fuchs's heterochromic iridocyclitis is a unilateral, nongranulomatous anterior uveitis commonly characterized by the triad of heterochromia, cataract, and glaucoma in the affected eye. Patients with this condition characteristically show stellate keratic precipitates distributed over the entire corneal endothelium (**A**). The iris heterochromia and cataract in the left eye are a result of the chronic unilateral inflammation in the left eye (**B**).*

flare that is characteristic of other types of uveitis. Posterior lens implantation is considered to be safe. The glaucoma associated with Fuchs's heterochromic iridocyclitis closely resembles the course of primary open-angle glaucoma.

Management Despite the presence of a chronic anterior uveitis, aggressive topical therapy with corticosteroids and the use of systemic immunosuppressive therapy are not recommended for the treatment of Fuchs's heterochromic iridocyclitis because of the poor response to treatment. In fact, the use of topical steroids may be contraindicated because they may accelerate the development of cataract and glaucoma. Medical therapy is recommended for the control of the glaucoma; however, as many as 66% of patients may require surgical management.[23] The best surgical procedure for patients with Fuchs's heterochromic iridocyclitis is unknown. Argon laser trabeculoplasty is not effective because of the formation of a hyaline membrane over the trabecular meshwork and should not be used.

Glaucomatocyclitic Crisis (Posner-Schlossman Syndrome)

Glaucomatocyclitic crisis is a syndrome of recurrent episodes of mild, idiopathic, unilateral, nongranulomatous anterior uveitis accompanied by marked elevation in the intraocular pressure. Although this syndrome was probably first described in 1929, it carries the eponym of Posner and Schlossman who reported the syndrome in 1948.[4]

Epidemiology Glaucomatocyclitic crisis typically occurs in patients between the ages of 20 and 50 years of age. Although bilateral cases are reported, it is a unilateral disease in the overwhelming majority of cases.

Etiology The cause of glaucomatocyclitic crisis is unclear. The increased intraocular pressure, however, is believed to result from an acute decrease in the aqueous outflow during the attack. Prostaglandins have been demonstrated to play a role in the disease pathogenesis,

with elevated levels in the aqueous humor correlating with the increase in intraocular pressure during an acute attack.[24] Prostaglandins break down the blood-aqueous barrier, resulting in an influx of proteins and inflammatory cells that can impair aqueous outflow and increase the intraocular pressure. Some patients with glaucomatocyclitic crisis have abnormal aqueous humor dynamics between episodes and may have an underlying primary open-angle glaucoma.

History Patients have a history of recurring symptoms of mild ocular pain or discomfort and blurred vision without ocular injection. Some patients may also describe halos that may indicate the presence of corneal edema.

Ophthalmic Examination External ocular examination is frequently normal. Anterior segment examination typically reveals few keratic precipitates distributed over the inferior corneal endothelium. In some cases, particularly if the intraocular pressure is sufficiently elevated, the cornea may show microcystic edema. Keratic precipitates may occasionally be seen on gonioscopy, suggesting the presence of a trabeculitis. The anterior chamber characteristically shows only mild aqueous cells and flare. If pressure is significantly elevated, the pupil may be slightly dilated; however, peripheral anterior synechiae and posterior synechiae do not occur. Infrequently, heterochromia may be noted as a result of stromal atrophy caused by the recurrent unilateral inflammatory attacks. The intraocular pressure is generally much greater than would be expected for the degree of intraocular inflammation, typically measuring greater than 30 mm Hg, often in the 40- to 60-mm Hg range. The fundus examination is typically normal.

Differential Diagnosis Diseases to be considered in the differential diagnosis of glaucomatocyclitic crisis include Fuchs's heterochromic iridocyclitis, herpes simplex or zoster uveitis, sarcoidosis, HLA-B27–associated anterior uveitides, and idiopathic anterior uveitis.

Laboratory Studies Glaucomatocyclitic crisis is a clinical diagnosis, and there are no laboratory studies that are specific for the diagnosis.

Course Posner-Schlossman syndrome is a self-limited ocular hypertension that resolves spontaneously regardless of treatment. The recurrent inflammatory attacks tend to occur at intervals of a few months to years and may last from several hours to a few weeks before spontaneously resolving. The development of optic nerve damage and visual field defects in glaucomatocyclitic crisis may occur as a result of the repeated bouts of extremely elevated intraocular pressure superimposed on an underlying primary open-angle glaucoma.[25]

Management Posner-Schlossman syndrome is treated initially with topical corticosteroids to control the anterior uveitis. If the intraocular pressure does not respond to topical antiinflammatory therapy, antiglaucoma medications may be required to lower the intraocular pressure. Mydriatic and cycloplegic agents are not commonly needed as ciliary muscle spasm is uncommon and synechiae rarely form. Oral indomethacin, 75 to 150 mg daily—a prostaglandin antagonist—has been reported to lower the intraocular pressure in patients with glaucomatocyclitic crises faster than standard antiglaucoma medications.[24] Topical nonsteroidal antiinflammatory medications are likewise expected to be an effective treatment option for patients with ocular hypertension. Miotics and argon laser trabeculoplasty are generally not effective. Between attacks, prophylactic antiinflammatory therapy is not required. Surgical filtration procedures are rarely required and, if performed, do not prevent the recurrent inflammatory attacks.

Herpetic Keratouveitis

In the eye, infection with the herpes simplex virus (HSV) can manifest as several distinct, recurrent, unilateral ocular diseases such as blepharoconjunctivitis, epithelial keratitis, stromal keratitis, and uveitis. Although ocular involvement may occur with primary herpes zoster infection (chickenpox), it more commonly accompanies herpes zoster ophthalmicus, a reactivation of herpes zoster in older adults affecting distribution of the ophthalmic branch of cranial nerve V. Uveitis associated with both HSV and herpes zoster infections typically follows previous episodes of keratitis and accounts for about 5% of all uveitis cases seen in adults.[26] Elevated intraocular pressure that can progress to a secondary glaucoma is a prominent feature of recurrent herpetic uveitis.

Epidemiology Approximately 0.15% of the United States population has a history of external HSV infection.[27] Ocular involvement occurs in two thirds of all cases of herpes zoster ophthalmicus. Stromal keratitis and uveitis, which together account for the greatest visual morbidity from all forms of recurrent herpes simplex ocular disease, develop in fewer than 10% of patients with primary ocular herpes simplex infection.[26] Uveitis and ocular hypertension in patients with zoster may be associated with either epithelial or stromal keratitis. The incidence of increased intraocular pressure in patients with herpetic uveitis varies from 28% to 40%.[28] The incidence of secondary glaucoma in patients with herpes simplex uveitis and herpes zoster uveitis is about 10% and 16%, respectively.[28,29]

Etiology It remains unclear whether the uveitis associated with herpes simplex keratitis is a secondary inflammatory response to the corneal disease or whether it is induced by invasion of the virus into the anterior uvea. The elevated intraocular pressure in herpes simplex and herpes zoster uveitis is the result of normal aqueous secretion in eyes with impaired outflow resulting from trabeculitis, direct inflammation of the trabecular meshwork. In herpes zoster uveitis, ischemia resulting from an occlusive vasculitis may also contribute to the increased intraocular pressure.[30] Herpes simplex virus has been cultured from the anterior chamber of patients with herpetic uveitis, and its presence is positively correlated with ocular hypertension. Prolonged steroid use may also contribute to ocular pressure in patients with herpetic uveitis.

History Patients with herpetic uveitis typically present with a complaint of unilateral ocular redness, pain, photophobia, and, often, decreased vision. A prior history of recurrent keratitis is commonly given. Patients with uveitis related to herpes zoster are generally older and report a history of herpes zoster ophthalmicus. Ocular disease related to HSV is rarely bilateral, whereas herpes zoster ophthalmicus only occurs unilaterally.

Ophthalmic Examination External ocular examination may reveal evidence of previous cutaneous lesions with herpes zoster, conjunctival injection, and ciliary flush. Corneal sensation is often decreased in the affected eye. The cornea in patients with herpes keratouveitis may show a range of findings related to the prior epithelial or stromal disease, including epithelial dendrites, ghost dendrites, active disciform or necrotizing stromal keratitis, neovascularization, or scarring. Diffuse, nongranulomatous, stellate keratic precipitates or pigmented granulomatous precipitates can be found in both forms of herpetic uveitis. In severe cases of herpetic uveitis, posterior synechiae and angle closure may be found. Iris atrophy is a characteristic finding in uveitis resulting from both herpes simplex and zoster (Figure 13-11A,B). With HSV, the iris atrophy tends to occur more centrally closer to the pupil and is often described as patchy, whereas with herpes zoster, the iris atrophy is more segmental and located toward the peripheral iris. In patients with herpes zoster, the iris atrophy is thought to be the result of an occlusive vasculitis in the iris stroma.

Differential Diagnosis The differential diagnosis for herpetic uveitis includes Fuchs's heterochromic iridocyclitis, glaucomatocyclitic crisis, and sarcoidosis. The presence of corneal hypoesthesia may be helpful in the diagnosis of herpetic uveitis.

Laboratory Studies The diagnosis of herpetic uveitis is clinical and does not routinely rely on laboratory testing. Viral serologies for HSV and varicella zoster virus, if negative, exclude the diagnosis. The detection of viral DNA in the aqueous by polymerase chain reaction is supportive but not diagnostic of herpetic uveitis.

Course Similar to the other ocular manifestations of herpes eye disease, the uveitis is recurrent and may or may not be associated with recurrent keratitis. Elevated intraocular pressure is typically present during the course of the intraocular inflammation and may normalize or remain elevated after the uveitis has subsided. Approximately 12% of patients will have persistently elevated intraocular pressure that will require antiglaucoma therapy or filtering surgery.[28]

Management Uveitis associated with HSV and herpes zoster should be treated with topical corticosteroids. Cycloplegic agents may also be necessary if there is ocular pain resulting from ciliary spasm. An antiviral agent should be used with the topical steroids to lessen the likelihood of a reactivation of the epithelial keratitis. Oral acyclovir in patients with herpes zoster ophthalmicus has been found to ameliorate the incidence and severity of dendritic keratitis, stromal keratitis, and uveitis. Patients with increased intraocular pressure should be treated as needed with antiglaucoma therapy. Filtration surgery may occasionally be required. Argon laser trabeculoplasty is not considered effective in the management of herpetic uveitis.

Syphilitic Interstitial Keratitis

Ocular syphilis may occur congenitally or may be acquired by sexual transmission. Congenital syphilis mainly affects the anterior segment of the eye, causing interstitial keratitis and anterior uveitis, whereas acquired syphilis more frequently causes both anterior and posterior uveitis. With the advent of effective diagnostic tests and antibiotic therapy, syphilitic interstitial keratitis and secondary glaucoma have become rare.

Epidemiology Ocular involvement in both congenital and acquired syphilis can be associated with increased intraocular pressure and secondary glaucoma that may occur during the active inflammatory stage or many years after the intraocular inflammation has become quiescent. Secondary glaucoma has been reported in 15% to 20% of adults with a history of interstitial keratitis caused by congenital syphilis.[31] Secondary glaucoma is less common in patients with acquired syphilis.

Etiology The pathologic mechanism of the increased intraocular pressure during the active

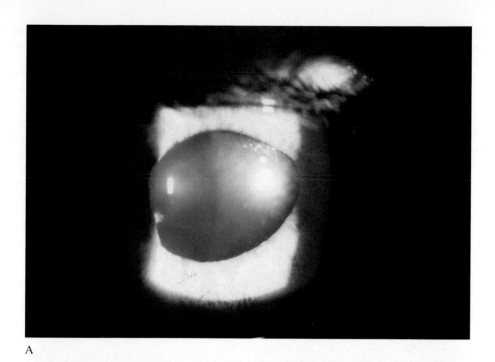

A

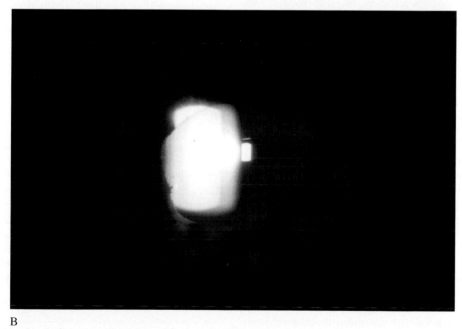

B

Figure 13-11A,B   Herpetic uveitis due to herpes simplex   *In patients presenting with unilateral anterior uveitis and elevated intraocular pressure, assessment of corneal sensation and transillumination of the pupil are helpful in making a clinical diagnosis of herpetic uveitis. Diffuse illumination of the iris (**A**) does not reveal the patchy atrophy of the iris stoma seen on transillumination (**B**). After the patient started oral acyclovir, he was able to discontinue topical antiglaucoma therapy.*

stage of the disease is likely obstruction to the aqueous outflow by inflammatory cells and aqueous proteins. Synechiae formation, ocular maldevelopment, and lens subluxation may contribute to the development of narrow-angle or angle-closure glaucoma. Endothelialization of the angle demonstrated by histopathology is believed to be the underlying mechanism of the late-onset glaucoma in patients with congenital syphilis.

History Patients with ocular disease resulting from congenital syphilis typically present in the first or second decade of life with acute symptoms of ocular pain, photophobia, tearing, and decreased vision. The condition is bilateral in 90% of cases. Nonocular signs of congenital syphilis that may be present include dental deformities such as notched incisors and mulberry molars; skeletal abnormalities including a saddle nose, palatal perforation, saber shins, and frontal bossing; deafness; rhagades; and mental retardation. Patients with acquired ocular syphilis are more likely to present with unilateral symptoms.

Ophthalmic Examination Ocular examination of patients with congenital syphilis may show a variety of findings, including acute and chronic anterior uveitis, cataracts, chorioretinitis, retinal vasculitis, optic neuritis, and scleritis. Of these, interstitial keratitis is the most characteristic manifestation. The cornea in patients with active interstitial keratitis typically shows sectoral edema, opacification, and deep stromal vascularization that may be so pronounced as to give the cornea a pink salmon patch appearance. Anterior uveitis commonly accompanies syphilitic interstitial keratitis and is often associated with elevated intraocular pressure. Ocular findings in patients with acquired syphilis frequently include anterior uveitis, chorioretinitis, and optic neuritis. Interstitial keratitis rarely develops in patients with acquired syphilis and when it occurs is typically unilateral. Nodular iris lesions often accompany the anterior uveitis in patients with acquired syphilis.

Differential Diagnosis The differential diagnosis for the active stage of ocular syphilis characterized by interstitial keratitis and anterior uveitis includes diseases such as herpes simplex and zoster infections, *Mycobacterium tuberculosis* and *leprae,* Lyme disease, rubeola (measles), Epstein-Barr virus (infectious mononucleosis), leishmaniasis and onchocerciasis, sarcoidosis, and Cogan's syndrome.

Laboratory Studies Ocular syphilis is diagnosed on the basis of a positive serology. The nontreponemal tests such as the venereal disease research lab (VDRL) or the rapid plasma reagin (RPR) alone are insufficient and a treponemal test, such as the fluorescent treponemal antibody absorption (FTA-ABS) test or the microhemagglutination test, *Treponema pallidum* (MHA-TP), must be obtained. Any patient with syphilitic uveitis should have a spinal fluid examination to rule out asymptomatic neurosyphilis.

Course The interstitial keratitis and anterior uveitis typically persist for several weeks to months before spontaneously resolving, leaving ghost vessels in the deep corneal stroma. Glaucoma is a late complication of patients with congenital syphilis that typically develops in eyes without evidence of ongoing intraocular inflammation decades after the interstitial keratitis has subsided. Both open-angle and narrow-angle glaucoma have been described in these patients with equal frequency.

Management During the active stage of the disease, management of the increased intraocular pressure relies on topical corticosteroids, cycloplegic agents, and antiglaucoma medications as needed. Systemic syphilis should be treated with an appropriate antibiotic course. Laser iridotomy or surgical iridectomy should be performed in patients with narrow-angle or closed-angle glaucoma. Patients with late-onset open-angle glaucoma are less responsive to antiglaucoma medications and may require a filtering procedure. Argon laser trabeculoplasty is of little benefit because of the angle endothelialization.

Juvenile Rheumatoid Arthritis

Juvenile rheumatoid arthritis (JRA) is a common cause of pediatric uveitis often complicated by increased intraocular pressure and glaucoma. Three subtypes of JRA with different risks for the development of uveitis can be diagnosed based on the extent of articular and systemic involvement within the first 3 months of presentation. Systemic-onset JRA, or Still's disease, is commonly seen in boys younger than 4 years of age and is an acute systemic disease consisting of a cutaneous rash, fever, polyarthritis, hepatosplenomegaly, leukocytosis, and polyserositis. Young girls more commonly present with the oligoarticular or pauciarticular (fewer than five joints) and polyarticular (five or more joints) forms of JRA that lack the systemic features.

Epidemiology   The incidence of uveitis in JRA varies from 2% to 21%.[4] Uveitis is typically not associated with Still's disease or systemic-onset JRA, seen more frequently in boys. Anterior uveitis is more common in patients with the pauciarticular form (19% to 29%) than in those with the polyarticular form (2% to 5%) of JRA.[32,33] Children with the pauciarticular or monoarticular onset of joint involvement account for more than 90% of the JRA patients with uveitis. Secondary glaucoma is seen in approximately 14% to 22% of patients with chronic anterior uveitis associated with JRA.[4]

Etiology   The development of increased intraocular pressure and glaucoma in patients with JRA is most often caused by progressive angle closure as a result of synechiae. Open-angle glaucoma also occurs and may be the result of chronic inflammatory damage to the trabecular meshwork or steroid-induced glaucoma resulting from prolonged topical steroid treatment.

History   Anterior uveitis develops after the arthritis in 90% of the patients with JRA. Because the anterior uveitis associated with JRA is mild, asymptomatic, and rarely causes ocular redness, the disease may go unnoticed for a long period of time until visual loss cataract or an irregular pupil is noted. The uveitis in patients with JRA is bilateral in almost all cases.

Ophthalmic Examination   Band keratopathy is a found in up to 50% of children with anterior uveitis, and its presence is thought to be associated with the chronicity of the disease.[4] The anterior uveitis in patients with JRA is non-granulomatous in the vast majority of cases. Infrequently, however, mutton fat keratic precipitates and Koeppe nodules may be observed. Keratic precipitates are generally distributed over the inferior half of the cornea. Mitotic pupils resulting from posterior synechiae or pupillary membranes, iris bombé, and peripheral anterior synechiae are frequent findings in affected patients that can contribute to the development of glaucoma. Anterior and posterior subcapsular cataracts are present in up to one third of affected patients. Posterior segment examination in patients with JRA may show papillitis and cystoid macular edema, which can contribute to visual loss.

Differential Diagnosis   The differential diagnosis for chronic anterior uveitis in children includes sarcoidosis, pars planitis, HLA-B27–associated diseases, and idiopathic anterior uveitis.

Laboratory Studies   Up to 80% of patients with anterior uveitis and JRA are antinuclear antibody positive and rheumatoid factor negative.

Course   The uveitis associated with JRA is a chronic disease that is difficult to control despite treatment. In patients with JRA, there is no direct correlation between the activity of the ocular disease and the joint disease. The incidence of secondary complications, such as band keratopathy, cataract, and glaucoma, increases with the duration of the disease. The prognosis for children with uveitic glaucoma, previously considered poor, is improving with more effective surgical management.

Management   The initial treatment approach for the management of intraocular inflammation in patients with JRA includes topical corticosteroids and cycloplegic agents to prevent the formation of synechiae. Often, periocular steroid injections and even systemic steroids are necessary to control anterior uveitis. Oral nonsteroidal agents are also used in JRA patients. Methotrexate alone or in combination with other immunosuppressive agents such as prednisone or cyclosporine has been used to treat the ocular and joint manifestations of JRA. Newer biologic agents such as etanercept

(Enbrel) and infliximab (Remicade), shown to be of benefit for the joint disease in JRA, are currently being evaluated for their efficacy in the treatment of uveitis.

Elevated intraocular pressure in JRA is treated initially with antiglaucoma medications. Medical management is initially effective in only about 50% of JRA patients, with only 30% of patients being controlled medically over the long term.[33] Laser iridotomy or surgical iridectomy may be necessary to relieve the pupillary block in patients with posterior synechiae. Surgical management is required for patients who are unresponsive to medical therapy. To increase the likelihood of a good outcome, if possible, surgical intervention should be deferred until the intraocular inflammation has been adequately controlled for a period of at least 3 months. Operative procedures most commonly used in children with JRA include trabeculectomy and tube shunts (see Figure 13-8). Improved success has been reported with the use of antimetabolites in patients undergoing trabeculectomy.[4] Trabeculodialysis in a small case series has been shown to be safe and effective for controlling the pressure in patients with JRA for up to 2 years.[34]

Lens-induced Uveitis and Glaucoma

The liberation of lens proteins through an intact or disrupted lens capsule into the anterior chamber or vitreous cavity can trigger a severe intraocular inflammatory reaction that may impair aqueous outflow and cause an acute elevation in the intraocular pressure or glaucoma. Leakage of lens proteins is typically the result of accidental or surgical trauma to the lens capsule or may be associated with cataract progression. Clinical entities characterized by lens-induced uveitis and glaucoma include phacoantigenic uveitis, phacolytic glaucoma, lens particle glaucoma, and phacomorphic glaucoma. Uveitis and glaucoma may also be a complication of intraocular lens placement.

Epidemiology   Although the condition is well described, the exact incidence of glaucoma due to various forms of lens-induced uveitis is not known. In one study of patients with phacoanaphylactic uveitis (phacoantigenic uveitis), 17% of patients were diagnosed with glaucoma.[35]

History   Phacoantigenic uveitis, also referred to as phacoanaphylactic uveitis or phacoanaphylactic endophthalmitis, is initiated by the release of lens proteins though a ruptured lens capsule. The onset of the inflammation is days to weeks after the traumatic or surgical injury to the lens. Patients present with a red, painful eye. Rarely, phacoantigenic uveitis is associated with sympathetic ophthalmia and the development of an inflammatory reaction in the fellow eye.[36]

Phacolytic glaucoma typically seen in older patients arises when lens proteins leak from a mature or hypermature cataract through an intact but permeable lens capsule. Patients with phacolytic glaucoma commonly present with the abrupt onset of ocular pain and redness in a poorly seeing eye with a known cataract.

Lens particle glaucoma, also known as phacotoxic uveitis, occurs following any ocular injury that results in the liberation of lens cortical material into the anterior chamber. In most cases, the onset of increased intraocular pressure is detected days or weeks after the inciting injury.

In cases of phacomorphic glaucoma, the lens capsule is not typically violated and the eye generally does not show significant intraocular inflammation. Patients typically present with a redness and pain from angle closure in an eye with decreased vision caused by a cataract.

The uveitis-glaucoma-hyphema (UGH) syndrome was a frequent cause of postoperative intraocular inflammation and glaucoma in patients following implantation with the first generation of rigid, anterior chamber intraocular lenses. The syndrome was attributed to poor intraocular lens size selection or manufacturing defects in the lens material, causing mechanical irritation to anterior chamber structures. Chronic or severe postoperative inflammation can also result in pseudophakic inflammatory glaucoma in patients with posterior chamber intraocular lens implants.

Etiology   Obstruction of aqueous outflow at the level of the trabecular meshwork is the common mechanism in the lens-induced glaucomas.

In phacoantigenic uveitis, there is a granulomatous inflammatory response to the elaborated lens proteins that can induce the formation of synechiae and blockage of the trabecular meshwork. In phacolytic glaucoma, the released lens proteins and macrophages engorged with lens proteins obstruct the trabecular meshwork, whereas in lens particle glaucoma, it is the actual fragments of lens cortical material that are believed to injure the trabecular meshwork. Unlike the other lens-induced glaucomas, in which the anterior chamber angle is typically open, in phacomorphic glaucoma the intumescent lens can cause pupillary block or dislocate the iris forward, resulting in a shallowed anterior chamber or acute angle closure. In pseudophakic eyes, intraocular inflammation may be the result of a previous uveitis, a delayed onset postsurgical endophthalmitis, or irritation of the uveal tissue by the intraocular lens. Glaucoma may arise because of damage to the trabecular meshwork or formation of synechiae on the lens implant, causing pupillary block, and peripheral anterior synechiae formation, resulting in angle closure.

Ophthalmic Examination External examination of patients with acute lens-induced uveitis and glaucoma commonly reveals conjunctival injection and ciliary flush. There may also be external evidence of a prior ocular injury. If the pressure is significantly elevated, the cornea is often edematous. The anterior chamber typically contains anterior chamber cells and flare, with granulomatous or nongranulomatous keratic precipitates. White, flocculent material and fragments of lens cortex may be seen circulating within the aqueous and in the anterior chamber angle, which may be open, narrowed, or closed. Peripheral anterior and posterior synechiae are not uncommon. In cases of phacoantigenic uveitis and lens particle glaucoma, evidence of injury to the native lens or retained lens material can usually be found. In cases of phacolytic and phacomorphic glaucoma, examination reveals a hypermature or intumescent cataract, respectively, and in cases of pseudophakic inflammatory glaucoma, an intraocular lens is present. Posterior segment examination may show vitreous cells and haze,

lens material in the vitreous cavity, and other findings related to the ocular injury.

Differential Diagnosis The main differential diagnoses for phacoantigenic and lens particle glaucoma are posttraumatic and postsurgical endophthalmitis. Other causes of acute angle closure should be considered in patients with phacomorphic glaucoma.

Laboratory Studies The diagnosis of lens-induced uveitis and glaucoma is clinical and does not rely on laboratory testing. Histopathologic examination of the lens in patients with phacoantigenic uveitis reveals a zonal granulomatous inflammation centered at the site of lens injury.

Course The clinical course of the lens-induced glaucomas tends to be relatively brief because they are effectively managed with surgical intervention.

Management Cataract extraction or removal of the retained lens material or lens implant is the definitive therapy for lens-induced uveitis and glaucoma. Prior to surgical intervention, the intraocular inflammation is treated with topical corticosteroids and the increased intraocular pressure is controlled with antiglaucoma medications. In patients with phacomorphic glaucoma, after the intraocular pressure is lowered medically laser iridotomy can be used to temporize the condition if cataract extraction needs to be delayed or cannot be performed.

Sarcoidosis

Sarcoidosis is a systemic disease characterized by noncaseating, granulomatous, inflammatory infiltrates affecting the lungs, skin, liver, spleen, central nervous system, and eyes. Ocular disease occurs in 10% to 38% of patients with systemic sarcoidosis.[37] Sarcoidosis, which can present as anterior, intermediate, posterior, or panuveitis, is the prototype for a chronic, granulomatous uveitis.

Epidemiology Sarcoidosis is eight to ten times more frequent among African Americans than whites, having an estimated prevalence of

82 per 100,000 in this population.[37] Although sarcoidosis can develop at any age, the disease is typically diagnosed in adults between 20 and 50 years of age. Sarcoidosis accounts for 5% of all uveitis cases in adults but about 1% of uveitis cases in children.[38] Sarcoidosis involves the anterior segment in up to 70% of cases with ocular involvement, whereas the posterior segment is affected in less than 33% of cases.[39] Secondary glaucoma occurs in approximately 11% to 25% of all patients with sarcoidosis and is more commonly a complication of the anterior segment disease.[40] African-American patients with sarcoidosis have a higher incidence of uveitic glaucoma and blindness.

Etiology Ocular hypertension and glaucoma in patients with sarcoidosis results from obstruction of the trabecular meshwork by the chronic granulomatous inflammation and angle closure caused by the formation of peripheral anterior and posterior synechiae with iris bombé. Anterior segment neovascularization and the prolonged use of steroids can also contribute to the impairment of aqueous outflow.

History Most adult patients with sarcoidosis present with pulmonary involvement that may manifest as cough, shortness of breath, wheezing, or dyspnea on exertion. Another common presentation of sarcoidosis is with generalized symptoms such as fever, fatigue, and weight loss. Many patients, however, may be asymptomatic at the time of diagnosis. Patients with ocular involvement typically present with complaints of ocular pain, redness, photophobia, floaters, and blurred or decreased vision.

Ophthalmic Examination The ocular disease of sarcoidosis is typically bilateral, although it may be unilateral or very asymmetric. Most frequently a cause of granulomatous uveitis, sarcoidosis may also cause a nongranulomatous uveitis. Ophthalmic findings in the anterior segment include orbital and cutaneous granulomas, enlarged lacrimal glands, and palpebral and bulbar conjunctival nodules. The cornea most commonly shows large, mutton fat keratic precipitates, with nummular corneal infiltrates and inferior areas of endothelial opacification being noted less frequently. Posterior and peripheral anterior synechiae, when extensive, result in elevated intraocular pressure or secondary uveitic glaucoma caused by angle closure or iris bombé. Koeppe and Busacca-type iris nodules are often seen in the more severe cases of anterior segment disease (see Figure 13-5).

Posterior segment involvement in sarcoidosis occurs less frequently than anterior segment disease. The vitreous frequently shows a vitritis with vitreous snowballs and inferior inflammatory debris. Examination of the posterior pole may reveal a variety of findings, including peripheral retinal vasculitis, peripheral exudates similar to snowbanks, hemorrhages, retinal exudates, and perivascular nodular granulomatous lesions, Dalen-Fuchs's nodules, and retinal, subretinal, or disc neovascularization. Granulomas in the retina, choroid, and optic nerve may also be seen. Visual loss in sarcoidosis is most often a result of cystoid macular edema, optic neuritis caused by granulomatous infiltration of the optic nerve, and secondary glaucoma.

Differential Diagnosis The differential diagnosis of sarcoidosis includes the other causes of granulomatous panuveitis such as the Vogt-Koyanagi-Harada syndrome, sympathetic ophthalmia, and tuberculosis. Syphilis, Lyme disease, primary intraocular lymphoma, and pars planitis should also be considered.

Laboratory Studies The diagnosis of sarcoidosis is confirmed with a tissue biopsy showing noncaseating or nonnecrotizing granulomas or granulomatous inflammation in a patient in whom all other causes of granulomatous disease, such as tuberculosis and fungal infections, have been excluded. An initial diagnostic evaluation for sarcoidosis should include a chest x-ray and serum angiotensin-converting enzyme (ACE) level. Serum lysozyme levels may be elevated in patients with sarcoidosis but are less specific than serum ACE as a marker for the disease. Additional studies that may be useful in confirming the diagnosis include anergy testing, pulmonary function testing, gallium scan, computed tomographic scan of the thorax, bronchoalveolar lavage, and transbronchial biopsy. Because ACE levels may be high in normal children, serum ACE level is a less useful diagnostic test for sarcoidosis in children. Elevated ACE levels have been reported in the aqueous humor and cerebrospinal fluids of patients with ocular and central nervous system sarcoid uveitis and neurosarcoidosis, respectively.

Course The clinical course of ocular sarcoidosis can be acute and self limited or chronic, recurrent, and relentless. The chronic form of sarcoid uveitis has the worse prognosis because of the onset of complications such as glaucoma, cataract, and macular edema.

Management The mainstay of therapy for both systemic and ocular sarcoidosis is corticosteroids. Anterior segment disease may be managed with topical or periocular corticosteroid injections. Systemic therapy is typically required for bilateral posterior segment uveitis. Other immunosuppressive agents such as cyclosporine and methotrexate have demonstrated therapeutic benefit in the management of sarcoidosis and should be considered early for patients with chronic sarcoidosis requiring prolonged steroid therapy. The glaucoma should be treated medically with aqueous suppressants for as long as possible. Argon laser trabeculoplasty is frequently ineffective. Laser iridotomy and surgical iridectomy are the treatments of choice for patients with pupillary block. If the intraocular pressure remains uncontrolled, surgical intervention with either a filtering procedure or a tube shunt is required. Surgical success is improved if the intraocular inflammatory disease can be controlled prior to the surgical procedure. The use of antimetabolites is recommended for patients undergoing trabeculectomy, particularly African-American patients.

REFERENCES

1. Baarsma GS. The epidemiology and genetics of endogenous uveitis: A review. *Curr Eye Res* 11 Suppl:1–9, 1992.
2. Cunningham ET Jr. Uveitis in children. *Ocul Immunol Inflamm* 8:251–261, 2000.
3. Tran VT, Mermoud A, Herbort CP. Appraisal and management of ocular hypotony and glaucoma associated with uveitis. *Int Ophthalmol Clin* 40:175–203, 2000.
4. Moorthy RS, Mermoud A, Baerveldt G, Minckler DS, Lee PP, Rao NA. Glaucoma associated with uveitis. *Surv Ophthalmol* 41:361–394, 1997.
5. Kanski JJ, Shun-Shin GA. Systemic uveitis syndromes in childhood: An analysis of 340 cases. *Ophthalmology* 91:1247–1252, 1984.
6. Peretz WL, Tomasi TB. Aqueous humor proteins in uveitis. Immunoelectrophoretic and gel diffusion studies on normal and pathological human aqueous humor. *Arch Ophthalmol* 65:20–23, 1961.
7. Beitch BR, Easkins KE. The effects of prostaglandins on the intraocular pressure of the rabbit. *Br J Pharmacol* 37:158–167, 1969.
8. Bhattacherjee P. The role of arachidonate metabolites in ocular inflammation. *Prog Clin Biol Res* 312:211–227, 1989.
9. Weinreb RN, Mitchell MD, Polansky JR. Prostaglandin production by human trabecular cells: In vitro inhibition by dexamethasone. *Invest Ophthalmol Vis Sci* 24:1541–1545, 1983.
10. Jabs DA, Rosenbaum JT, Foster CS, Holland GN, Jaffe GJ, Louie JS, Nussenblatt RB, Stiehm ER, Tessler H, Van Gelder RN, Whitcup SM, Yocum D. Guidelines for the use of immunosuppressive drugs in patients with ocular inflammatory disorders: Recommendations of an expert panel. *Am J Ophthalmol* 130:492–513, 2000.
11. Larkin G, Lightman S. Mycophenolate mofetil. A useful immunosuppressive in inflammatory eye disease. *Ophthalmology* 106:370–374, 1999.
12. Akingbehin T, Villada JR. Metipranolol-associated granulomatous anterior uveitis. *Br J Ophthalmol* 75:519–523, 1991.
13. Whitcup SM, Csaky KG, Podgor MJ, Chew EY, Perry CH, Nussenblatt RB. A randomized, masked, cross-over trial of acetazolamide for cystoid macular edema in patients with uveitis. *Ophthalmology* 103:1054–1062, 1996.
14. Warwar RE, Bullock JD, Ballal D. Cystoid macular edema and anterior uveitis associated with latanoprost use. Experience and incidence in a retrospective review of 94 patients. *Ophthalmology* 105:263–268, 1998.
15. Da Mata A, Burk SE, Netland PA, Baltatzis S, Christen W, Foster CS. Management of uveitic glaucoma with Ahmed glaucoma valve implantation. *Ophthalmology* 106:2168–2172, 1999.
16. Prata JA Jr, Neves RA, Minckler DS, Mermoud A, Heuer DK. Trabeculectomy with mitomycin C in glaucoma associated with uveitis. *Ophthalmic Surg* 25:616–620, 1994.
17. Hill RA, Nguyen QH, Baerveldt G, Forster DJ, Minckler DS, Rao N, Lee M, Heuer DK. Trabeculectomy and Molteno implantation for glaucomas associated with uveitis. *Ophthalmology* 100:903–908, 1993.
18. Skuta GL, Parrish RK 2nd. Wound healing in glaucoma filtering surgery. *Surv Ophthalmol* 32:149–170, 1987.
19. Wolner B, Liebmann JM, Sassani JW, Ritch R, Speaker M, Marmor M. Late bleb-related endophthalmitis after trabeculectomy with adjunctive 5-fluorouracil. *Ophthalmology* 98:1053–1060, 1991.
20. Schuman JS, Bellows AR, Shingleton BJ, Latina MA, Allingham RR, Belcher CD, Puliafito CA. Contact transscleral Nd:YAG laser cyclophotocoagulation. Midterm results. *Ophthalmology* 99:1089–1094, 1992.
21. O'Connor GR. Doyne lecture. Heterochromic iridocyclitis. *Trans Ophthalmol Soc U K* 104:219–231, 1985.
22. Bloch-Michel E. Physiopathology of Fuchs's heterochromic cyclitis. *Trans Ophthalmol Soc U K* 101:384–386, 1981.
23. Liesegang TJ. Clinical features and prognosis in Fuchs' uveitis syndrome. *Arch Ophthalmol* 100:1622–1626, 1982.
24. Masuda K, Izawa Y, Mishima SS. Prostaglandins and glaucomato-cyclitis crisis. *Jpn J Ophthalmol* 19:368, 1975.
25. Kass MA, Becker B, Kolker AE. Glaucomatocyclitic crisis and primary open-angle glaucoma. *Am J Ophthalmol* 75:668–673, 1973.
26. Barron BA, Gee L, Hauck WW, Kurinij N, Dawson CR, Jones DB, Wilhelmus KR, Kaufman HE, Sugar J, Hyndiuk RA, et al. Herpetic Eye Disease Study. A controlled trial of oral acyclovir for herpes simplex stromal keratitis. *Ophthalmology* 101:1871–1882, 1994.

27. Parrish CM. Herpes simplex virus eye disease. In: *Focal Points: Clinical Modules for Ophthalmologists.* San Francisco: American Academy of Ophthalmology; 15:2, 1997.

28. Falcon MG, Williams HP. Herpes simplex keratouveitis and glaucoma. *Trans Ophthalmol Soc U K* 98:101–104, 1978.

29. Panek WC, Holland GN, Lee DA, Christensen RE. Glaucoma in patients with uveitis. *Br J Ophthalmol* 74:223–227, 1990.

30. Johns KJ, O'Day DM, Webb RA, Glick A. Anterior segment ischemia in chronic herpes simplex keratouveitis. *Curr Eye Res* 10 Suppl: 117–124, 1991.

31. Lichter PR, Shaffer RN. Interstitial keratitis and glaucoma. *Am J Ophthalmol* 68:241–248, 1969.

32. Calabro JJ, Parrino GR, Atchoo PD, Marchesano JM, Goldberg LS. Chronic iridocyclitis in juvenile rheumatoid arthritis. *Arthritis Rheum* 13:406–413, 1970.

33. O'Brien JM, Albert DM. Therapeutic approaches for ophthalmic problems in juvenile rheumatoid arthritis. *Rheum Dis Clin North Am* 15:413–437, 1989.

34. Kanski JJ, McAllister JA. Trabeculodialysis for inflammatory glaucoma in children and young adults. *Ophthalmology* 92:927–930, 1985.

35. Thach AB, Marak GE Jr, McLean IW, Green WR. Phacoanaphylactic endophthalmitis: a clinicopathologic review. *Int Ophthalmol* 15:271–279, 1991.

36. Allen JC. Sympathetic uveitis and phacoanaphylaxis. *Am J Ophthalmol* 63:280–283, 1967.

37. Nussenblatt RB, Whitcup SM, Palestine AG. Sarcoidosis. In: Nussenblatt RB, Whitcup SM, Palestine AG, eds. *Uveitis: Fundamentals and Clinical Practice.* St Louis, MO: Mosby; 289–98, 1996.

38. Hoover DL, Khan JA, Giangiacomo J. Pediatric ocular sarcoidosis. *Surv Ophthalmol* 30:215–228, 1986.

39. Jabs DA, Johns CJ. Ocular involvement in chronic sarcoidosis. *Am J Ophthalmol* 102:297–301, 1986.

40. Obenauf CD, Shaw HE, Sydnor CF, Klintworth GK. Sarcoidosis and its ophthalmic manifestations. *Am J Ophthalmol* 86:648–655, 1978.

Chapter 14

LENS-ASSOCIATED OPEN-ANGLE GLAUCOMAS

Michele C. Lim, MD

Lens-associated open-angle glaucomas are composed of three separate diagnoses with similar clinical presentations. Lens protein glaucoma, lens particle glaucoma, and lens-associated uveitis (LAU) may each present with intraocular inflammation, an abnormal lens, and elevated intraocular pressure, although hypotony may commonly occur in the latter. Distinguishing among the three entities requires careful examination and an understanding of the mechanisms that define each diagnosis (Table 14-1).

TABLE 14-1   **CLINICAL PRESENTATION OF LENS-ASSOCIATED OPEN-ANGLE GLAUCOMAS**

	Lens Particle Glaucoma	Lens Protein Glaucoma	LAU
Mechanism	Lens material obstructs TM	HMW lens proteins obstruct TM	Loss of immune tolerance
IOP	Elevated	Elevated	Low or elevated
Gonioscopy	Open angle	Open angle	Open angle
Lens status	Disruption to lens capsule with release of lens particles	Mature or hypermature cataract	Disruption to lens capsule; exposure of large lens fragments
Management	Antiglaucoma medication, steroids, surgical removal of lens material	Antiglaucoma medication, topical steroids, cataract removal	Antiglaucoma topical medication, topical steroids, removal of lens fragments

HMW = heavy-molecular-weight proteins; IOP = intraocular pressure; LAU = lens-associated uveitis; TM = trabecular meshwork.

LENS PROTEIN OR PHACOLYTIC GLAUCOMA

Lens protein glaucoma occurs in the presence of a mature or a hypermature cataract (Figure 14-1). Soluble lens proteins seep into the anterior chamber and obstruct the trabecular meshwork, causing an elevation in intraocular pressure.

Pathophysiology

In lens protein glaucoma, heavy-molecular-weight (HMW) proteins (greater than 150×10^6 daltons) obstruct trabecular meshwork outflow, causing a rise in intraocular pressure. Previously, it was thought that the rise in pressure resulted exclusively from macrophage outflow obstruction, based on the fact that they were identified in the aqueous humor and in the trabecular meshwork of patients with lens protein glaucoma[1,2] (Figure 14-2). However, Epstein et al[3,4] suggested that HMW proteins obstruct the trabecular meshwork based on the

following experimental evidence:

1. Epstein sampled aqueous fluid of patients with phacolytic glaucoma and showed an abundance of HMW proteins, which increase in concentration as the cataract matures.
2. In vitro perfusion of cadaver eyes with HMW soluble proteins caused a 60% decrease in outflow facility after 1 hour.
3. The HMW proteins were present in high-enough concentrations in the aqueous humor of patients with lens protein glaucoma to cause obstruction of outflow.
4. Several of the eyes with phacolytic glaucoma had a paucity of macrophages.

Lens proteins can induce the migration of peripheral blood monocytes,[5] and macrophages probably function as scavengers to remove soluble lens proteins and fragments from the anterior chamber and trabecular meshwork.

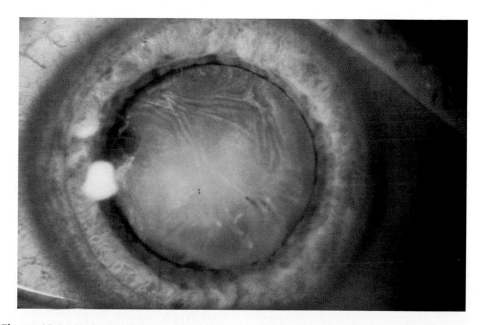

Figure 14-1   Mature cataract   *Mature cataract with folds in the anterior capsule. (Courtesy of Donald L. Budenz, MD, Bascom Palmer Eye Institute, Miami, FL)*

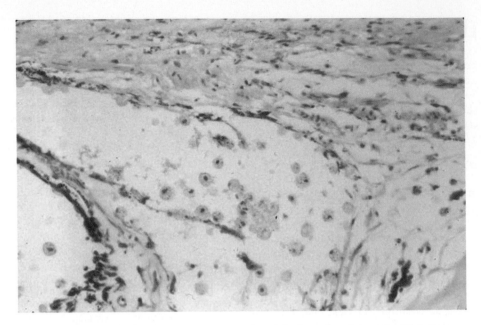

Figure 14-2 **Lens protein glaucoma** *Macrophages in the trabecular meshwork in lens protein glaucoma. (Courtesy of Donald L. Budenz, MD, Bascom Palmer Eye Institute, Miami, FL)*

History

Patients report gradually diminishing vision from the mature or hypermature cataract and pain from inflammation and elevated intraocular pressure.

Clinical Examination

Lens protein glaucoma occurs in the presence of a mature or hypermature cataract. These patients have an acutely elevated intraocular pressure, ocular redness, and pain. There is intense flare, which correlates with soluble proteins released from the mature cataract (Figure 14-3). A cellular response composed mostly of macrophages is present, and the cells appear larger and more translucent than lymphocytes. Hypopyon is uncommon. White patches may be observed on the lens and are thought to correspond to aggregates of macrophages phagocytosing lens proteins at leakage sites on the capsule. Gonioscopy reveals open angles. A retinal perivasculitis has been observed in some cases.[6]

Special Tests

Samples taken from the aqueous humor and concentrated via Millipore filtration may reveal macrophages and an amorphous substance corresponding to lens protein. The diagnosis is usually made on clinical observation alone.

Management

Management of lens protein glaucoma should start with medical therapy to temporize the elevated intraocular pressure. Beta-blockers, prostaglandin analogues, alpha-adrenergic drugs, and carbonic anhydrase inhibitors are the mainstays of medical therapy. Topical steroids to reduce the inflammation and cycloplegics to stabilize the blood-aqueous barrier and to reduce pain may also be used. Medical therapy may help to partially lower the pressure, but definitive treatment can only be obtained by removal of the cataract.

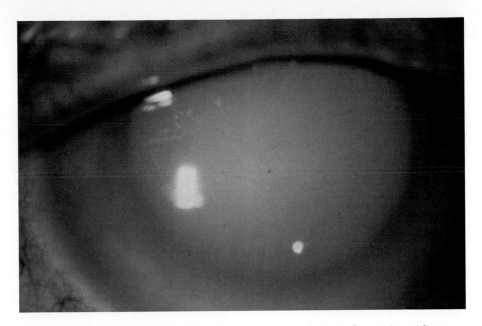

Figure 14-3   Lens protein glaucoma   *Intense anterior chamber inflammation with mature cataract in lens protein glaucoma. (Courtesy of Donald L. Budenz, MD, Bascom Palmer Eye Institute, Miami, FL)*

LENS PARTICLE GLAUCOMA

Lens particle glaucoma occurs when the lens capsule is disrupted and lens cortex and proteins are released into the anterior chamber. This may occur after extracapsular cataract surgery, lens trauma with capsular disruption, and neodymium (Nd):YAG posterior capsulotomy in which liberated lens particles obstruct the trabecular meshwork, reducing aqueous outflow. Lens particle glaucoma after subluxation of a posterior chamber intraocular lens in a patient with pseudoexfoliation syndrome has also been reported[7] (Figure 14-4).

Pathophysiology

The elevated intraocular pressure in lens particle glaucoma can be caused by:

- Lens particles obstructing the trabecular meshwork
- Inflammatory cells
- Peripheral anterior synechiae and angle closure related to the inflammation
- Pupillary block from posterior synechiae

Epstein et al[4] perfused whole enucleated human eyes with particulate lens material as well as with HMW soluble lens proteins. Aqueous outflow facility decreased in a stepwise fashion as the concentration of lens particles increased. Not all patients undergoing cataract surgery with lens particles in the anterior chamber develop elevated pressures. This suggests that a dynamic state exists between lens particle obstruction of the trabecular meshwork and lens particle clearance by phagocytic

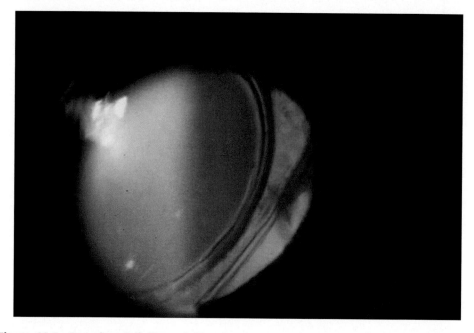

Figure 14-4 Pseudoexfoliation *Subluxed posterior chamber intraocular lens (PCIOL) in a patient with pseudoexfoliation. This patient developed lens particle glaucoma as a result of released lens cortex after the PCIOL dislocation.*

cells. Phagocytic cells in the trabecular meshwork can ingest lens particles and clear the outflow pathways. Macrophages have been observed to contain lens proteins and lens particles. Perhaps, in patients who develop lens particle glaucoma, the mechanism of meshwork clearance becomes overloaded or that phagocytic cells or the meshwork itself are abnormal.

Elevated intraocular pressure can occur after Nd:YAG capsulotomy. Smith[8] has shown that the aqueous outflow facility after Nd:YAG capsulotomy decreases. One hour after the laser procedure, the aqueous outflow facility decreased by an average of 43% and the intraocular pressure increased by an average of 38%. At 24 hours and 1 week after the laser procedure, outflow facility drifted back to normal values. After Nd:YAG capsulotomy, lens debris consisting of lens capsule fragments and fragments of cortex can be seen on slit-lamp examination. It was suggested that this is one of the mechanisms for the decrease in outflow facility.

History

Patients have decreased vision resulting from corneal edema and pain if the intraocular pressure is extremely high. In some cases, a recent history of trauma, cataract surgery, or laser procedure to the eye exists, though pressure rise can also occur years after cataract surgery.[9]

Clinical Examination

The rise in intraocular pressure seen with lens particle glaucoma may correlate with the amount of lens particles circulating in the anterior chamber. There can be a delay of days to weeks between the release of the material and the onset of elevated intraocular pressure. Small white fragments of the lens cortex can be seen circulating in the anterior chamber and can deposit on the corneal endothelium. Elevated intraocular pressure can cause corneal edema, and inflammation can be marked, as evidenced by flare and cell. A hypopyon may be present. Early in the process the angle is open on gonioscopy, although peripheral anterior synechiae may develop.

Special Tests

The diagnosis is made by the observation of free lens particles floating around in the anterior chamber and an elevated intraocular pressure. If the appearance is atypical or if there is a paucity of lens particles, an aqueous sample can be taken to identify lens material histologically (Figure 14-5).

Management

Glaucoma medications mentioned previously for treatment of lens protein glaucoma should be used in conjunction with the degree of pressure elevation. A cycloplegic agent may be used to prevent posterior synechiae. Topical corticosteroids should be used, but the inflammation should not be completely suppressed or lens absorption will be delayed. If medical therapy is not effective, the lens particles should be removed surgically by aspiration. If surgery is delayed, the persistent inflammation may cause peripheral anterior synechiae, pupillary block, and inflammatory membranes that may extend posteriorly, placing tension on the retina. At this stage, membranes and debris must be cut out with vitrectomy instruments.

Usually, surgical aspiration of the material is enough to bring about control of intraocular pressure and inflammation.

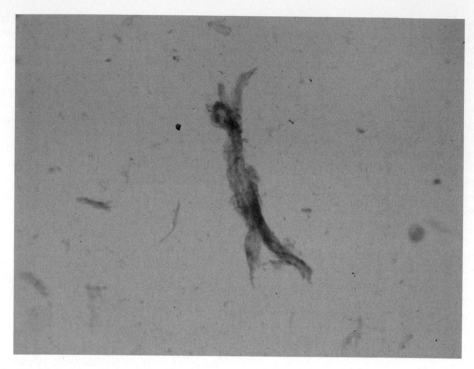

Figure 14-5 Lens fiber *Lens fiber recovered from aqueous aspirate of the eye shown in Figure 14-4.*

LENS-ASSOCIATED UVEITIS (PHACOANAPHYLAXIS)

Lens-associated uveitis (LAU), formerly known as phacoanaphylactic uveitis, can be confused with the previous two entities although it is usually associated with hypotony. This is a rare granulomatous inflammation that develops in situations in which the immune system is exposed to lens proteins:

- After cataract extraction
- After traumatic rupture of the lens capsule
- After cataract extraction in one eye followed by cataract extraction or leaking mature cataract in the other eye

Pathophysiology

Lens-associated uveitis was once thought to represent an immune rejection of previously sequestered lens proteins. However, lens proteins are found in the aqueous of normal eyes. It is now thought that an alteration in immune tolerance to lens proteins occurs, because not all eyes with disrupted lens capsules develop LAU. Cousins and Kraus-Mackiw[10] speculate that LAU is a spectrum of diseases that may be explained by autoimmune, infectious, and toxic mechanisms. The autoimmune theory has never been proven in human eyes, but experimental lens-induced granulomatous endophthalmitis in rats closely resembles LAU. The animals are sensitized to lens homogenates and, upon surgical injury to the lens, develop uveitis with histology similar to LAU. The infectious mechanism postulates that an inflammatory response is mounted against indolent bacteria such as *Propionibacterium acnes* that are found in lens material or that bacteria instigate a loss of immune tolerance in the eye. Finally, the theory of lens toxicity may be described as lens material that directly triggers an inflammatory reaction without previous immunity. All three entities are possibilities in the explanation of LAU, but none has been proven thus far.

Unfortunately, LAU is often diagnosed after enucleation when histology can be examined. The histology of LAU may be described as a zonal granulomatous inflammation with three populations of cell types found in layers around the lens material (Figure 14-6):

Zone 1—Neutrophils closely surround and infiltrate the lens

Zone 2—A secondary zone of monocytes, macrophages, epithelioid cells, and giant cells surround the neutrophils

Zone 3—A nonspecific mononuclear cell infiltrate forms the outer zone of inflammation

History

Patients have pain, decreased vision, and red eye.

Clinical Examination

The presentation can be variable and may present as a low-grade anterior segment inflammation, especially after cataract surgery. Once remaining lens material is resorbed, the inflammation resolves. Panuveitis with a hypopyon

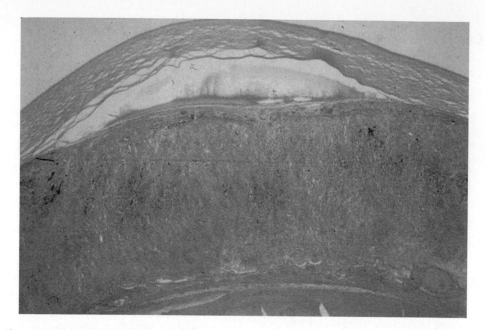

Figure 14-6   Lens-associated uveitis *Zonal granulomatous formation in a patient with lens-associated uveitis. (Courtesy of Donald L. Budenz, MD, Bascom Palmer Eye Institute, Miami, FL)*

represents a more severe presentation that is difficult to distinguish from endophthalmitis (Figure 14-7). There is usually a history of retained lens fragments in the vitreous. The granulomatous inflammatory reaction can occur within days or months after disruption of the lens. Lens-associated uveitis is usually associated with hypotony rather than with elevated intraocular pressure, although high pressures may occur. Keratic precipitates are present, and synechiae can lead to pupillary block or angle-closure glaucoma.

Special Tests

Aspirates of aqueous or vitreous with negative bacterial cultures may help differentiate LAU from bacterial endophthalmitis, but cytology is rarely helpful. Ultrasound may help locate large lens fragments in the vitreous chamber in the setting of cataract surgery or trauma.

Management

If left untreated, a relentless uveitis can lead to phthisis. Topical, sub-Tenon's, and oral steroids may be used as a temporizing measure, but definitive treatment results from removal of lens fragments, optimally by pars plana vitrectomy. Historically, the prognosis of severe cases of LAU has been very poor, but currently, with better surgical techniques and equipment, the possibility of retaining good vision is improving.[11]

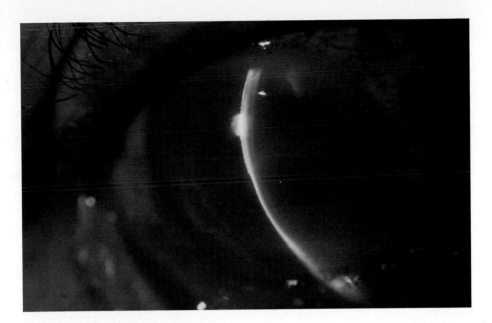

Figure 14-7   Lens-associated uveitis   *Severe anterior chamber inflammation, hypopyon, and corneal edema in a patient with lens-associated uveitis. (Courtesy of Donald L. Budenz, MD, Bascom Palmer Eye Institute, Miami, FL)*

PHACOMORPHIC GLAUCOMA

Phacomorphic glaucoma results from angle closure secondary to a mature or hypermature lens. It may be distinguished from the previous entities by the clinical appearance of an intumescent lens, shallow anterior chamber, and angle closure.

Pathophysiology

Phacomorphic glaucoma is a direct sequela of a mature or hypermature lens that has become intumescent, causing crowding of the anterior segment structures.[12] In the early stage, pupillary block may cause high intraocular pressure. Later, the growing size of the lens presses forward on the iris in the periphery, blocking off outflow through the trabecular meshwork. Phacomorphic glaucoma is a common condition in developing countries in which cataract surgery is delayed. The visual prognosis is poor, with one study reporting that only 57% of 49 patients with phacomorphic glaucoma attained visual acuity of 6/12 or better.[13]

History

Patients have chronic or acute decrease in vision, ocular pain, headache, and photophobia.[14]

Clinical Examination

The crux of the problem is the mature or hypermature cataract causing a shallow anterior chamber. The pupil may be mid-dilated with or without iris bombé, and gonioscopy reveals angle closure. The intraocular pressure is high from obstruction of aqueous outflow and as a result, the cornea may be edematous (Figure 14-8A,B).

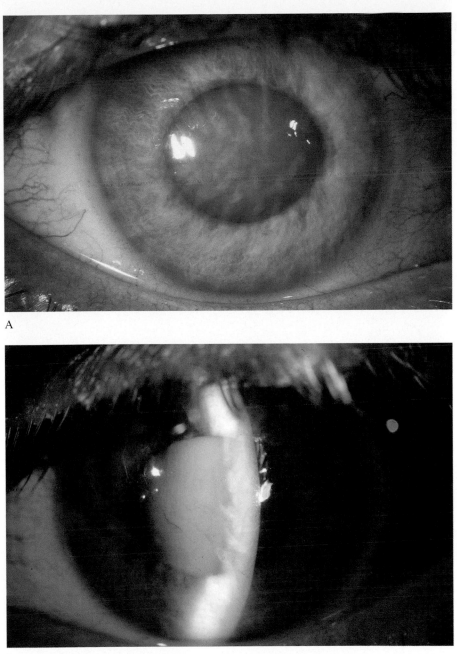

A

B

Figure 14-8A,B Phacomorphic glaucoma *A. Slit-lamp photograph of an eye with phacomorphic glaucoma. Descemet's folds from an edematous cornea and darkly brunescent cataract are seen. **B.** Slit-beam photograph of the same eye shows the corneal swelling and narrow anterior chamber. (Courtesy of Douglas J. Rhee, MD, Wills Eye Hospital, Philadelphia, PA.)*

Management

Medical therapy to suppress aqueous formation is the first line of treatment. Miotics may increase contact between the lens and iris and should not be used.[12] Laser iridotomy should be performed to alleviate any component of pupillary block. Iridotomy may open up the angle, lower the intraocular pressure, and allow the eye to quiet before cataract removal. It may also give the clinician an opportunity to examine the angle for peripheral anterior synechiae.[14] The degree of scarring in the angle may signal the need for glaucoma surgery either at the time of cataract removal or in the future. The definitive treatment for phacomorphic glaucoma is removal of the intumescent lens. Capsulorrhexis in the setting of a dense lens may be facilitated by the use of indocyanine green staining of the anterior capsule.

REFERENCES

1. Hogan M, Zimmerman L. *Ophthalmic Pathology: An Atlas and Textbook.* Philadelphia: Saunders; 797, 1962.
2. Irvine S, Irvine A. Lens-induced uveitis and glaucoma. 35:489, 1952.
3. Epstein D, Jedziniak J, Grant W. Identification of heavy-molecular-weight soluble protein in aqueous humor in human phacolytic glaucoma. *Invest Ophthalmol Vis Sci* 17:398–402, 1978.
4. Epstein D, Jedziniak J, Grant W. Obstruction of aqueous outflow by lens particles and by heavy-molecular-weight soluble lens proteins. *Invest Ophthalmol Vis Sci* 17:272–277, 1978.
5. Rosenbaum J. Chemotactic activity of lens proteins and the pathogenesis of phacolytic glaucoma. *Arch Ophthalmol* 105:1582, 1987.
6. Uemura A, Sameshima M, Nakao K. Complications of hypermature cataract: Spontaneous absorption of lens material and phacolytic glaucoma-associated retinal perivasculitis. *Jpn J Ophthalmol* 32:35–40, 1988.
7. Lim MC, Doe EA, Vroman DT, Robert H, Rosa J, Richard K, Parrish I. Late onset lens particle glaucoma as a consequence of spontaneous dislocation of an intraocular lens in pseudoexfoliation syndrome. *Am J Ophthalmol* 132:261–263, 2001.
8. Smith C. Effect of neodymium:YAG posterior capsulotomy on outflow facility. *Glaucoma* 6:171, 1984.
9. Barnhorst D, Meyers S, Meyers T. Lens-induced glaucoma 65 years after congenital cataract surgery. *Am J Ophthalmol* 188:807–808, 1994.
10. Cousins SW, Kraus-Mackiw E. Ocular infection and immunity. In: Pepose JS, Holland GN, Wilhelmus, KR, eds. St. Louis, MO: Mosby; 1552, 1996.
11. Oruc S, Kaplan H. Outcome of vitrectomy for retained lens fragments after phacoemulsification. *Ocul Immunol Inflamm* 9:41–47, 2001.
12. Liebmann JM, Ritch R. Glaucoma associated with lens intumescence and dislocation. In: Ritch R, Shields MB, Krupin T, eds. *The Glaucomas,* vol 2. St. Louis, MO: Mosby-Year Book; 1033–1053, 1996.
13. Prajna N, Ramakrishnan R, Krishnadas R, Manoharan N. Lens induced glaucomas—visual results and risk factors for final visual acuity. *Indian J Ophthalmol* 44:149–155, 1996.
14. Tomey K. Neodymium:YAG laser iridotomy in the initial management of phacomorphic glaucoma. *Ophthalmology* 99:660–665, 1992.

Chapter 15

TRAUMATIC GLAUCOMA

Mary Jude Cox, MD and John B. Jeffers, MD

Following blunt or penetrating trauma to the globe, patients often develop difficulties with intraocular pressure control. Intraocular pressure may be elevated, or the eye may be hypotonous. Patients may have difficulty acutely or many years following the injury. In either case, a thorough history and examination often will determine the cause and severity of the intraocular damage and the appropriate course of treatment. Blunt and penetrating trauma can result in injury to any of the ocular structures. This chapter focuses on traumatic hyphemas, angle recession, and cyclodialysis clefts.

TRAUMATIC HYPHEMA

Definition

The term *hyphema* refers to blood in the anterior chamber. The amount of blood may be microscopic, termed *microhyphema,* visible only at the slit lamp as nonlayering red blood cells in the aqueous, or the red blood cells may layer in the anterior chamber (Figures 15-1A,B through 15-3). A *total hyphema* refers to layered blood filling the entire anterior chamber (Figure 15-5). A total hyphema that has clotted and appears black in color is referred to as an *eight-ball hyphema* (Figure 15-6). A traumatic hyphema can result from either blunt or penetrating injury to the globe. The majority of hyphemas resolve gradually without sequelae; however, complications such as rebleeding, increased intraocular pressure, and corneal blood staining can occur (Figure 15-7).

Epidemiology

A traumatic hyphema may follow either blunt or penetrating trauma. Traumatic hyphemas are most common in young active men, with a male-to-female ratio of approximately three to one. In general, the risk of complications such as rebleeding, uncontrolled intraocular pressure, or corneal blood staining increases with the size of the hyphema. Patients with sickling hemoglobinopathies, however, are the exception. These patients are at increased risk for complications regardless of the size of the hyphema.

Rebleeding occurs in up to 35% of patients. The majority of rebleeding episodes take place within 2 to 5 days postinjury. Rebleeding is often larger than the original hyphema and more prone to complications.

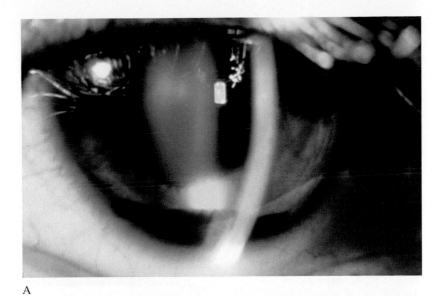

A

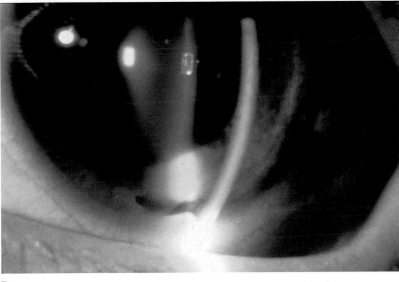

B

Figure 15-1A,B   Small hyphema   *A. This small hyphema shows blood layering in the anterior chamber. Most hyphemas resorb gradually. **B.** The same eye 4 days later has a much smaller clot in the anterior chamber.*

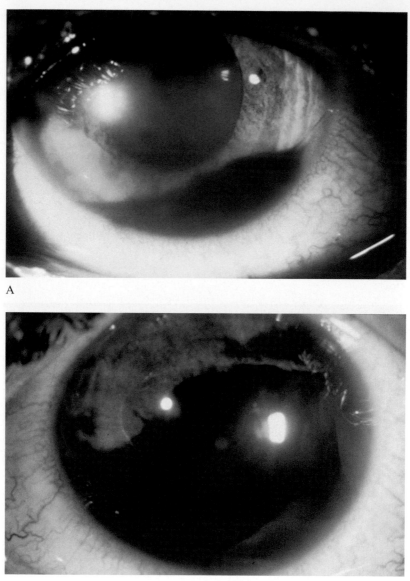

A

B

Figure 15-2A,B   Traumatic hyphema   *A. Blood layers in the anterior chamber of this eye with a traumatic hyphema. **B.** The same eye rebleeds 24 hours later, demonstrating an increase in the amount of blood in the anterior chamber.*

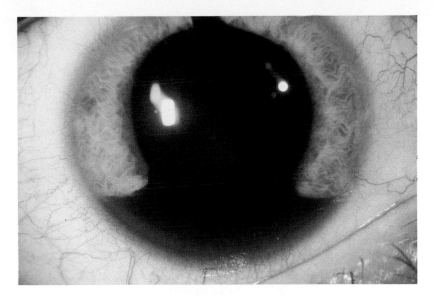

Figure 15-3　Hemorrhage in new hyphema　*The hemorrhage in this new hyphema is settling into the inferior anterior chamber. Patients are instructed to keep their head elevated to assist this process.*

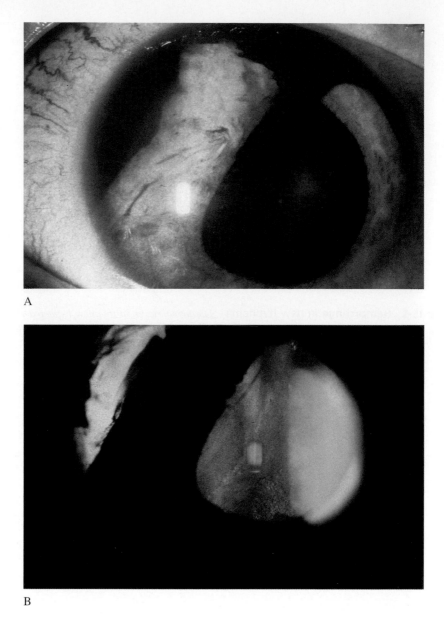

A

B

Figure 15-4A,B Iridodialysis *A. Blunt trauma can result in tears at the iris root (iridodialysis) and cataract formation in addition to traumatic hyphema. **B.** Retroillumination demonstrates the large iridodialysis in this trauma patient.*

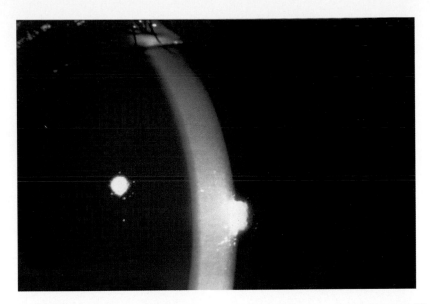

Figure 15-5 Total hyphema *A total hyphema is present following a baseball injury. The anterior chamber is filled with bright red blood.*

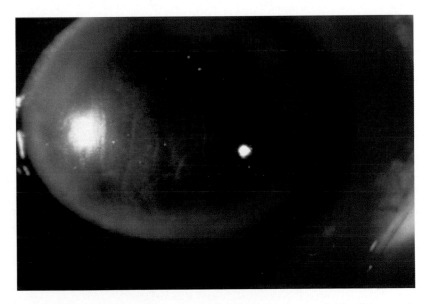

Figure 15-6 Eight-ball hyphema *An eight-ball hyphema is a total clot of the anterior chamber that gets its black appearance from decreased oxygenation as a result of impaired aqueous circulation.*

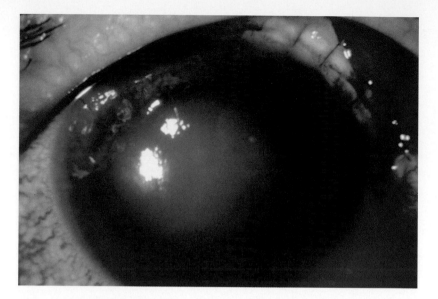

Figure 15-7 Corneal blood staining *Corneal blood staining persists in this eye following surgical evacuation of the hyphema.*

Pathophysiology

Blunt trauma causes compressive forces that result in the rupture of iris and ciliary body vessels. Tears in the ciliary body result in damage to the major arterial circle of the iris. Penetrating injuries can cause direct damage to blood vessels. Clotted blood plugs these damaged blood vessels. Rebleeding occurs as these clots retract and lyse (see Figures 15-2A,B and 15-3).

Intraocular pressure rises acutely as red blood cells, inflammatory cells, and debris obstruct the trabecular meshwork. Elevated intraocular pressure can also be the result of pupillary block caused by the clot in the anterior chamber or mechanical blocking of the trabecular meshwork. Eight-ball hyphemas often cause this form of pupillary block. An eight-ball hyphema is a clotted total hyphema, which impairs aqueous circulation (see Figure 15-6). The impaired aqueous circulation causes a decrease in oxygen concentration in the anterior chamber and the black appearance of the clot.

In patients with sickle cell disease or trait, sickling causes the red blood cells to be rigid and easily trapped in the trabecular meshwork, leading to elevated intraocular pressure even in the presence of a small hyphema. Sickle cell patients are subject to vascular occlusion and optic nerve damage at lower intraocular pressures as the result of microvascular compromise.

History and Clinical Examination

Patients present with a history of trauma. A thorough evaluation of the timing and nature of the trauma is important to determine the likelihood of additional injuries and the need for close observation and treatment. Patients may be asymptomatic or have decreased vision, photophobia, and pain. Nausea and vomiting may accompany a rise in intraocular pressure. There may be evidence of orbital trauma or damage to other ocular tissues.

Slit Lamp Slit-lamp examination may show circulating red blood cells alone or in combination with a layered hyphema in the anterior chamber. There may be evidence of trauma to other ocular structures such as cataract (Figure 15-8A,B), phacodenesis, subconjunctival hemorrhage, foreign bodies, lacerations, iris sphincter tears, or tears at the iris root (iridodialysis). Figure 15-4.

Gonioscopy Gonioscopy should be delayed until the risk for rebleeding has passed. When performed 3 to 4 weeks posttrauma, the angle may appear undamaged or, more often, may show evidence of angle recession. A cyclodialysis cleft may be present.

Posterior Pole The posterior pole may show evidence of blunt or penetrating trauma. Commotio retina, choroidal ruptures, retinal detachments, intraocular foreign bodies, or vitreous hemorrhage may be present. Scleral depression should be delayed until the risk for rebleeding has passed.

Special Tests

B-scan ultrasonography should be performed in any patient in whom there is no view of the posterior pole. Computed tomographic scan of the orbits should be performed if the clinical examination indicates orbital fractures or intraocular foreign bodies.

Any black or Hispanic patients or any patient with a positive family history should undergo sickle prep or hemoglobin electrophoresis to determine the presence of sickling hemoglobinopathies.

Management

The affected eye is shielded, and the patient is typically placed on bedrest with the head of the bed elevated (see Figure 15-3). Aspirin and nonsteroidal agents should be avoided. Topical cycloplegics and steroids are given. Aminocaproic acid, an antifibrinolytic, can be given orally to prevent rebleeding. Aminocaproic acid may cause postural hypotension, nausea, and vomiting and should be avoided in pregnant patients and those with cardiac, hepatic, or renal disease.

Elevated intraocular pressure is treated topically with beta-blockers, alpha-agonists, or carbonic anhydrase inhibitors (CAIs). Miotics may increase inflammation and should be avoided. Oral or intravenous CAIs may also be given. However, CAIs should be avoided in patients with sickling hemoglobinopathies because these agents increase the pH of the aqueous, resulting in increased sickling. In addition, hyperosmotics should be used with care in sickle

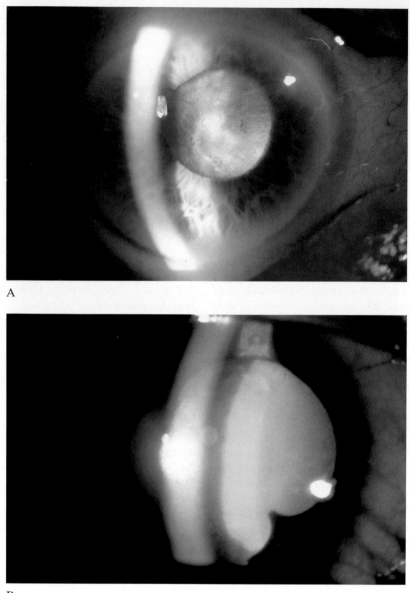

A

B

Figure 15-8A,B   Traumatic cataracts   *A. Traumatic cataracts often result from blunt trauma. Cataracts may appear acutely or weeks to months following trauma. This cataract resulted from disruption of the lens capsule and caused a phacolytic glaucoma. **B.** This eye with an old traumatic cataract shows synechiae formation at 11 o'clock. (adherence of the iris to the anterior lens capsule).*

cell patients because hemoconcentration may also lead to increased sickling.

Surgical intervention is indicated in patients with large, nonclearing hyphemas, early corneal blood staining (Figure 5-7), and uncontrolled intraocular pressure. The timing of surgical intervention for intraocular pressure control depends on the individual patient. In a patient with a healthy optic nerve, an intraocular pressure of 50 mm Hg for 5 days or an intraocular pressure greater than 35 mm Hg for 7 days requires surgical intervention. Patients with compromised optic nerves or corneal endothelium require earlier intervention, as do patients with sickle cell disease or trait. Surgical intervention is indicated in sickle cell patients with an intraocular pressure greater than 24 mm Hg for more than 24 hours.

Surgical options to remove the hyphema include anterior chamber washout, clot expression at the limbus, or removal with anterior vitrectomy instrumentation. If possible, clot removal should be performed 4 to 7 days posttrauma in order to prevent new bleeding. In most cases, a guarded filtration procedure is usually performed to control intraocular pressure.

ANGLE RECESSION

Definition

Angle recession refers to a tear in the ciliary body between the longitudinal and circular muscle layers. It occurs as the result of blunt or penetrating trauma to the globe.

Epidemiology

Angle recession occurs following blunt or penetrating trauma to the anterior segment. The risk of developing angle recession glaucoma is proportional to the extent of ciliary body damage, with an incidence as high as 10% in eyes with greater than 180 degrees of damage. Glaucoma may develop months to years after the original injury. Patients who develop angle recession glaucoma may be predisposed to open-angle glaucoma, as evidenced by the fact that up to 50% of these patients will develop elevated pressures in the contralateral eye.

Pathophysiology

Angle recession is caused by a tear between the circular and longitudinal muscle layers of the ciliary body. Angle recession glaucoma results from outflow obstruction. This outflow obstruction may occur as the result of direct damage to the trabecular meshwork or as the result of a Descemet-like endothelial proliferation over the trabecular meshwork.

History and Clinical Examination

Patients present with either a recent or remote history of trauma in the affected eye. Patients may be asymptomatic or present with pain, photophobia, and decreased vision as the result of elevated intraocular pressure. They may have evidence of visual field loss or an afferent pupillary defect from glaucomatous optic nerve damage. There may also be evidence on examination of damage to other ocular or orbital structures.

Slit Lamp Slit-lamp examination may show evidence of previous trauma. Corneal scarring or blood staining, cataract (see Figure 15-8A,B), phacodenesis, iris sphincter tears, or tears at the iris root (iridodialysis) (see Figure 15-4) may be present.

Gonioscopy Gonioscopy demonstrates an irregular widening of the ciliary body band (Figure 15-9). There may be evidence of torn iris processes or increased prominence of the scleral spur. The normal ciliary body should be roughly even in size around its circumference and not as wide as the trabecular meshwork. Comparison with the unaffected eye often aides in diagnosis.

Posterior Pole The posterior pole may show evidence of previous blunt or penetrating trauma. Choroidal ruptures, retinal detachments, or vitreous hemorrhage may be present. Asymmetric optic nerve cupping from elevated intraocular pressure in the affected eye may also be present.

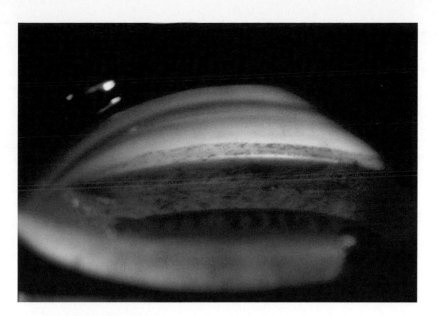

Figure 15-9 Angle recession *This eye with angle recession shows irregular widening of the ciliary body band on gonioscopy.*

Special Tests

Visual field testing may demonstrate glaucomatous field loss.

Management

Patients who demonstrate angle recession on gonioscopy following trauma need to be followed indefinitely for the development of glaucoma. If elevated intraocular pressures are found, they are often difficult to control. Initially they can be treated medically with aqueous suppressants. Hyperosmotics may be added if necessary. Miotics often make angle recession worse, because they decrease uveoscleral outflow in eyes that rely on uveoscleral outflow for intraocular pressure control. Laser trabeculoplasty has limited success in eyes with angle recession. A guarded filtration procedure is often required to control intraocular pressure in these patients.

CYCLODIALYSIS CLEFT

Definition

The term *cyclodialysis cleft* refers to a focal detachment of the ciliary body from its insertion at the scleral spur (Figure 15-10). It may occur as the result of blunt or penetrating trauma or as a complication of intraocular surgery, and leads to temporary or permanent hypotony.

Epidemiology

Cyclodialysis clefts that result from blunt or penetrating trauma are less common than angle recession. The presence of a cleft should be considered in any hypotonous eye with a history of trauma.

Pathophysiology

Trauma causes a separation of the ciliary body from its attachment to the scleral spur. This allows a direct passage of aqueous from the anterior chamber to the suprachoroidal space, leading to hypotony. Spontaneous or induced closure of the cleft results in elevation of the intraocular pressure as the primary outflow pathway of aqueous is disrupted.

History and Clinical Examination

Patients present with a history of trauma or intraocular surgery in the affected eye. They may be asymptomatic or have decreased vision. The affected eye may be hypotonous or have elevated intraocular pressure, pain, photophobia, and redness as a result of spontaneous closure of a previous cleft.

Slit Lamp Slit-lamp examination may show evidence of previous blunt or penetrating trauma such as corneal scarring or blood staining, cataract, disruption of the zonules supporting the lens (phacodenesis), iris sphincter tears, or tears at the iris root (iridodialysis) (Figure 4A,B). Evidence of previous intraocular surgery, such as posterior or anterior intraocular lens placement, may also be present. The affected eye can be hypotonous with corneal folds and a shallow anterior chamber when compared with the contralateral eye.

Gonioscopy Gonioscopy demonstrates a deep angle recess with a gap between the sclera and ciliary body. This is in contrast to angle recession, which appears as an irregular, widened ciliary body band. Angle recession may also be present in the affected eye as a result of trauma.

Posterior Pole Hypotony can result in bullous detachments and folds of the choroid. If these folds involve the macula, the condition is termed *hypotony maculopathy*. Evidence of previous trauma may also be present, such as choroidal rupture, posterior vitreous detachment, or macular hole.

Special Tests

B-scan ultrasonography should be performed in any hypotonous posttraumatic eye with a limited view of the posterior pole in order to rule out occult scleral rupture or retinal detachment.

Management

Occasionally, atropine may result in cyclodialysis cleft closure. Argon laser and cryotherapy may also be tried; however, most cyclodialysis clefts with persistent hypotony require surgical closure. Following closure of the cleft, the intraocular pressure often elevates dramatically and should be monitored closely. Medical treatment with aqueous suppressants and hyperosmotics may be initiated as necessary.

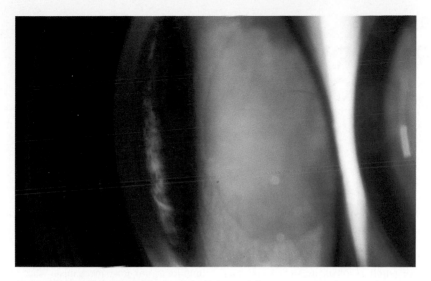

Figure 15-10 Cyclodialysis cleft *A cyclodialysis cleft appears as a deep angle recess with a gap between the sclera and ciliary body.*

Chapter 16

PRIMARY ANGLE-CLOSURE GLAUCOMA

Erin C. Doe, MD

Angle-closure glaucomas arising from a preexisting iris configuration are termed *primary angle closure*. This term encompasses acute, subacute, and chronic angle-closure secondary to relative pupillary block as well as plateau iris. The underlying mechanism in all forms of angle closure is the mechanical obstruction of outflow through the trabecular meshwork by peripheral iris. In acute, subacute, and chronic primary angle closure, the iris is pushed

forward by relatively higher pressure behind the iris. In plateau iris, the iris is pushed forward by anteriorly rotated ciliary processes.

The term *primary* is confusing, because it implies an unknown mechanism when in fact the mechanism is clear. However, this term continues to be used and differentiates these glaucomas from the *secondary* angle-closure glaucomas; that is, neovascular, tumor, and others.

PRIMARY ANGLE-CLOSURE GLAUCOMA WITH RELATIVE PUPILLARY BLOCK

Epidemiology

White patients have a 2% incidence of narrow angles and a 0.1% rate of acute angle-closure glaucoma (AACG). Eskimos have up to 40 times this rate. AACG is less common in blacks; rather, they are more likely to develop chronic angle-closure glaucoma. Asians have a rate of AACG that is higher than whites but not as high as that of Eskimos. Women develop AACG at a rate three to four times that of men. The highest incidence is in individuals between the ages of 55 and 65 years. Hyperopia, and usually a smaller anterior chamber, is also a risk factor.

Pathophysiology

The apposition of the iris sphincter to the anterior lens capsule may cause an increase in pressure

behind the iris (Figure 16-1A), causing the iris in susceptible individuals to bow forward (Figure 16-1B) and obstruct the trabecular meshwork (Figure 16-1C), leading to a rise in intraocular pressure. The apposition of the pupil to the lens and the subsequent increase in pressure behind the iris is termed *relative pupillary block*. If the relative pupillary block is large and the angle is already very narrow, then complete obstruction of the trabecular meshwork occurs, and the intraocular pressure rise may be precipitous—resulting in AACG. If the relative pupillary block is small, the angle is narrow but not occludable, and the trabecular meshwork is blocked only in small portions, then the intraocular pressure rises very slowly, often over many years. This process is termed *chronic primary angle closure*. Subacute angle-closure lies between acute and chronic with regard to the amount of time the intraocular pressure rises.

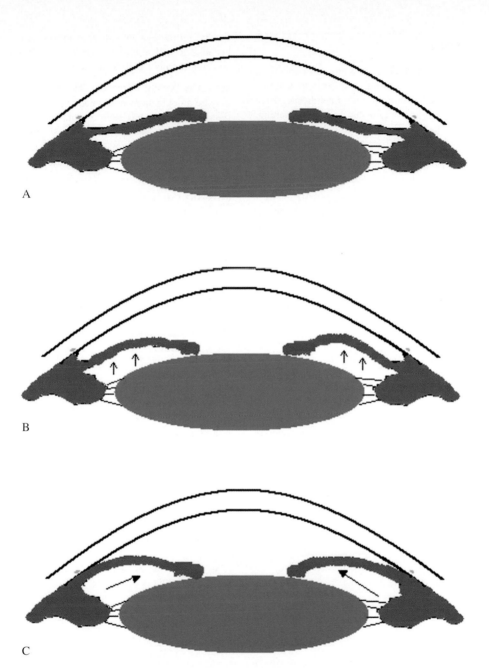

Figure 16-1A–C   Pathophysiology of primary angle closure   *Drawing of (A) apposition of iris margin to lens, (B) aqueous pressure developing behind iris and pushing iris forward, and (C) iris bombé causing obstruction of the trabecular meshwork.*

History

ACUTE ANGLE CLOSURE   Symptoms range from unilateral mild blurring and pain to extreme pain, nausea, vomiting, and diaphoresis. These symptoms commonly occur during the evening. Attacks may be associated with fatigue, dim illumination, stress, or prolonged near work.

SUBACUTE ANGLE CLOSURE   Symptoms of subacute angle closure include intermittent attacks of pain and possibly mildly blurry vision. Symptoms often occur with dim illumination, stress, fatigue, and near work. Sleep may break the attack. This may be confused with migraine headache.

CHRONIC ANGLE CLOSURE   Usually, there are no symptoms. Once the closure is complete, the pressure may rise acutely, and the patient may experience pain.

Clinical Examination

Slit Lamp and Gonioscopy

ACUTE ANGLE CLOSURE   The affected eye may show a mid-dilated pupil, intensive conjunctival hyperemia, corneal edema, and a shallow anterior chamber. The iris is often in a classic bombé pattern (Figures 16-2 and 16-3A,B). The intraocular pressure may be as high as 80 mm Hg. Mild cell and flare are often present. Gonioscopy is often difficult because of the corneal edema. If a view is available, the iris will obscure the trabecular meshwork.

The fellow eye should be examined closely because it will almost always have a shallow anterior chamber with a narrow angle.

SUBACUTE ANGLE CLOSURE   The affected eye may be quiet or show mild injection and cell and flare if an attack has been recent. The anterior chamber may be somewhat shallow (Figure 16-4A,B), and a mild form of iris bombé may be present. Gonioscopy demonstrates a narrow but nonoccluded angle.

CHRONIC ANGLE CLOSURE   The eye is usually quiet with a mildly shallow angle. Gonioscopy demonstrates a narrow angle with broad areas of peripheral anterior synechia. Advanced cases may have little trabecular meshwork visible.

Posterior Pole

ACUTE ANGLE CLOSURE   Early in the attack, the optic nerve head can show edema and hyperemia. A prolonged attack may produce a pale optic nerve head with visual field loss disproportionate to the disc cupping.

Arterial pulsations may be seen if the intraocular pressure is greater than the diastolic pressure at the optic nerve head. If the intraocular pressure exceeds the perfusion pressure of the central retinal artery, then ischemic retina will be seen.

SUBACUTE ANGLE CLOSURE   Optic nerve head cupping may be present if the attacks have been frequent and over a long period of time.

CHRONIC ANGLE CLOSURE   The optic nerve head may show typical changes associated with chronic, high intraocular pressure.

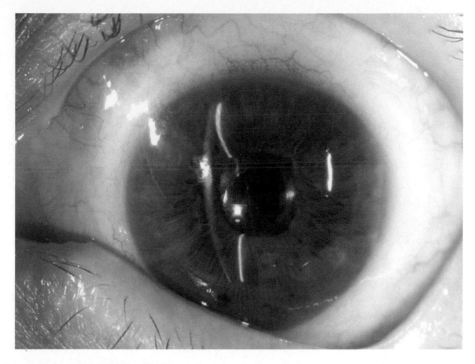

Figure 16-2   Iris bombé   *Slit-beam photograph showing the appearance of iris bombé. This eye has iris bombé from uveitis causing 360 of posterior synechiae (scarring between the pupillary margin and the anterior surface of the intraocular lens), causing secondary pupillary block by mechanically blocking aqueous flow through the pupil.*

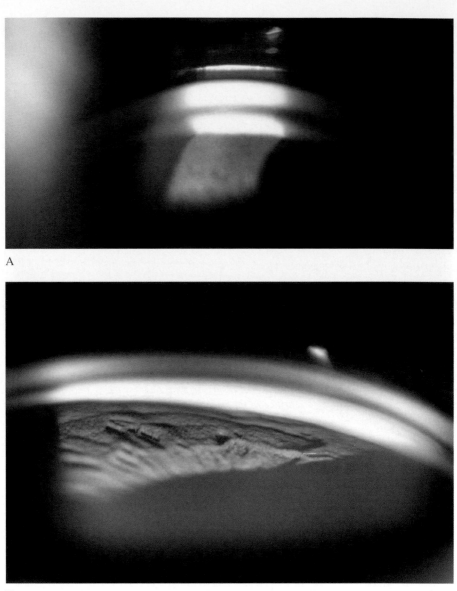

A

B

Figure 16-3A,B   Primary acute angle-closure glaucoma   *A patient with primary acute angle-closure glaucoma and a relatively clear cornea.* **A.** *The slit-beam photograph of the gonioscopic view shows the steep approach of the iris in this case of acute angle-closure glaucoma (iris bombé).* **B.** *The diffuse illumination of the gonioscopic view of the same eye shows no angle structures (i.e., an occluded angle).*

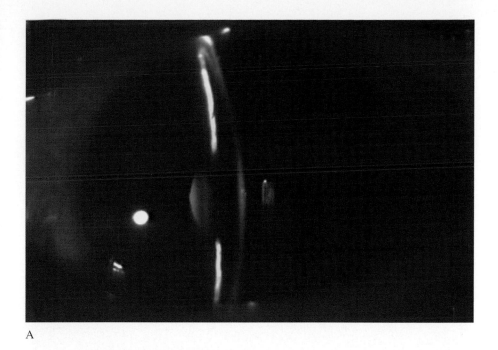

A

Figure 16-4A,B   Narrow anterior chamber angle   A. *Slit-beam photograph showing a narrow anterior chamber angle.* **B.** *The gonioscopic view of the same eye showing the absence of angle structures in an eye with normal intraocular pressure. This angle is occludable. (Courtesy of Douglas J. Rhee, MD, Wills Eye Hospital, Philadelphia, PA.)*

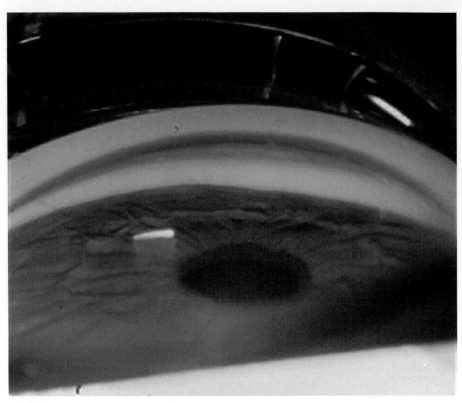

B

Figure 16-4A,B   Narrow anterior chamber angle   *(continued)*

Management

ACUTE ANGLE CLOSURE   Attacks of AACG require breaking of the relative pupillary block for resolution. The definite treatment is a peripheral iridectomy, which prevents further attacks.

The angle may occasionally be opened by pressure (indentation gonioscopy) on the central cornea with a Zeiss-type lens. This causes a transient increase in pressure in the anterior chamber and mechanically opens the angle.

Pharmacologic manipulation of the iris sphincter or dilator may also break the attack by moving the iris sphincter away from the lens surface at the critical 4- to 5-mm zone, although this has limited success and may make the situation worse by further increasing relative pupillary block. Aqueous suppressants and osmotic agents may also break the attack by lowering the intraocular pressure and dehydrating the vitreous, allowing the lens-iris diaphragm to move posteriorly and changing the fluid dynamics causing the relative pupillary block.

The most common treatment method is to first lower the pressure by aqueous suppressants and osmotic agents. Once the corneal edema has cleared, a laser peripheral iridotomy can be performed (Figures 16-5A,B through 16-8).

SUBACUTE ANGLE CLOSURE   Definitive management is a laser peripheral iridotomy.

CHRONIC ANGLE CLOSURE   Management includes a laser peripheral iridotomy to prevent further angle closure. The trabecular meshwork may have sustained enough damage that the intraocular pressure will still be elevated despite a patent iridotomy, necessitating continued use of medications to lower the intraocular pressure.

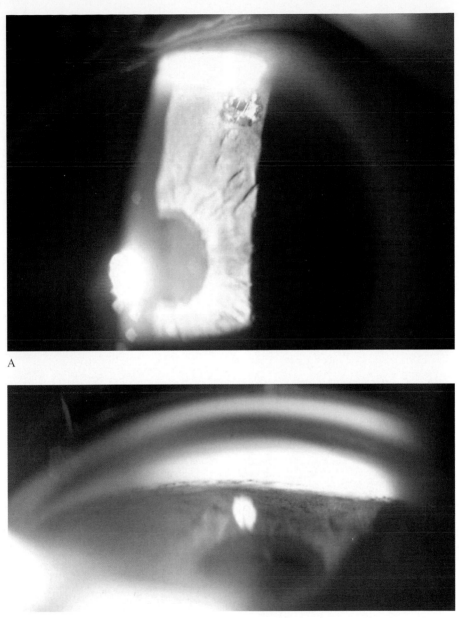

A

B

Figure 16-5A,B **Appearance after peripheral laser iridotomy** *A. Slit-lamp photograph of the same eye shown in* **Figure 16-3** *following peripheral laser iridotomy.* **B.** *Gonioscopic view following the laser iridotomy shows deepening of the anterior chamber. The angle structures are now visible. There is residual pigment deposition on the angle from the appositional closure.*

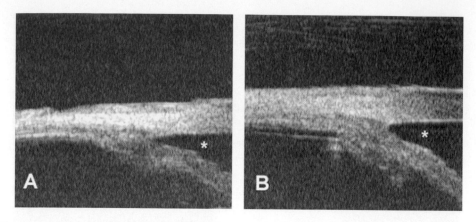

Figure 16-6A,B Appearance after laser iridotomy *A. Ultrasound biomicroscopy (UBM) of a narrow anterior chamber angle (star) before laser iridotomy. **B.** UBM of the same angle following laser iridotomy shows deepening of the anterior chamber angle.*

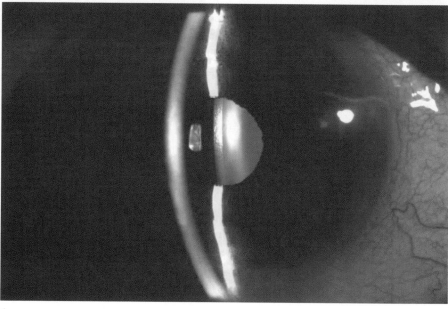

A

Figure 16-7A–C Plateau iris syndrome *A. Slit-beam photograph showing a relatively deep anterior chamber. There is a patent peripheral iridotomy superiorly.*

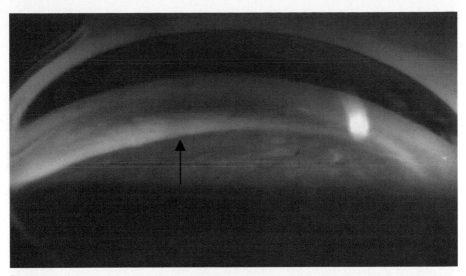

B

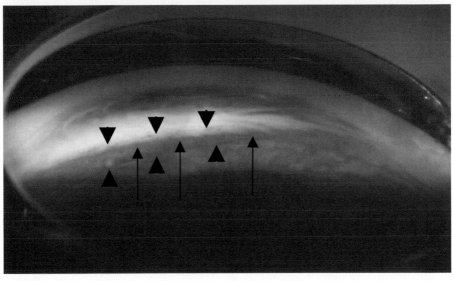

C

Figure 16-7A–C   Plateau iris syndrome   *(continued)*   *B. Gonioscopy with no pressure on the cornea; no angle structures are visible. The* white arrow *shows a prominent last iris fold.* *C. Indentation gonioscopy. The* arrow *pointing up shows the same prominent last iris fold seen in* *(B); the* arrow *pointing down points toward the trabecular meshwork now revealed behind the prominent iris fold. The image is distorted because of the corneal striae induced by the indentation. (Courtesy of Douglas J. Rhee, MD, Wills Eye Hospital, Philadelphia, PA.)*

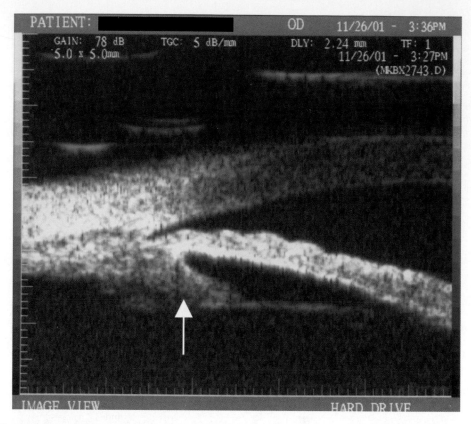

Figure 16-8 *UBM of the same eye shown in* **Figure 16-7.** *The* arrow *shows the anteriorly displaced ciliary body causing a prominent iris roll directly above it in this picture. (Courtesy of Douglas J. Rhee, MD, Wills Eye Hospital, Philadelphia, PA.)*

PLATEAU IRIS

Epidemiology

Plateau iris typically occurs in the fourth through sixth decades in women. Hyperopia is not as common in plateau iris as it is in angle closure secondary to relative pupillary block.

Pathophysiology

In plateau iris *configuration,* the iris is displaced anteriorly at its root by large or abnormally positioned ciliary processes. The trabecular meshwork may be occluded if the displacement is anterior enough. A component of relative pupillary block may also be present, particularly in older individuals.

Plateau iris *syndrome* is defined by having occlusion of the trabecular meshwork despite a patent laser peripheral iridotomy.

History

Symptoms, as with angle closure secondary to relative pupillary block, are dependent on the rapidity of the angle closure. An acute attack may occur if a component of relative pupillary block exists; the symptoms will mirror those of acute angle closure. In most cases, the angle closes slowly and there are no symptoms until the intraocular pressure is very elevated or the visual field loss is severe.

Clinical Examination

Usually, the eye is quiet and the central anterior chamber is deep. Compression gonioscopy demonstrates a prominent last roll of iris, pushed forward by the ciliary processes. Occasionally, individual processes can be seen with compression. Optic nerve changes reflect the chronicity and extent of the intraocular pressure elevation.

Management

No intervention is needed for plateau iris configuration if no obstruction of the trabecular meshwork is occurring. A laser peripheral iridotomy may be indicated if there is an element of relative pupillary block.

In plateau iris syndrome, iridoplasty may be useful to help "draw" the iris out of the angle. Typical treatment includes 16 spots of argon green laser placed in the far periphery. Spot size is usually 500 μm, 0.5 seconds, and 200 to 400 mJ.

Filtration surgery may ultimately become necessary in some patients.

Chapter 17

SECONDARY ANGLE-CLOSURE GLAUCOMA

Douglas J. Rhee, MD

Jamie E. Nicholl

NEOVASCULAR GLAUCOMA

Definition

Neovascular glaucoma (NVG) is a secondary closed-angle form of glaucoma. Initially, a fibrovascular membrane grows over the trabecular meshwork. This is an occluded but open angle. Within a short period of time, the fibrovascular membrane contracts, closing the anterior chamber angle. This often leads to a dramatic elevation of intraocular pressure, usually greater than 40 mm Hg.

Epidemiology and Pathophysiology

The exact incidence of all NVGs is not known. Neovascular glaucoma can occur as the sequela of several different possible conditions, most commonly, ischemic central retinal vein occlusions and proliferative diabetic retinopathy. Other predisposing factors include ischemic central retinal arterial occlusions, ocular ischemic syndrome, branch retinal arterial or vein occlusions, chronic uveitis, chronic retinal detachments, and radiation therapy.

Some of the best estimates of the incidence of NVG come from studies on central retinal vascular occlusions (CRVOs). Approximately one third of all CRVOs are ischemic. Between 16% and 60%, depending on the extent of capillary nonperfusion, of ischemic CRVOs will develop neovascularization of the iris. Approximately 20% of eyes with proliferative diabetic retinopathy will develop NVG. Approximately 18% of eyes with central retinal arterial occlusions will develop neovascularization of the iris (Figure 17-1). Eyes with neovascularization of the iris are at high risk for developing NVG.

History

Patients may be asymptomatic or may complain of pain, red eye, and decreased vision.

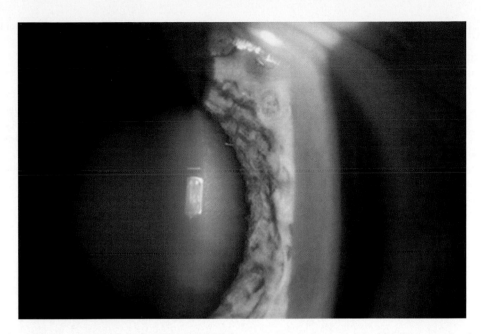

Figure 17-1   Neovascularization of the iris   *Neovascularization of the iris (fine, noncircular vessels) is seen near the papillary border extending onto the iris.*

Clinical Examination

Slit Lamp Corneal edema may be present in the anterior chamber from elevated intraocular pressure. The anterior chamber is usually deep with some flare. Hyphema and rare white cells may be present. Fine, nonradial vessels are present on the iris (Figure 17-1).

Gonioscopy If the cornea is clear, gonioscopy may show a vascular net over the angle in the early stages (Figure 17-2). Later, broad peripheral anterior synechiae occluding some or all of the angle may be seen.

Posterior Pole Retinal findings are consistent with the underlying pathology.

Management

Typically, medical management is not adequate in controlling the intraocular pressure. Surgical intervention is usually required. Options include trabeculectomy with an antifibrotic agent, a glaucoma drainage implant device, and cyclodestructive procedures.

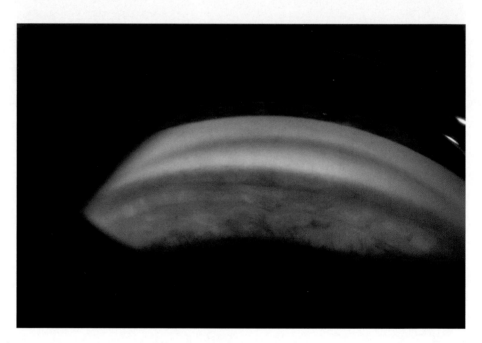

Figure 17-2 Neovascularization of the iris *Gonioscopic photo showing neovascularization (fine, nonradial vessels) over the trabecular meshwork before the fibrovascular membrane has contracted causing peripheral anterior synechiae.*

IRIDOCORNEAL SYNDROMES

Definition

The iridocorneal (ICE) syndrome is a group of secondary angle-closure glaucomas with overlapping features. There are three entities within this syndrome:

1. Essential iris atrophy (Figures 17-3A,B through 17-5A,B)
2. Chandler's syndrome (Figure 17-6A,B)
3. Cogan-Reese syndrome (iris nevus; Figure 17-7)

Epidemiology

Iridocorneal syndrome is rare; the exact incidence is not known. Typically, it affects middle-aged women in one eye.

Pathophysiology

All three of the ICE syndrome entities share a common pathophysiology. The corneal endothelium grows abnormally over the anterior chamber angle covering the iris, which gives the iris the characteristic findings. Initially, the anterior chamber angle is open but occluded. Over time, the endothelial membrane contracts, secondarily closing the angle and distorting the pupil and iris.

History

Patients are usually asymptomatic in the early stages. Later, the patient may notice decreased vision in one eye and irregular appearance of the iris. As the intraocular pressure rises, the patient may have pain or a red eye, or both.

Clinical Examination

Slit Lamp   The cornea has a fine, beaten-metal appearance in the endothelial layer unilaterally.

There are iris abnormalities that are more specific to the separate entities:

> *Essential iris atrophy*—there are areas of thinning and a displaced and distorted pupil as the endothelial membrane contracts, pulling on the iris.
>
> *Chandler's syndrome*—the iris changes are nearly identical to those of essential iris atrophy, but there is a greater degree of corneal edema, and the corneal findings are more apparent.
>
> *Cogan-Reese syndrome*—the iris has a flattened appearance with small nodules of normal iris tissue poking through holes in the endothelial layer, giving the appearance of a mushroom patch.

Gonioscopy   Early in the disease process, gonioscopy may show a normal-appearing anterior chamber angle. Later, broad and irregular peripheral anterior synechiae occluding some or all of the angle may be seen.

Posterior Pole   The appearance of the posterior pole is normal, aside from some degree of glaucomatous optic nerve cupping as the intraocular pressure rises.

Management

Typically, medical management is not adequate in controlling the intraocular pressure. Surgical intervention is usually required. Options include trabeculectomy with an antifibrotic agent, a glaucoma drainage implant device, and cyclodestructive procedures. Corneal transplantation is helpful once the corneal edema has significantly affected the patient's vision.

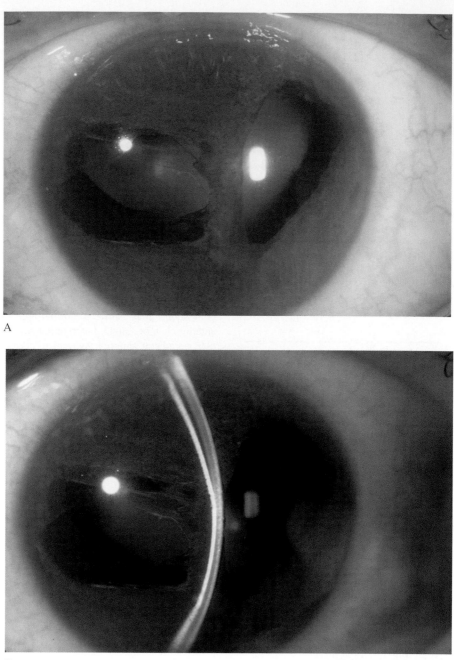

A

B

Figure 17-3A,B   Essential iris atrophy   *A. Essential iris atrophy showing pulling and distortion of the pupil. **B.** Slit-beam photograph of same eye as in (**A**).*

DISEASE SYNDROMES

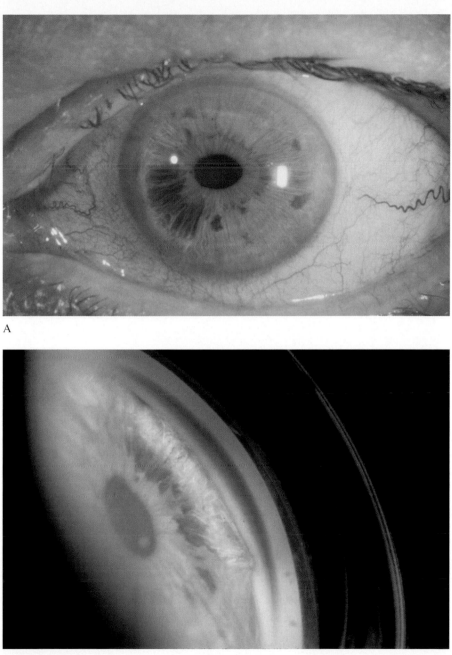

A

B

Figure 17-4A,B   Essential iris atrophy   *A. Another example of essential iris atrophy. B. Gonioscopic view of the same eye, showing peripheral anterior synechiae.*

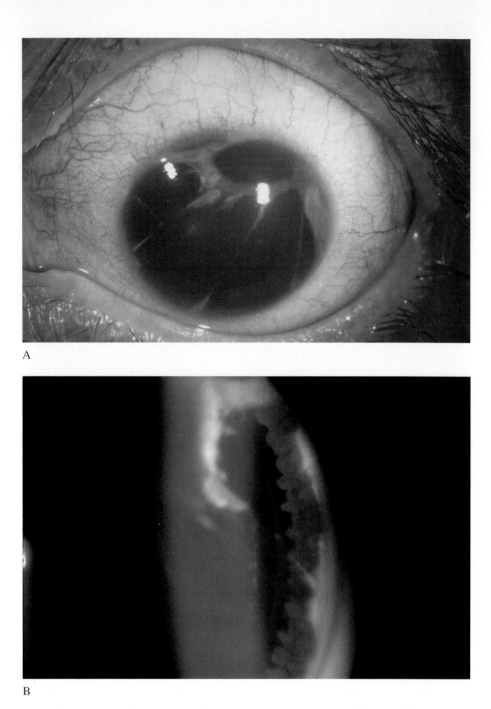

A

B

Figure 17-5A,B   Essential iris atrophy   *A. Extreme example of essential iris atrophy.*
B. Gonioscopic view of the same eye, showing peripheral anterior synechiae.

DISEASE SYNDROMES

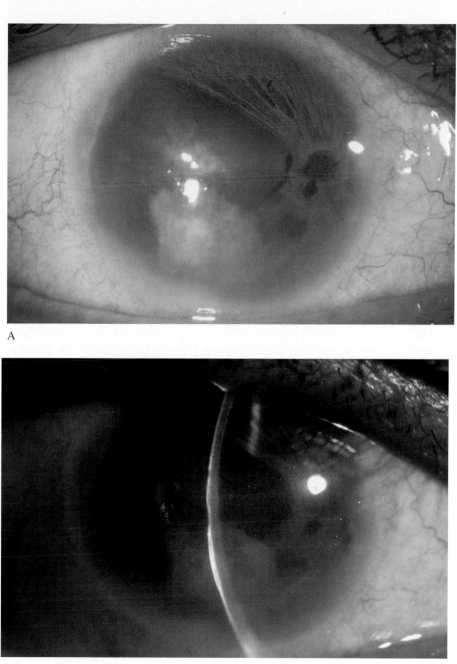

A

B

Figure 17-6A,B   Chandler's syndrome   *A. Chandler's syndrome the iris findings are similar to essential iris atrophy except that the corneal findings are more prominent.* ***B.*** *Slit-beam photograph of the same eye as in* ***(A).***

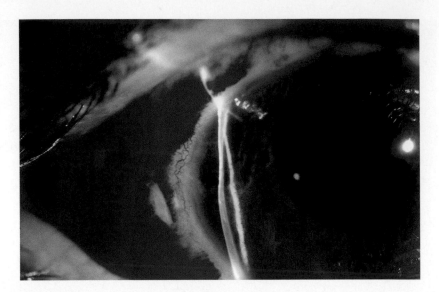

Figure 17-7 Advanced iris nevus syndrome *Slit-lamp photograph of an individual with an advanced case of iris nevus syndrome. The temporal aspect of the iris (clock hours 8 to 9) shows loss of the normal crypts of the iris. The small brown dots are tufts of normal iris tissue poking through the abnormal corneal endothelial membrane. From clock hours 9 to 11, the membrane has retracted, causing stretch tears in the iris. The subconjunctival hemorrhage is a result of this patient's recent guarded filtration surgery.*

AQUEOUS MISDIRECTION SYNDROME (MALIGNANT GLAUCOMA)

Definition

This syndrome usually occurs following penetrating surgery of the eye, although it has certainly been reported following laser procedures.

Epidemiology

In 1951, Chandler reported the incidence of malignant glaucoma to be 4% of eyes undergoing glaucoma surgery. Since then, filtering surgery has undergone some changes, and it is the impression of many clinicians that malignant glaucoma occurs less frequently in modern times.

Pathophysiology

It is believed that the intervention in the eye changes the direction of aqueous humor flow. Instead of moving forward around the pupil, the aqueous goes into the vitreous. This causes a flattening of the anterior chamber angle and a relatively high or frankly high intraocular pressure (Figures 17-8A–C and 17-9A,B). Relatively high can be considered greater than 8 mm Hg. Typically, a flat anterior chamber is the result of overfiltration causing hypotony and choroidal detachments. One would not expect an intraocular pressure greater than 10 mm Hg with a flat anterior chamber. Sometimes the pressure can be overtly elevated (more than 30 mm Hg).

History

Typically, there is a recent history of eye surgery. The patient has blurry vision from anterior movement of the iris or lens complex, but this may be difficult to distinguish from normal postoperative blurring of vision. Unless the intraocular pressure is frankly elevated, there is usually no pain.

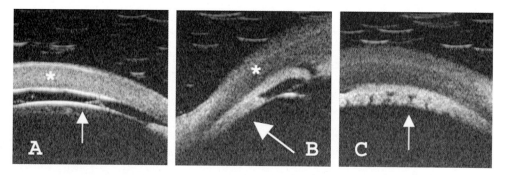

Figure 17-8A–C Aqueous misdirection following glaucoma drainage device implantation *Ultrasound biomicroscopy of a patient with aqueous misdirection syndrome following a glaucoma drainage device implantation procedure. In panels (A) and (B), the* star *indicates the cornea.* **A.** *The* arrow *shows the anterior lens capsule; this central view shows a shallow anterior chamber with iridocorneal touch to the papillary margin.* **B.** *The* arrow *shows the flattened ciliary body processes diagnostic of aqueous misdirection syndrome; this view of the angle also shows the iridocorneal touch.* **C.** *A magnified view of the flattened ciliary processes.*

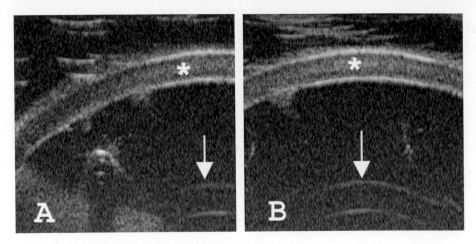

Figure 17-9A,B   Appearance after limited vitrectomy   *The same patient shown in Figure 17-8 following limited vitrectomy with disruption of the anterior hyaloid face. In panels (A) and (B), the* star *indicates the cornea while the* arrow *indicates the anterior capsule of the lens. A. Deepening of the anterior chamber angle; the tube can be seen lying flat on the iris. B. A central view showing the deep anterior chamber.*

Clinical Examination

Slit Lamp   The anterior chamber is evenly narrow. There is no iris bombé. If a glaucoma filtering procedure has been performed, the bleb is usually low with no evidence of wound leak. The intraocular pressure is as discussed earlier. Corneal edema may be present if the intraocular pressure is markedly elevated, or if there is lens-corneal contact.

Gonioscopy   Usually, gonioscopy is not possible secondary to obvious iridocorneal contact.

Posterior Pole   The hallmark of the disease is that there are no choroidals.

Special Studies

Ultrasound biomicroscopy can be quite helpful. It will typically show flattening of the ciliary body processes and no anterior choroidals.

Management

Often, the episode can be treated medically with topical cycloplegics and aqueous suppressants. Surgical intervention may be required if medical management fails. The key component to resolving the attack is disruption of the anterior hyaloid face. Sometimes this can be done using lasers if the anterior hyaloid face can be visualized peripheral to the lens or intraocular lens implant. If this is not possible, then a pars plana vitrectomy may be required. During the pars plana vitrectomy, the retinal surgeon must be aware of the need to break the anterior hyaloid face.

BIBLIOGRAPHY

Chandler PA. Malignant glaucoma. *Am J Ophthalmol* 34:993, 1951.

Diabetic Retinopathy Study Research Group. Preliminary report on effects of photocoagulation therapy. *Am J Ophthalmol* 81:383, 1976.

Hayreh SS, Podhajsky P. Ocular neovascularization with retinal vascular occlusion II. Occurrence in central and branch retinal artery occlusion. *Arch Ophthalmol* 100:1585, 1982.

Laatikainen L, et al. Panretinal photocoagulation in central retinal vein occlusion: A randomized controlled clinical study. *Br J Ophthalmol* 61:741, 1977.

Magargal LE, et al. Efficacy of panretinal photocoagulation in preventing neovascular glaucoma following ischemic central retinal vein obstruction. *Ophthalmology* 89:780, 1982.

Nielsen NV. The prevalence of glaucoma and ocular hypertension in type 1 and 2 diabetes mellitus: An epidemiological study of diabetes mellitus on the island of Falster, Denmark. *Acta Ophthalmol Scand* 27:662, 1983.

Chapter 18

LATE COMPLICATIONS OF GLAUCOMA SURGERY

Francisco Fantes, MD

Paul F. Palmberg, MD, PhD

In the majority of cases, glaucoma filtering surgery is safe and effective at lowering intraocular pressure. However, this treatment is not always perfect. Many of the undesired outcomes of filtering surgery are caused by technical failures or by an undesirable wound healing response (Table 18-1). Reproducible, methodical, and safe surgical techniques combined with attempted modulation of the biologic response may minimize some of these undesired outcomes. Despite our best efforts, however, delayed problems can occur (Table 18-2).

The goal of this chapter is to review some of the more common delayed complications of glaucoma filtering surgery and discuss possible treatment strategies. Some of the treatment strategies are more strongly established and have passed the test of time. Other procedures and alternatives are newer and may have helped one or more of the authors to solve some individual problems. The newer or somewhat infrequent procedures may not yet have passed the tests of rigorous research and time because of the rarity of the situations in which they have been applied.

TABLE 18-1 FACTORS THAT CAN INFLUENCE WOUND HEALING

Impeccable and precise surgical techniques
Use of antimetabolites
Etiology of glaucoma, such as uveitic or neovascular cause
Use of postoperative antiinflammatory medications
Other biologic factors, such as genetics, age, and race

TABLE 18-2 UNDESIRABLE OUTCOMES AS A RESULT OF A VIGOROUS OR INADEQUATE HEALING RESPONSE

Vigorous Healing Response
  Loss of filter due to scarring
  Inadequate filtration
  Bleb encapsulation

Inadequate Healing Response
  Hypotony
  Choroidal effusion
  Macular folds
  Flat chambers
  Bleb leaks
  Bleb-related infections
  Giant blebs

HYPOTONY

Hypotony can result in maculopathy, choroidal effusion, and delayed suprachoroidal hemorrhages. Hypotony is often the result of insufficient scleral flap resistance that many times will require resuturing the flap in trabeculectomies performed with antimetabolites. Alternative therapies have also been described.[1–4] However, these therapies are probably less likely to be successful in cases in which antimetabolites were used or a rapid result is needed, such as patients with a flat chamber, maculopathy, or so-called kissing choroidals. When there is overfiltration with a necrotic-looking scleral flap, sutures may not provide enough resistance to flow. In these cases, donor tissue may be needed as a roof to the flap to achieve the desired resistance. It is advisable to have donor tissue available whenever one is attempting to revise a scleral flap or to repair a leaking bleb.

Hypotony Maculopathy

Hypotony maculopathy is a condition in which folds in the choroid or retina, or both, involving the foveal region cause blurred vision in the setting of hypotony. The mechanism is probably scleral contraction. The maculopathy does not occur in all cases of hypotony, but is more likely to occur in eyes of patients who are young and myopic, and those with marked reductions in intraocular pressure. It is best to treat this condition quickly, because it can become permanent, although there are reports of success after years of involvement[5] (Figure 18-1A).

The best therapy is prevention, such as the cornea safety-valve incision as devised by Palmberg.[6] Palmberg also described a technique for bleb revisions to fix maculopathies whereby two sets of sutures are added. The first set of two sutures adjusts the outflow from the flap to an intraocular pressure of 8 to 12 mm Hg. The second set is adjusted to an intraocular pressure of 20 to 25 mm Hg.[6] It is important to keep in mind the possibility that donor tissue may be needed when revising a flap (see Figure 18-1A,B).

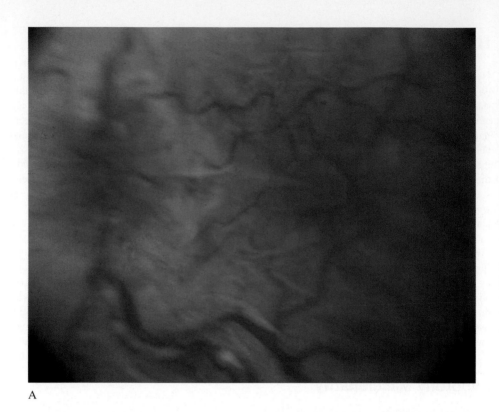

A

Figure 18-1A–C   Hypotony   *A. Dramatic example of hypotony causing optic disc edema, hemorrhages, and folds in the choroid and retina involving the foveal region.*

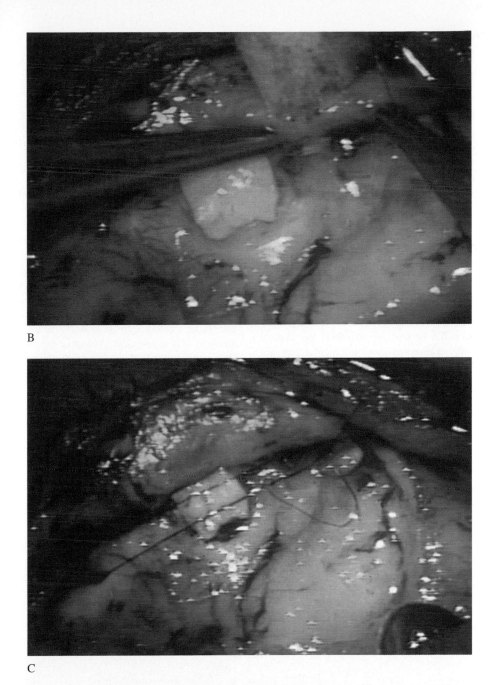

B

C

Figure 18-1A–C Hypotony (continued) *B. Intra-operative video still-frame showing a cut piece of donor sclera being used to cover a flap. C. Intraoperative video still-frame showing a compression suture of 10-0 nylon being used over the piece of donor sclera to increase the scleral resistance to aqueous outflow.*

High Intraocular Pressure and Flat Chamber
Aqueous misdirection syndrome (i.e., malignant glaucoma)
Suprachoroidal hemorrhage
Pupillary block

Low Intraocular Pressure and Flat Chamber
Overfiltration caused by insufficient flap resistance
Uveal-scleral outflow tract due to choroidal detachment
Cyclodialysis cleft
A true flat chamber with lens-cornea or intraocular lens–cornea touch (should be fixed immediately)

Shallow and Flat Anterior Chamber

Depending on the etiology, flat chambers can be associated with high or low intraocular pressures (Table 18-3; Figure 18-2). With a postoperative flat or shallow chamber, the clinical history, examination, and intraocular pressure guide the examiner in making the diagnosis.

The indications for draining a choroidal effusion include (1) flat chamber resulting in lens-corneal contact, (2) so-called kissing choroidals (retina-retina contact between the choroidal swellings) to avoid fibrin adherence between the overlying retina, and (3) persistence (after treating with cycloplegics or topical steroids). It is appropriate to observe these eyes for several weeks so long as neither of the first two conditions is present.

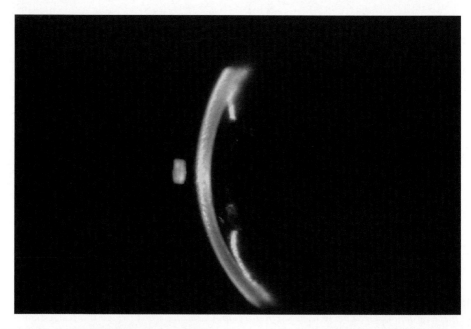

Figure 18-2 Shallow anterior chamber *Slit-beam photograph showing a shallow anterior chamber. There is significant iridocorneal touch; however, neither the pupillary border nor intraocular lens is in contact with the cornea.*

Strategies for Reformation of the Anterior Chamber

Tamponade via pressure or Simmon's shell—the strategy is likely to be more successful in surgeries without antimetabolites, and is to be used in situations of overfiltration.

Viscoelastic injection into the anterior chamber—this strategy is also likely to have success in filters without antimetabolites.

Resuturing the flap—this may end up being the solution when antimetabolites were used.

Draining Choroidal Effusions (Figure 18-3)

1. A paracentesis is placed temporally (Figure 18-4A).
2. Conjunctival incisions are made at 4:30 and 7:30 o'clock meridians from 2 to 7 mm from the limbus, or a limbal peritomy from the 4 to 8 o'clock positions.
3. A half-thickness radial incision of 2 mm is made, beginning 3 mm from the limbus as measured by calipers.
4. The edge of the flap is grasp by a toothed forceps for countertraction.
5. With a sharp blade, the incision is slowly and carefully deepened until the suprachoroidal space is opened (Figure 18-4B).
6. The incision is enlarged with a Kelly punch (Figure 18-4C).
7. If the incision is over a pocket of fluid, it will begin the outflow, which can be helped by infusing BSS through the paracentesis, lifting the edges of the flap, and rolling a cotton-tipped swap along the scleral surface.
8. If the incision is not over a pocket of fluid and fluid is not mobilized to the incision, a cyclodialysis spatula can be used to separate the choroids gently from the scleral wall to obtain communication to an adjacent pocket of fluid. This dissection should be done extremely carefully, and not more than a few millimeters from the incision.
9. Indirect ophthalmoscopy could be used at this time to look at the flattened retina. The anterior chamber should be deep, as well.
10. The conjunctival incisions should be closed, leaving the punched incisions open (Figure 18-4D).

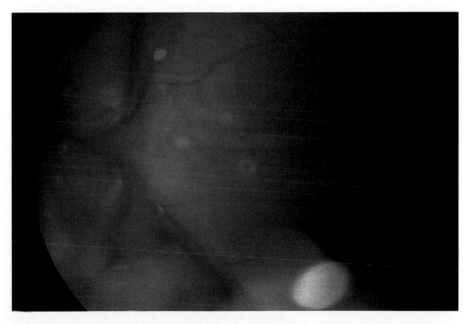

Figure 18-3   Peripheral choroidal effusions *Fundus photograph showing peripheral choroidal effusions* (left).

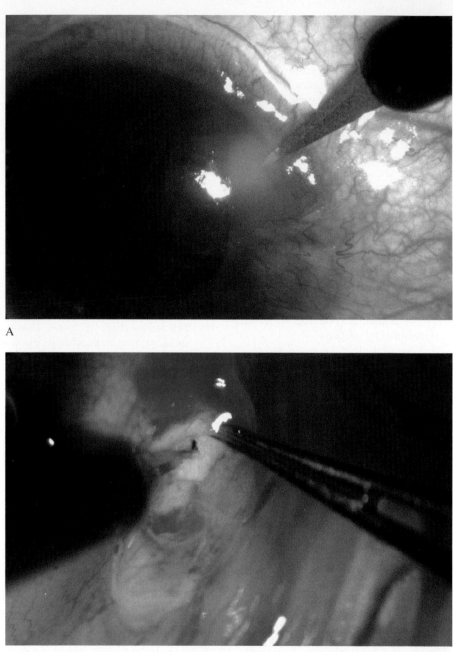

A

B

Figure 18-4A–D   Repair of choroidal effusion   *Intraoperative video still-photographs of a repair of choroidal effusion.* **A.** *Paracentesis side-port using a sharp point number 75 blade is made at the corneoscleral limbus.* **B.** *A sharp blade is used to gently enter the suprachoroidal space at the base of the partial-thickness radial scleral incision.*

DISEASE SYNDROMES

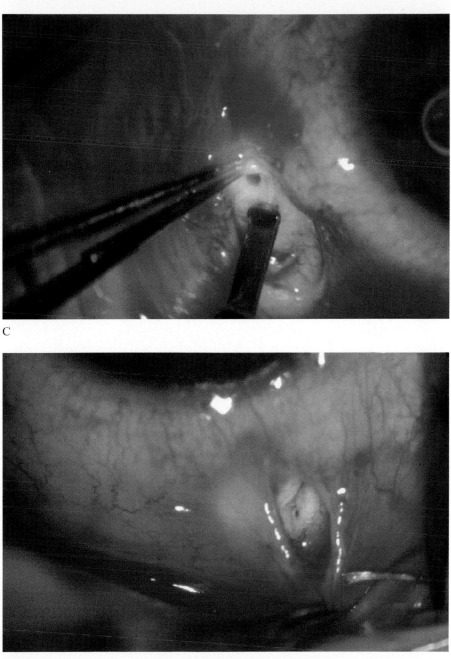

C

D

Figure 18-4A–D Repair of choroidal effusion *(continued) C. Once the suprachoroidal space is entered, the incision is widened using a Kelly punch; at the base of the incision, a hole created by the punch can be seen. **D.** The conjunctival incision is closed using 7-0 Vicryl sutures; the sclerotomy is left open.*

Delayed Suprachoroidal Hemorrhages

A suprachoroidal hemorrhage is a condition in which bleeding occurs in the suprachoroidal space separating the uvea from the sclera. These hemorrhages can occur intraoperatively as well as in the postoperative period. If bleeding occurs intraoperatively, the posterior pressure can cause extrusion of the contents of the eye (e.g., expulsive hemorrhage). The delayed suprachoroidal hemorrhages can be the result of de novo bleeding into the suprachoroidal space or of bleeding into a preexisting choroidal effusion. The risk factors include marked decompressions of the intraocular pressure, multiple previous eye surgeries, myopia, previous vitrectomy, and systemic hypertension.

A suprachoroidal hemorrhage often presents as sudden, severe pain associated with a brown-colored choroidal elevation in one side of the vitreous cavity. It is advisable to manage the patient with vitreoretinal surgery if possible. Serial B-scan ultrasounds are helpful to show the location of the hemorrhage and monitor the clot for lysis; this usually occurs between 5 and 10 days after the onset of the hemorrhage. Many surgeons prefer waiting until the clot liquefies (lyses) before draining the hemorrhage. The technique is the same as described earlier for drainage of a choroidal effusion. Smaller suprachoroidal hemorrhages may reabsorb spontaneously in about 1 month with good visual results. While the clot is liquefying, the intraocular pressure should be controlled medically to the best degree possible. An extremely elevated intraocular pressure could force an earlier intervention.

BLEB LEAKS

A bleb leak is a tiny hole in the wall of the bleb causing leakage of aqueous. This is a direct communication between the exterior world and the interior of the bleb. Use of intraoperative antimetabolites is a risk factor for the development of a bleb leak.

The mechanism of a bleb leak is thought to be as follows. Ischemic blebs are stretched and surrounded by heavily scarred tissue, which limits the ability of the aqueous to flow beyond the scarred tissue. The bleb expands locally, producing a tractional hole when the tissue overreaches its maximal stretch.

The bleb leaks are best detected by applying fluorescein to the surface of the bleb and viewing it under a slit lamp with a cobalt blue filter in place. A positive Seidel test consists of change in color of the dye to green-yellow, in response to the outflow of aqueous from the leak. Sometimes a leak can only be detecting after applying gentle pressure to the globe.

Leaks increase the risk of infection and endophthalmitis; therefore, early detection and management could be critical.[11-14] Careful surgical techniques during surgery are critical in decreasing the risk of bleb leaks. Special attention has to be paid to technique in the trabeculectomy; in suturing the conjunctiva; in the time, area, and washout of the antimetabolites; and to being methodical when applying laser suturelysis.[6]

Management

Conservative Management Following are some of the techniques described to manage wound healing. These techniques have the advantage of sparing the patient from surgery. The disadvantage is that they are not always successful and leaks can recur. Although these treatments are not operative procedures, each has its own set of risks.

1. Use of 18-mm soft contact lenses for 2 weeks[6]

2. Use of butyryl methacrylate glue and a silicon disk[6]
3. Infusion of autologous blood into the bleb[2]
4. Application of compression sutures[6]

Surgical Treatment Options include:

1. *Conjunctival advancement*—this has been demonstrated to be highly successful. Patients with late bleb leaks managed with conjunctival advancement were more likely to have successful outcomes and less likely to have serious intraocular infections than those managed more conservatively.[15-19]
2. *Free conjunctival graft*[20]—free conjunctival autologous graft is a safe and successful procedure for bleb repair and bleb reduction. However, patients should be aware of the possibility of requiring postoperative medical or surgical intervention for intraocular pressure control after the revision.
3. *Amniotic membrane*[19]—in cases in which the conjunctival tissue available is considered by the surgeon to be very limited (e.g., as a result of thinning or scarring), or there is already some degree of ptosis present, an amniotic membrane graft could be an alternative. The technique described next is slightly different than the one described by Budenz et al.[19] In this technique, the graft is folded upon itself, leaving the basement layer outward, and the stromal layer covered (Figure 18-5).

The technique of suturing amniotic membrane (AM) is as follows:

1. The conjunctiva surrounding the ischemic bleb is freed (Figure 18-6A,B).
2. The old ischemic bleb is excised (Figure 18-6C).
3. The donor AM is removed and folded upon itself (see Figure 18-5).
4. The anterior edges of the graft are sutured at the corners to corneal limbus using 9-0 nylon.

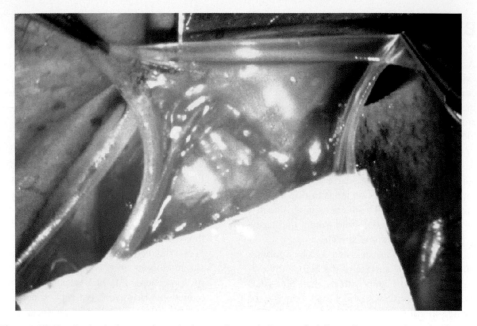

Figure 18-5 *A single layer of amniotic membrane being peeled from the supporting membrane. The stromal layer is against the paper, facing away from the paper.*

5. The posterior edge of the amniotic membrane underneath the free undermined anterior conjunctiva (Figure 18-6D).
6. The graft is tightly sutured to the anterior edge of the patient's free conjunctiva using a running 8-0 Vicryl suture (Figure 18-6E).
7. A 9-0 nylon compression suture is placed at the anterior edge of the graft, at the level of the limbus (Figure 18-6F).
8. The site is checked for wound leaks with fluorescein strips.
9. The anterior compression suture can be removed after 1 month (Figure 18-7).

A variation of this technique could be applied to free conjunctival grafts as well, adding the steps of cutting the tissue from the selected site, and without folding the free graft.

Budenz et al's[19] study of amniotic membrane transplantation does not offer an effective alternative to conjunctival advancement for repair of leaking glaucoma filtering blebs. The cumulative survival rate for amniotic membrane transplant was 81% at 6 months, 74% at 1 year, and 46% at 2 years. The cumulative survival rate was 100% for conjunctival advancement throughout follow-up.

Although Budenz et al's study showed that amniotic membrane grafts were less successful than results of the standard conjunctival advancement, their study showed that they could be successful in certain situations, providing an alternative treatment for bleb leaks in special circumstances.

In addition, if an amniotic membrane graft fails, conjunctival advancement is still a possibility. It may even be possible to make modifications in the surgical technique that could alter the outcomes. This last point is only speculative; it will need to be proven by a randomized clinical trial comparable to the Budenz et al trial and, of course, by the final test of time.

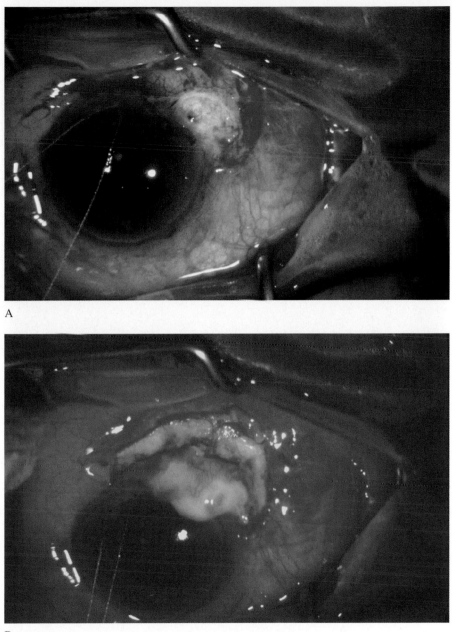

A

B

Figure 18-6A–F Amniotic membrane graft technique *A. The conjunctival tissue surrounding the ischemic bleb has been cut along the margins of the bleb; a superiorly placed 7-0 Vicryl corneal traction suture is also seen.* **B.** *The conjunctival-Tenon's flap has been bluntly undermined to mobilize the tissue.*

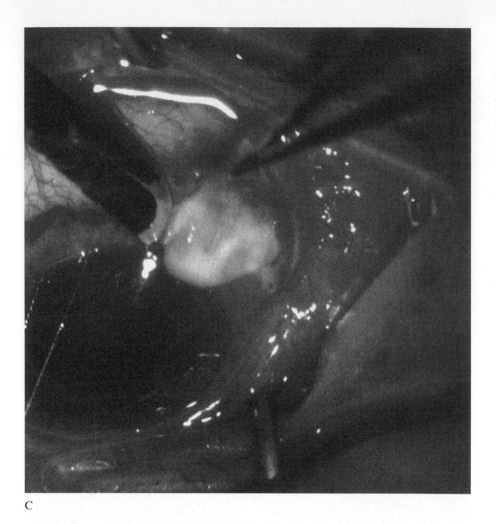

C

Figure 18-6A–F   Amniotic membrane graft technique *(continued)*   *C. The ischemic bleb is excised using a number 67 blade.*

DISEASE SYNDROMES

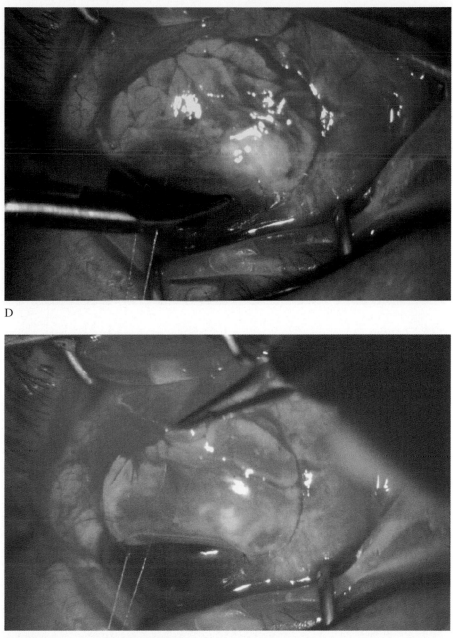

D

E

Figure 18-6A–F   Amniotic membrane graft technique   *(continued)*   **D.** *The posterior layer of the amniotic membrane sandwich is pushed and now lying underneath the conjunctival-Tenon's flap.* **E.** *The conjunctival-Tenon's flap and amniotic membrane sandwich are sutured together using a running 8-0 Vicryl suture.*

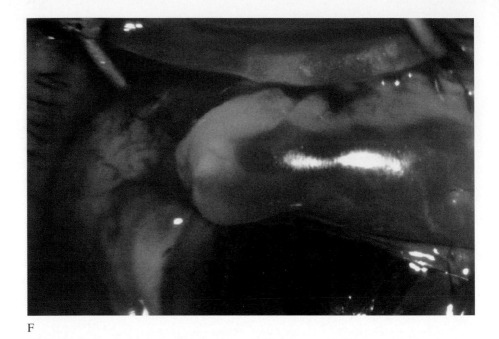

F

Figure 18-6A–F   Amniotic membrane graft technique *(continued)* *F. At the corneal edge of the graft, a 9-0 nylon compression suture is used to obstruct flow from underneath the amniotic membrane graft at the limbus.*

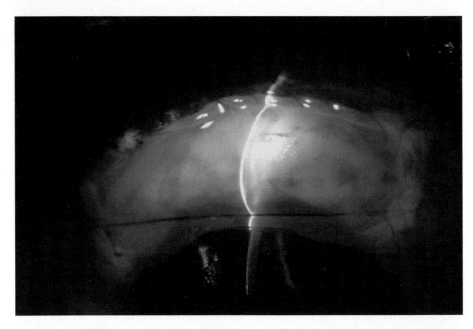

Figure 18-7   Appearance after bleb revision *Postoperative appearance of the same eye shown in* **Figure 18-6** *following bleb revision using a double-layer amniotic membrane graft.*

DISEASE SYNDROMES

GIANT BLEBS

Giant blebs can grow over the cornea, creating dellen and producing irregular astigmatism and loss of best-corrected visual acuity. The management of a giant bleb should be in a stepwise fashion, moving from the simplest to more complex solutions.

Management

1. *Cleavage and pushing technique*—a cleavage plane of the hanging bleb is found using a dull spatula; this is then pushed back posterior to the limbus.
2. *Same technique with compression stitch*—the same technique is followed, placing a compressive stitch as the limbus that will encourage permanent contraction.
3. *Amputation of the corneal portion in spongy looking blebs*—this approach is useful for spongy looking blebs over the cornea. The exuberant portion is cut with Vannas scissors.
4. *Amputation of the whole bleb*—this is generally unnecessary.

There are always exceptions. The following clinical study describes an exceptional case. The patient was a 55-year-old African-American man, who had only one functioning eye in which multiple surgeries had been performed, including the latest, a successful mitomycin C trabeculectomy for advanced glaucoma. The other eye had been lost to glaucoma.

The patient developed corneal edema and underwent cornea transplant when his visual acuity decreased from 20/30 to 20/200 in the functional eye. We performed a corneal transplant, and his visual acuity improved to a baseline of 20/30 after 6 months.

The trabeculectomy also remained functional and kept the intraocular pressure controlled throughout the postoperative course. After 1 year, the patient began to develop a larger bleb that invaded the cornea, significantly reducing his visual acuity (Figure 18-8A).

The patient was managed as previously described, but the bleb always returned, growing larger. Eventually his visual acuity worsened to 20/400, resulting in an eye that was barely functional. In response to the patient's frustration, and after a long discussion with him about the risks of surgery, we decided to take the unusual step of revising the whole bleb.

In this case, the patient had another problem—a lack of free, unscarred conjunctiva surrounding the bleb, or in that eye, for that matter. As a result, we decided to excise the bleb and to rebuild it with a double layer of amniotic membrane donor graft. A small bleb with minimal vascularization formed, and this has maintained the intraocular pressure under good control for over 4 years (Figure 18-8B).

Bleb-related Infections and Use of Corneal Patches

Bleb leaks and inferior blebs are risk factors for infections. The infections can be localized to the bleb (Figure 18-9), produce necrosis of the surrounding tissue (Figure 18-10), or progress to full-blown endophthalmitis. Inferior location of the bleb should be considered a high risk factor for infections, so consideration should be made to their closure, especially when there has been a history of infection or leaks.

Corneal Patch Corneal tissue that is not of transplant quality can be preserved in glycerin and use for patching, as follows:

1. The donor cornea is cut to the needed size.
2. Descemet's membrane is peeled off with two large, toothed forceps.
3. The bed is cleaned of necrotic tissue.
4. The cornea patch is sutured with 9-0 nylon sutures and compressive sutures, as needed.
5. The patch is covered by conjunctiva. If little conjunctiva is available, the surgeon may consider covering it with amniotic membrane, with the stromal layer inside, in direct contact with patch.

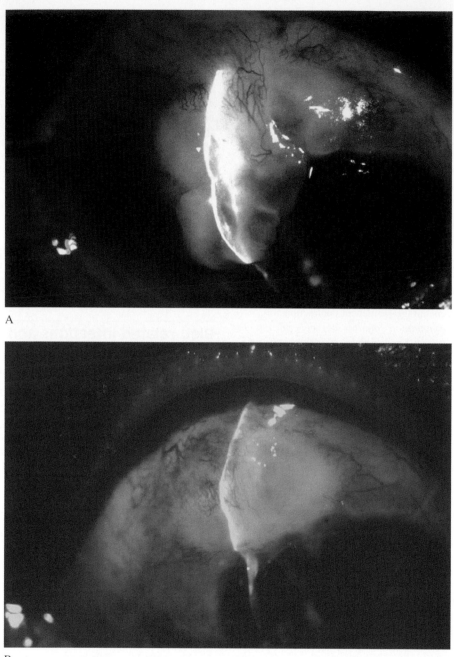

A

B

Figure 18-8A,B Giant bleb *A. An ischemic, giant cystic bleb can be seen overhanging onto the cornea. A dell can be seen at the anterior edge of the overhanging bleb. **B.** Postoperative appearance of the eye following bleb revision.*

DISEASE SYNDROMES

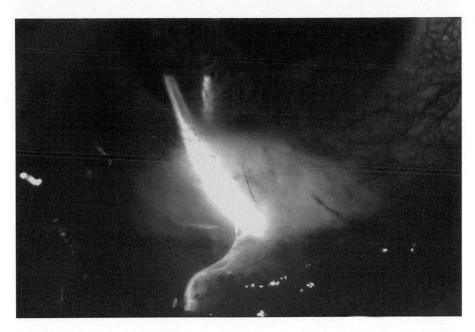

Figure 18-9   Bleb-related infection   *An inferiorly located bleb with blebitis. The overlying conjunctival tissue is clear, showing hazy bleb fluid beneath.*

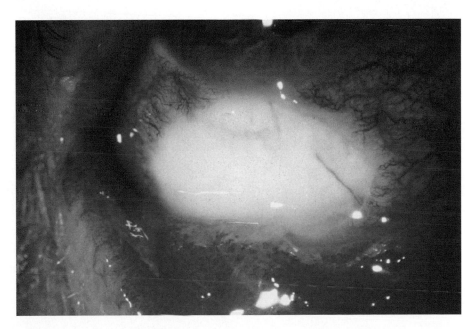

Figure 18-10   Bleb-related infection   *An inferiorly located bleb, which is ischemic, and a necrotic bleb with opaque conjunctival tissue overlying the bleb.*

6. To close the filtration permanently, the surgeon can consider placing more than one tight compression stitch, and leaving the stitches in place until they become loose, or for 6 to 8 weeks if they are reasonably well tolerated.

In one case, a patient developed necrotizing blebitis (see Figure 18-9), which required use of a corneal patch graft, covered by an amniotic membrane graft. At the same time, a glaucoma drainage device was placed superiorly (Figure 18-11A–C).

Bleb Dysesthesia

On occasion, blebs can be associated with a certain degree of discomfort. The etiology of the pain is attributed to the height and shape of the bleb, which disturbs the spread of the tear film, producing dellen.[21,22] This condition has been associated with the presence of bubbles at the slit-lamp examination, by the capture of air bubbles within the tears as the upper eyelid moves over the irregular bleb (Figure 18-12).

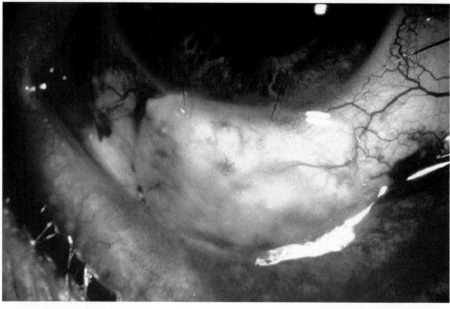

A

Figure 18-11A–C Corneal patch *A. Postoperative appearance at 6 weeks; the clear corneal tissue gives the illusion that a bleb is present.*

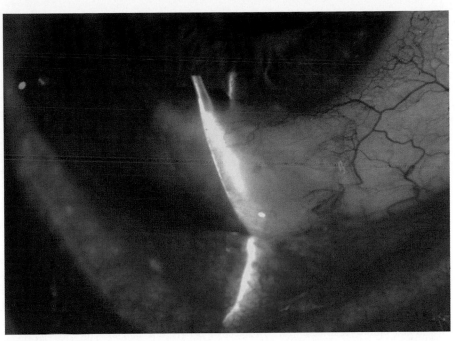

B

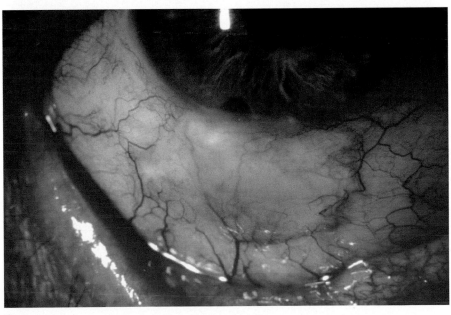

C

Figure 18-11A–C Corneal patch *(continued)* *B. Slit-beam photograph shows that there is no fluid beneath the conjunctiva C. Postoperative appearance at 1 year.*

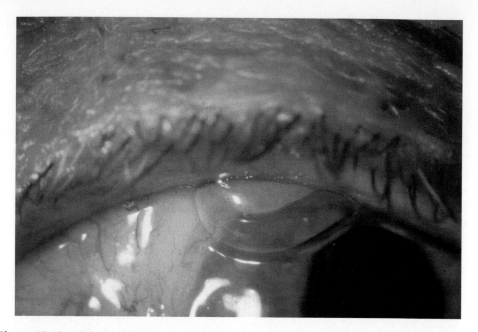

Figure 18-12   Bleb dysesthesia   *An air bubble can be seen extending from the bleb and upper lid.*

Eyes with glaucoma filtering blebs experience more dysesthesia than eyes without filtering blebs. Budenz et al identified young age, supranasal bleb location, poor lid coverage, and bubble formation as being associated with glaucoma filtering bleb discomfort.[21]

Some blebs that produce dysesthesia have been described as ischemic, thin-walled, and associated with low-normal pressures. Palmberg described a technique in which, by using compressing stitches for 3 weeks over the bleb, there is a change in the offending profile of the bleb, thereby reducing discomfort for up to 83% of patients tested with this technique.[6] The technique is as follows:

1. If the bleb is very thin, and the sutures could traumatize the surface, the surgeon may consider aspirating a small amount of aqueous with a 30-gauge needle from the anterior chamber to decompress the bleb (Figure 18-13A).

2. One or more 9-0 nylon mattress sutures are anchored in the cornea.

3. Sutures are passed posteriorly over the portion of the bleb to be compressed, and passed again over the bleb to tie the knot (Figure 18-13B).

4. The knot is tied tightly and rotated into the cornea, making sure that the area targeted is well compressed.

5. Sutures are left in place from 1 to 4 weeks, and then removed (Figure 18-13C).

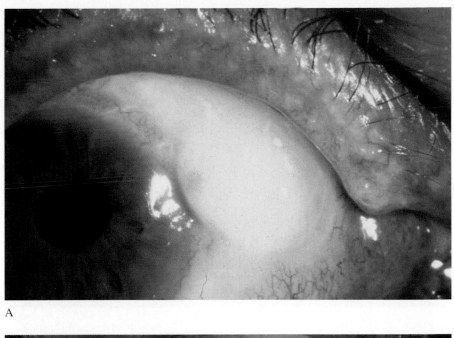

A

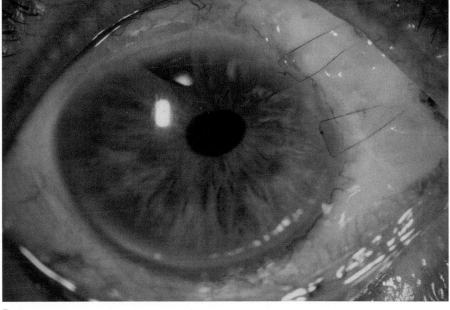

B

Figure 18-13A–C   Dysesthetic bleb   *A. Preoperative appearance of a large dysesthetic bleb.*
***B.** Two 9-0 nylon mattress sutures (or compression sutures) can be seen delimiting the size and
height of the bleb.*

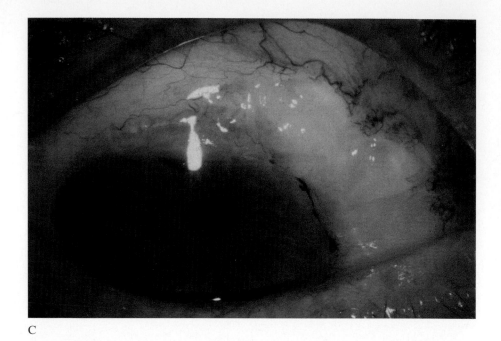

C

Figure 18-13A–C Dysesthetic bleb *(continued)* *C. Postoperative appearance of the eye following removal of the compression sutures; the bleb is smaller.*

THE FAILING BLEB: ENCAPSULATION

There are many reasons why trabeculectomies fail. The filter may stop functioning for external causes, such as encapsulation (Figure 18-14) or scarring. It may fail because of internal causes, as when the ostium becomes occluded as a result of different etiologies, such as membrane formation, iris clot, or iris vitreous.

Management

Medical management may prove to be successful in such cases. This management consists simply of antiglaucoma medications, topical steroids, and digital compression. Mandal, in a retrospective study of 503 patients, noted that 18 patients developed encapsulation and 15 of those patients responded well to conservative treatment alone. Three who did not respond underwent excisional bleb revision with mitomycin.[23] Ophir's findings emphasize inflammation as the etiology of encapsulation.[24]

Bleb needling is an alternative that can be successful. Meyer et al showed that needling was effective in reducing intraocular pressure in one third of cases for more than 6 months. They also showed that reneedlings are as successful as the first one.[25]

Finally, excisional bleb revision may possibly be augmented with antimetabolites. This could be a last alternative in cases where medical management and needling prove unsuccessful.

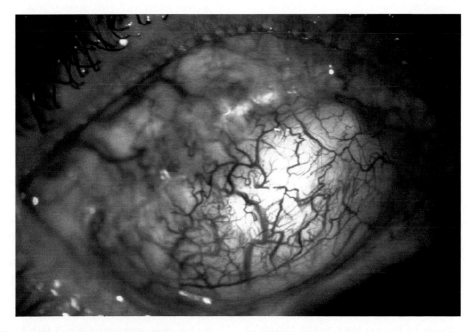

Figure 18-14 Encapsulated bleb *An encapsulated bleb; the tense appearance and thickened appearance of the wall of the "cyst" can be seen. Also note the increased vascularization of the overlying conjunctiva.*

REFERENCES

1. Yieh FS, Lu DW, Wang HL, Chou PI. The use of autologous fibrinogen concentrate in treating ocular hypotony after glaucoma filtration surgery. *J Ocul Pharmacol Ther* 17(5):443–448, 2001.
2. Okada K, Tsukamoto H, Masumoto M, Jian K, Okada M, Mochizuki H, Mishima HK. Autologous blood injection for marked overfiltration early after trabeculectomy with mitomycin C. *Acta Ophthalmol Scand* 79(3):305–308, 2001.
3. Marzeta M, Toczolowski J. [Administration of autologous blood to a patient via intrableb injection as a method for treating hypotony after trabeculectomy]. *Klin Oczna* 102(3):199–200, 2000; in Polish.
4. Akova YA, Dursun D, Aydin P, Akbatur H, Duman S. Management of hypotony maculopathy and a large filtering bleb after trabeculectomy with mitomycin C: Success with argon laser therapy. *Ophthalmic Surg Lasers* 31(6):491–494, 2000.
5. Delgado MF, Daniels S, Pascal S, Dickens CJ. Hypotony maculopathy: Improvement of visual acuity after 7 years. *Am J Ophthalmol* 132(6): 931–933, 2001.
6. Palmberg P. Surgery for complications. In: Albert DM, ed. *Ophthalmic Surgery: Principles and Techniques,* vol 1. London: Blackwell Science; 476–491, 1999.
7. Tuli SS, WuDunn D, Ciulla TA, Cantor LB. Delayed suprachoroidal hemorrhage after glaucoma filtration procedures. *Ophthalmology* 108(10):1808–1811, 2001.
8. Stamper R. Bilateral chronic hypotony following trabeculectomy with mitomycin-C. *J Glaucoma* 10(4):325–328, 2001.
9. Schwenn O, Kersten I, Dick HB, Muller H, Pfeiffer N. Effects of early postfiltration ocular hypotony on visual acuity, long-term intraocular pressure control, and posterior segment morphology. *J Glaucoma* 10(2):85–88, 2001.
10. Sihota R, Dada T, Gupta SD, Sharma S, Arora R, Agarwal HC. Conjunctival dysfunction and mitomycin C-induced hypotony. *J Glaucoma* 9(5):392–397, 2000.
11. Lehmann OJ, Bunce C, Matheson MM, Maurino V, Khaw PT, Wormald R, Barton K. Risk factors for development of post-trabeculectomy endophthalmitis. *Br J Ophthalmol* 84(12):1349–1353, 2000.
12. Liebmann JM, Ritch R. Bleb related ocular infection: A feature of the HELP syndrome. Hypotony, endophthalmitis, leak, pain. *Br J Ophthalmol* 84(12):1338–1339, 2000.
13. Jampel HD, Quigley HA, Kerrigan-Baumrind LA, Melia BM, Friedman D, Barron Y. Risk factors for late-onset infection following glaucoma filtration surgery. *Arch Ophthalmol* 119(7): 1001–1008, 2001.
14. Soltau JB, Rothman RF, Budenz DL, Greenfield DS, Feuer W, Liebmann JM, Ritch R. Risk factors for glaucoma filtering bleb infections. *Arch Ophthalmol* 118(3):338–342, 2000.
15. Budenz DL, Chen PP, Weaver YK. Conjunctival advancement for late-onset filtering bleb leaks: Indications and outcomes. *Arch Ophthalmol* 117(8):1014–1019, 1999.
16. Burnstein AL, WuDunn D, Knotts SL, Catoira Y, Cantor LB. Conjunctival advancement versus nonincisional treatment for late-onset glaucoma filtering bleb leaks. *Ophthalmology* 109(1):71–75, 2002.
17. Wadhwani RA, Bellows AR, Hutchinson BT. Surgical repair of leaking filtering blebs. *Ophthalmology* 107(9):1681–1687, 2000.
18. O'Connor DJ, Tressler CS, Caprioli J. A surgical method to repair leaking filtering blebs. *Ophthalmic Surg Lasers* 23(5):336–338, 1992.
19. Budenz DL, Barton K, Tseng SC. Amniotic membrane transplantation for repair of leaking glaucoma filtering blebs. *Am J Ophthalmol* 130(5):580–588, 2000.
20. Schnyder CC, Shaarawy T, Ravinet E, Achache F, Uffer S, Mermoud A. Free conjunctival autologous graft for bleb repair and bleb reduction after trabeculectomy and nonpenetrating filtering surgery. *J Glaucoma* 11(1):10–16, 2002.
21. Budenz DL, Hoffman K, Zacchei A. Glaucoma filtering bleb dysesthesia. *Am J Ophthalmol* 131(5):626–630, 2001.
22. Soong HK, Quigley HA. Dellen associated with filtering blebs. *Arch Ophthalmol* 101(3):385–387, 1983.
23. Mandal AK. Results of medical management and mitomycin C-augmented excisional bleb revision for encapsulated filtering blebs. *Ophthalmic Surg Lasers* 30(4):276–284, 1999.
24. Ophir A. Encapsulated filtering bleb. A selective review—new deductions. *Eye* 6(Pt 4): 348–352, 1992.
25. Meyer JH, Guhlmann M, Funk J. [How successful is the filtering bleb "needling"?] *Klin Monatsbl Augenheilkd* 210(4):192–196, 1997; in German.

Section 4
IMAGING TECHNOLOGIES

Douglas J. Rhee, MD

INTRODUCTION

As stated earlier, the goal for the treatment of glaucoma is to prevent (further) symptomatic visual loss for the patient while minimizing the side effects or complications incurred by the interventions. In terms of pathophysiology, that translates to lowering the intraocular pressure to the point at which the retinal ganglion cell axons are no longer stressed. At this time, the gold standard for determining the functional status of the ganglion cell axons (i.e., their stress) is the automated static monochromatic visual field test. The information provided by this test is used for both diagnosis and determination of treatment adequacy (i.e., absence or presence of progression of damage). However, the test has limitations with regard to degree of axonal loss required before the test detects an abnormality for diagnosis and variability of measurement for determination of progression.

The first chapter in this section demonstrates the clinical utility of ultrasound biomicroscopy for the diagnosis and management of various conditions in glaucoma. The second chapter describes some of the newer technologies that are being evaluated for their ability to both diagnose glaucoma and determine the adequacy of treatment. Some of these technologies try to determine whether there is axonal loss at an earlier stage of disease. Others may be more sensitive at determining morphologic change in the anatomic structures important in glaucoma—nerve fiber layer or optic nerve cupping—than the methods currently in use. The final chapter describes the methods used to measure optic nerve blood flow. Many feel that this component is important to the pathogenesis of glaucomatous optic nerve damage. This area is still in a relative infancy of development.

Chapter 19

ULTRASOUND BIOMICROSCOPY IN GLAUCOMA

H. Viet Tran, MD

Hiroshi Ishikawa, MD

Celso Tello, MD

Jeffrey M. Liebmann, MD

Robert Ritch, MD

Anterior segment ultrasound biomicroscopy (UBM) uses high-frequency transducers (50 MHz) to provide high-resolution (approximately 50 μm), in vivo imaging of the anterior segment (penetration depth of 5 mm). The structures surrounding the posterior chamber, hidden from clinical observation, can be imaged and their anatomic relationships assessed.

Ultrasound biomicroscopy has been used to investigate both normal structure and pathophysiology of ocular disease in numerous areas of ophthalmology, including glaucoma, cornea, lens, congenital abnormalities, effects and complications of surgical procedures, anterior segment trauma, cysts and tumors, and uveitis. It has been useful in understanding the mechanisms and pathophysiology of angle closure, malignant glaucoma, pigment dispersion syndrome, and filtration blebs. Studies using UBM remain primarily qualitative. Quantitative and three-dimensional analysis of UBM images are still in their infancy.

ANGLE-CLOSURE GLAUCOMA

Because of its ability to image the ciliary body, posterior chamber, iris-lens relation, and angle structures simultaneously, UBM is ideally suited to the study of angle closure. When assessing an eye with a narrow angle clinically for occludability, gonioscopy in a completely darkened room, using the smallest square of light for a slit beam to avoid stimulating the pupillary light reflex, is of the utmost importance. The effect of ambient light on the angle configuration is well illustrated by performing UBM under illuminated and darkened conditions (Figure 19-1A,B).

Although the trabecular meshwork itself cannot be visualized with UBM, identification of the scleral spur during imaging localizes its posterior extent. In a UBM image, the scleral spur can be seen as the innermost point of the line separating the ciliary body and the sclera at its point of contact with the anterior chamber. The trabecular meshwork is located directly anterior to this structure and posterior to Schwalbe's line (Figure 19-2).

We classify the angle-closure glaucomas on the basis of the site of the anatomic structure or force causing iris apposition to the trabecular meshwork. These are defined as block originating at the level of the iris (pupillary block), ciliary body (plateau iris), lens (phacomorphic glaucoma), and forces posterior to the lens (malignant glaucoma).

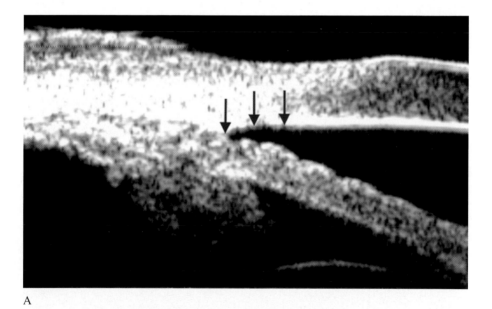

A

Figure 19-1A,B   Effect of ambient light on angle configuration   *A. Under light conditions the angle is open. Aqueous has access to the trabecular meshwork* (arrows).

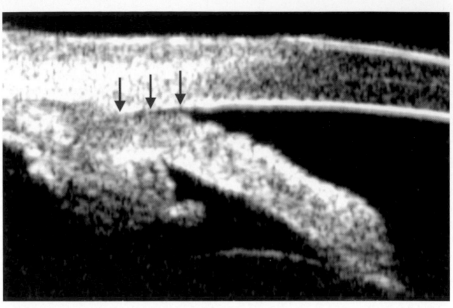

B

Figure 19-1A,B Effect of ambient light on angle configuration *(continued)* ***B.*** *In the dark, the angle is capable of occlusion* (arrows).

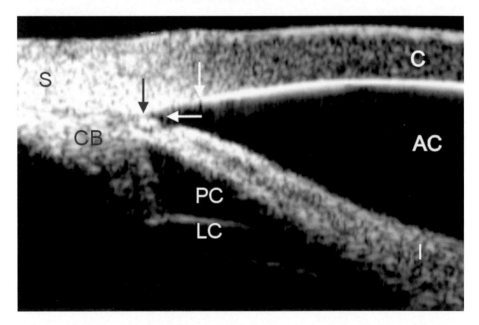

Figure 19-2 Anatomy of normal eye *Normal eye showing anterior chamber (AC), cornea (C), ciliary body (CB), iris (I), lens capsule (LC), posterior chamber (PC), sclera (S), scleral spur* (black arrow), *Schwalbe's line* (vertical white arrow), *and angle recess* (horizontal white arrow).

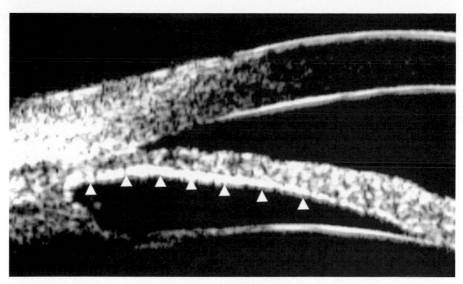

A

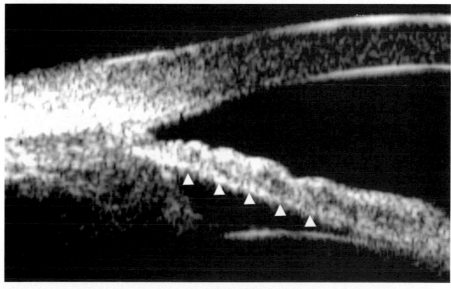

B

Figure 19-3A,B   Iris configuration before and after laser iridotomy   *Convex iris configuration* (arrowhead) *before (A) and planar configuration after (B) laser iridotomy in an eye with relative pupillary block.*

Relative Pupillary Block

Pupillary block is the most common cause of angle-closure glaucoma and is responsible for more than 90% of cases. In pupillary block, flow of aqueous is limited because of resistance to aqueous flow from the posterior to the anterior chamber through the pupil. Increased aqueous pressure in the posterior chamber forces the iris anteriorly (Figure 19-3A), causing anterior iris bowing, narrowing of the angle, and acute or chronic angle-closure glaucoma.

Pupillary block may be absolute, if the iris is completely bound to the lens by posterior synechiae, but most often is a functional block, termed *relative pupillary block*. Relative pupillary block usually causes no symptoms. However, if it is sufficient to cause appositional closure of a portion of the angle without elevating intraocular pressure, peripheral anterior synechiae may gradually form and lead to chronic angle closure (Figure 19-4). If the pupillary block becomes absolute, the pressure in the posterior chamber increases and pushes the peripheral iris farther forward to cover the trabecular meshwork and close the angle with an ensuing rise of intraocular pressure (acute angle-closure glaucoma).

Laser iridotomy eliminates the pressure differential between the anterior and posterior chambers and relieves the iris convexity. This results in several changes in anterior segment anatomy. The iris assumes a flat or planar configuration (see Figure 19-3B), and the iridocorneal angle widens. The region of iridolenticular contact actually increases, as aqueous flows through the iridotomy rather than the pupillary space.

Plateau Iris

In plateau iris, the ciliary processes are either large or anteriorly situated, or both, so that the ciliary sulcus is obliterated and the ciliary body supports the iris against the trabecular meshwork. The anterior chamber is usually of medium depth and the iris surface only slightly convex. Argon laser peripheral iridoplasty contracts and compresses the peripheral iris, pulling it away from the trabecular meshwork (Figure 19-5A,B).

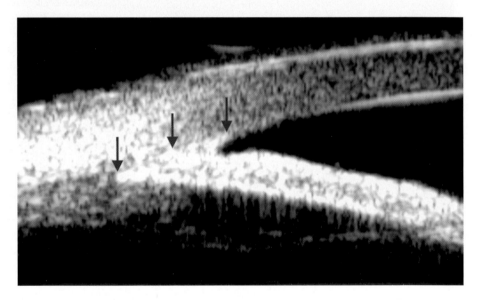

Figure 19-4   Peripheral anterior synechiae (arrows)

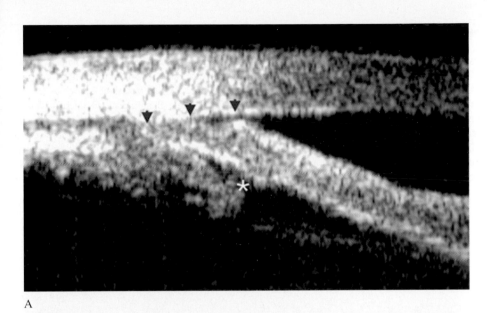

A

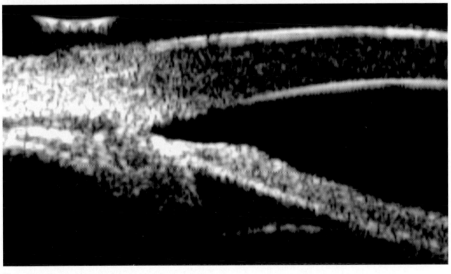

B

Figure 19-5A,B   Plateau iris syndrome   A. *In plateau iris syndrome, the angle remains* closed (arrowhead) *after laser iridotomy because the ciliary processes are anteriorly positioned. The ciliary sulcus is absent* (asterisk). ***B.*** *Following peripheral iridoplasty, the appositional angle closure is relieved.*

Phacomorphic Glaucoma

Swelling of the lens causes marked shallowing of the anterior chamber and may precipitate acute angle-closure glaucoma from pressure of the lens against the iris and ciliary body, forcing them anteriorly. Miotic treatment increases the axial length of the lens and causes the lens to move anteriorly, which further shallows the anterior chamber, and may paradoxically worsen the situation (Figure 19-6).

Malignant Glaucoma

Malignant (ciliary block) glaucoma is a multifactorial disease in which the following components may play varying roles: (1) previous acute or chronic angle-closure glaucoma, (2) shallowness of the anterior chamber, (3) forward movement of the lens, (4) pupillary block by the lens or vitreous, (5) slackness of the zonules, (6) anterior rotation or swelling of the ciliary body, or both, (7) thickening of the anterior hyaloid membrane,

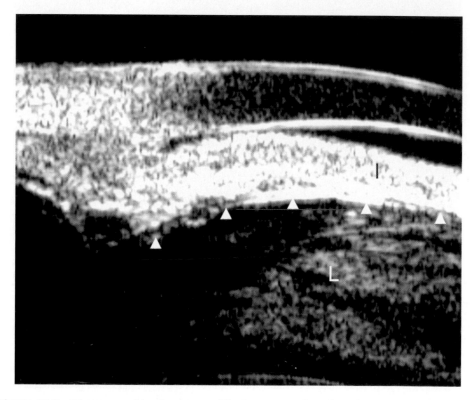

Figure 19-6　Phacomorphic glaucoma　*The intumescent lens (L and* arrowhead*) pushes the iris (I) and ciliary body into the angle.*

(8) expansion of the vitreous, and (9) posterior aqueous displacement into or behind the vitreous.

Ultrasound biomicroscopy reveals a shallow supraciliary detachment, not evident on routine B-scan or clinical examination. This effusion appears to be the cause of the anterior rotation of the ciliary body. Aqueous humor is secreted posterior to the lens (posterior aqueous displacement), increasing vitreous pressure, pushing the lens-iris diaphragm forward, and causing angle closure and shallowing of the anterior chamber (Figure 19-7).

Pseudophakic Pupillary Block

Anterior chamber inflammation after cataract extraction can lead to posterior synechiae between the iris and a posterior chamber intraocular lens, producing absolute pupillary block and angle closure. Anterior chamber lenses can also produce pupillary block (Figure 19-8A,B).

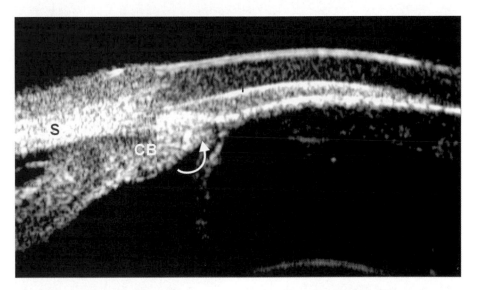

Figure 19-7   Malignant glaucoma   *Malignant glaucoma can result from aqueous misdirection or from annular ciliary body detachment. The ciliary body (Cb) is rotated anteriorly* (white arrow). *Fluid is visible in the supraciliary space* (asterisk); *S = sclera; I = iris.*

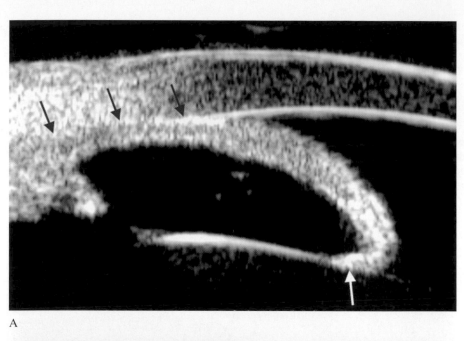

A

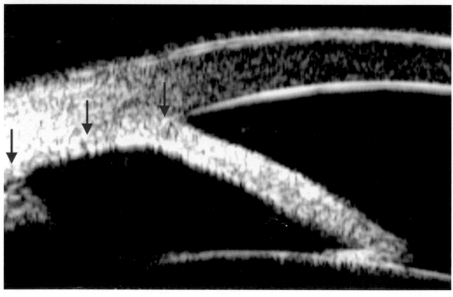

B

Figure 19-8A,B   Pseudophakic pupillary block   *A. This eye shows peripheral anterior* (black arrows) *and posterior synechiae* (white arrows), *resulting in an iris bombé configuration.* *B. After laser iridotomy, the iris configuration is flat while the peripheral anterior synechiae* (black arrows) *still hold the iris root to the trabecular meshwork.*

Pseudophakic Malignant Glaucoma

Malignant glaucoma may occur after cataract surgery with posterior chamber intraocular lens implantation. Forward displacement of the vitreous into apposition with the iris and ciliary body, possibly associated with thickening of the anterior hyaloid, has been proposed as the mechanism to account for the posterior diversion of aqueous flow. Ultrasound biomicroscopy reveals marked anterior displacement of the intraocular lens. Neodymium (Nd):YAG hyaloidotomy is curative (Figure 19-9).

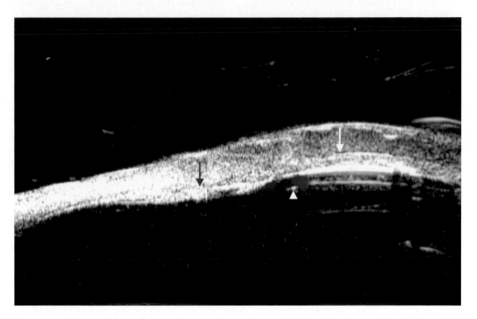

Figure 19-9 Pseudophakic malignant glaucoma *Peripheral iridocorneal touch* (white arrow) *with angle closure is visible (scleral spur at* black arrow). *The haptic is visible beneath the iris* (arrowhead).

OPEN-ANGLE GLAUCOMA

Pigment Dispersion Syndrome and Pigmentary Glaucoma

Ultrasound biomicroscopy illustrates a widely open angle. The midperipheral iris characteristically assumes a concave configuration (reverse pupillary block), presumably bringing the iris into contact with the anterior zonular bundles, and iridolenticular contact is greater than in a normal eye. The latter is thought to prevent equilibration of aqueous between the two chambers, leading to a greater pressure in the anterior chamber than in the posterior chamber. The concave configuration is accentuated by accommodation.

When blinking is inhibited, the iris assumes a convex configuration which is immediately reversed upon blinking, suggesting that the act of blinking acts as a mechanical pump to push aqueous from the posterior to the anterior chamber. Laser iridotomy eliminates the pressure differential between the anterior and posterior chambers and relieves the iris concavity. The iris assumes a flat or planar configuration (Figure 19-10A,B).

Exfoliation Syndrome

Exfoliation material may be detected earliest on the ciliary processes and zonules. Ultrasound biomicroscopy may demonstrate a granular pattern, reflecting well-defined zonules coated with exfoliation material (Figure 19-11A,B).

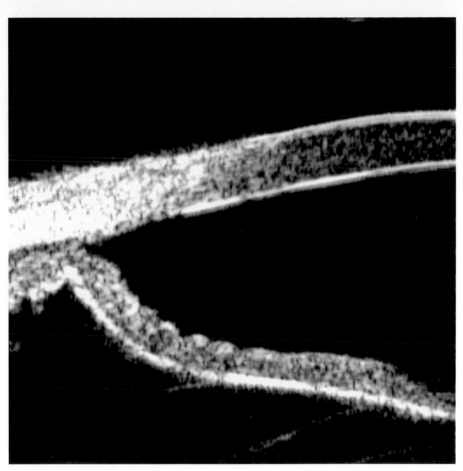

A

Figure 19-10A,B Pigment dispersion syndrome *A. Concave iris configuration.*

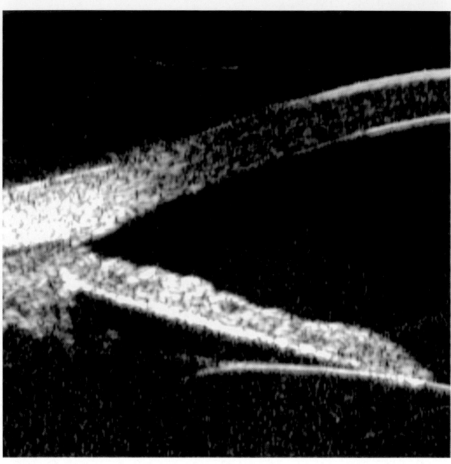

B

Figure 19-10A,B   Pigment dispersion syndrome   *(continued)*   *B. Planar configuration after laser iridotomy.*

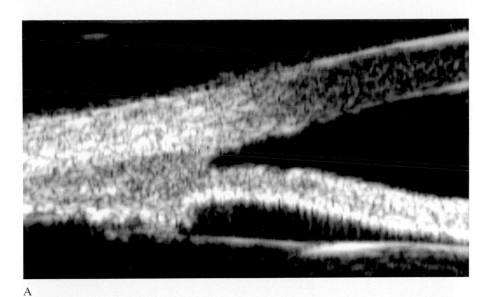

A

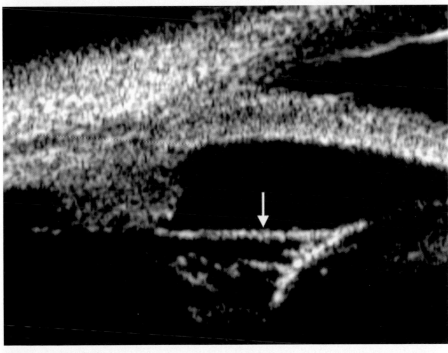

B

Figure 19-11A,B Exfoliation syndrome *A. Normal zonules.* ***B.*** *Deposited exfoliation material produces a diffuse patchy granular appearance to the zonules* (arrow).

OTHER CONDITIONS

Multiple Iridociliary Cysts

A situation similar to plateau iris is often present, the cysts functioning similarly to enlarged, anteriorly positioned ciliary processes. These are easily diagnosed with UBM (Figure 19-12).

Ciliary Body Tumors

Ultrasound biomicroscopy can be used to differentiate solid from cystic lesions of the iris and ciliary body. The dimensions of tumors can be measured and the extent to which they do or do not invade the iris root and ciliary face determined (Figure 19-13).

Iridoschisis

Iridoschisis is a separation of the anterior and posterior iris stromal layers. Angle closure may occur (Figure 19-14).

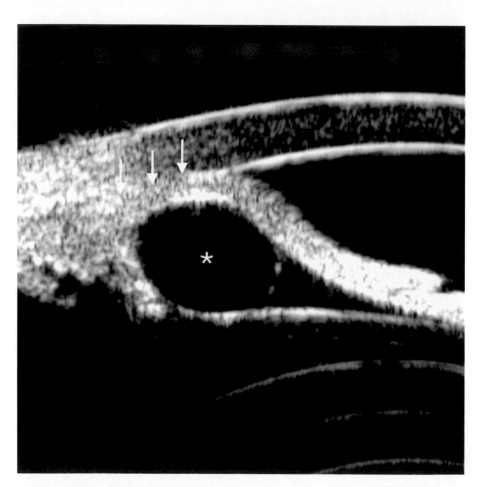

Figure 19-12   Iridociliary cysts   *Iridociliary cysts* (asterisk) *are characterized by an echolucent lumen. The angle is focally closed* (arrows).

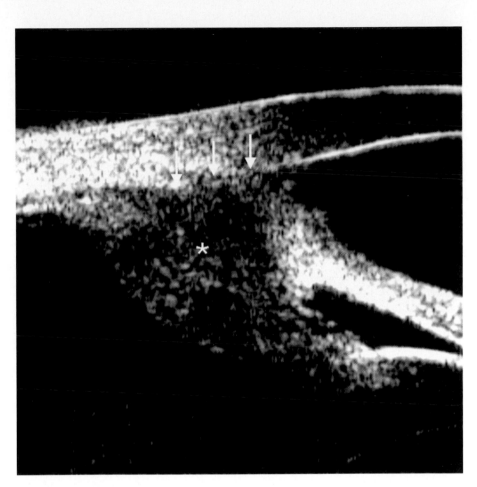

Figure 19-13 Ciliary body melanoma *In this eye with ciliary body melanoma* (asterisk), *the angle is focally closed* (arrows).

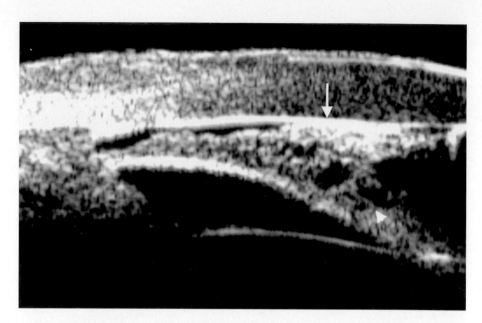

Figure 19-14 **Iridoschisis** *Extensive stromal separation* (arrowhead) *reaches the cornea and compromises aqueous outflow* (vertical arrow).

SURGERY AND GLAUCOMA

Filtering Bleb

Successful blebs have a diffuse, spongy appearance. Blebs following surgery with adjunctive antimetabolites are often thin walled and cystic. Encapsulated blebs tend to be elevated and localized, with or without prominent vessels. Failed blebs are often flat and may be vascularized.

However, the clinical appearance of a bleb is not always an accurate predictor of functional status.

The UBM appearance of a functioning bleb shows a fluid track from the anterior chamber, through the internal ostium, beneath the scleral flap, and into the subconjunctival space (Figure 19-15). Accurate localization of the site of obstruction to fluid flow can be facilitated by

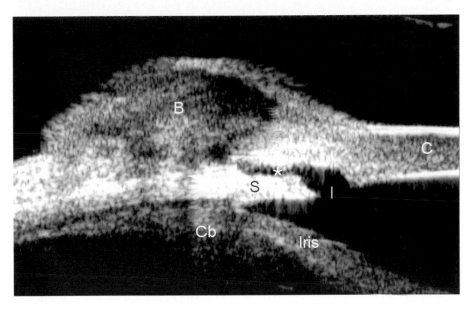

Figure 19-15   Functioning filtering bleb   *The internal ostium (I), intrascleral fluid pathway (asterisk), and scleral flap (S) are seen. The bleb (B) is thick and homogeneously spongy, with thin walls and fluid-filled spaces separated by septa; C = cornea; Cb = ciliary body.*

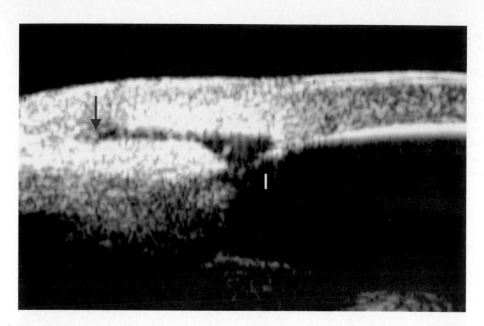

Figure 19-16   Failed bleb   *The internal ostium (I) and intrascleral fluid pathway are patent, but the scleral pathway for aqueous is closed* (arrow).

UBM. Eyes with flat blebs have no evidence of subconjunctival filtration and demonstrate blockage to flow at the level of the episclera (Figure 19-16). Tenon cysts demonstrate a non-patent scleral flap with a lumen filled with fluid and a thick conjunctival wall (Figure 19-17). Usually, eyes with encapsulated blebs normalize their intraocular pressure after needling.

Glaucoma Drainage Implants

Implants are considered in eyes in which filtering surgery has failed to control intraocular pressure. The position and course of drainage tubes can be ascertained using the UBM (Figure 19-18). The anatomic relationships can be assessed, as can compression of the tube at the scleral entry site.

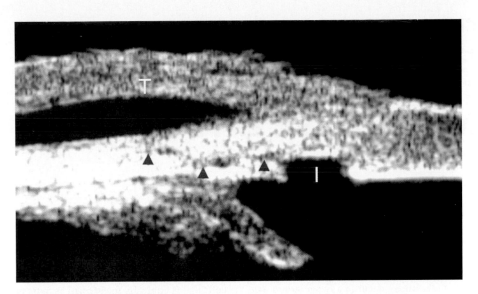

Figure 19-17 Bleb encapsulation *Tenon cyst wall (T) is thicker due to fibroblastic proliferation. The intrascleral pathway is closed* (arrowhead); *I = internal ostium.*

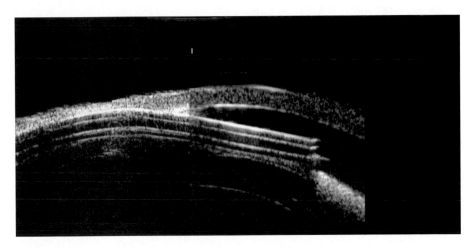

Figure 19-18 Glaucoma drainage implant *The path of the tube can be imaged in the anterior chamber.*

Chapter 20

EVALUATION OF THE OPTIC NERVE AND NERVE FIBER LAYER

Zinaria Y. Williams, MD

Joel S. Schuman, MD

Glaucoma is a common cause of blindness worldwide. It may occur in any age group, but is especially common after 40 years of age. Elevated intraocular pressure is the most important causal risk factor for glaucoma, but high intraocular pressure is not necessary for glaucomatous damage to occur. The physical impact of glaucomatous optic neuropathy includes an irreversible loss of retinal ganglion cells that is clinically manifested as optic nerve head cupping and localized or diffuse defects of the retinal nerve fiber layer. Because glaucomatous damage is irreversible but largely preventable, early and accurate diagnosis is important.

FUNCTIONAL TESTS

Evaluation of the optic nerve and nerve fiber layer includes examinations that test their structure and function. Glaucomatous retinal ganglion cell loss results structurally in nerve fiber layer and optic nerve defects, and functionally in visual field changes that can be assessed by automated perimetry and electrophysiologic testing. Glaucomatous visual field defects include localized paracentral scotomas, arcuate defects, nasal steps, and more uncommonly temporal defects (Figure 20-1A–D). The most common location of visual field defects related to glaucoma is within an arcuate area commonly referred to as Bjerrum's region, which extends from the blind spot to the median raphe.

Automated Perimetry

Automated perimeters test the visual field by presenting static stimuli of constant size and varying light intensity at specific locations for a short period of time while recording the patient's response at each location. The Humphrey Field Analyzer (HFA) 24-2 standard achromatic full threshold examination (Humphrey Systems, Dublin, CA) uses a white stimulus with white

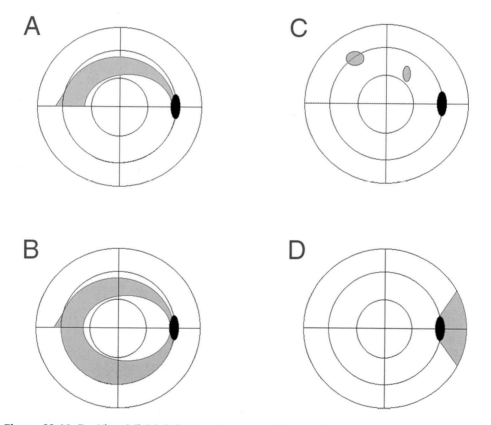

Figure 20-1A–D   Visual field defects   *A. Arcuate defect in Bjerrum's region. **B.** Double arcuate defect. **C.** Paracentral scotomas. **D.** Temporal wedge defect. (Adapted with permission from Epstein DL.* Chandler and Grant's Glaucoma, *4th ed. Baltimore: Williams & Wilkins, 1997.)*

---

background illumination; similar programs are present on other automated perimeters. Standard achromatic automated perimetry, along with clinical examination, has been the gold standard for following glaucoma; however, this early automated testing strategy is time-consuming, often resulting in patient fatigue and patient errors. Recent advances in automated perimetry have aimed at reducing testing time and at developing strategies for earlier detection of visual damage in glaucoma. Glaucoma hemifield testing is a strategy that compares specified regions

of the visual field above and below the horizontal midline (Figure 20-2). This test is present in the software of most automated perimeters.

Swedish Interactive Threshold Algorithms (SITA)

Swedish interactive threshold algorithms (Humphrey Systems, Dublin, CA) are a family of test algorithms developed to significantly

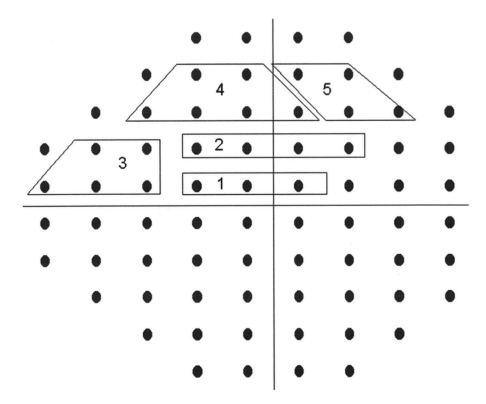

Figure 20-2 Glaucoma hemifield testing *Superior visual field zones used in the glaucoma hemifield test. Each zone is compared with its mirror zone below the horizontal meridian. (Adapted with permission from Epstein DL.* Chandler and Grant's Glaucoma, *4th ed. Baltimore: Williams & Wilkins, 1997.)*

reduce the testing time without a reduction in data quality[1] (Figures 20-3A,B and 20-4A,B).

How SITA Works SITA uses information gained throughout the program to determine the threshold strategy for adjacent points. SITA measures the response time of each patient and uses the information to set the pace of the test. These SITA strategies are fast and accomplish the

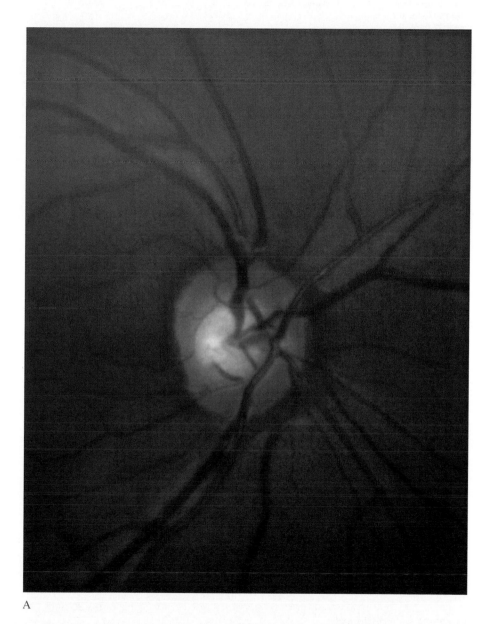

A

Figure 20-3A,B Swedish interactive threshold algorithms (SITA), normal eye *A. Normal optic nerve head (ONH) photograph. **B.** Normal SITA visual field.*

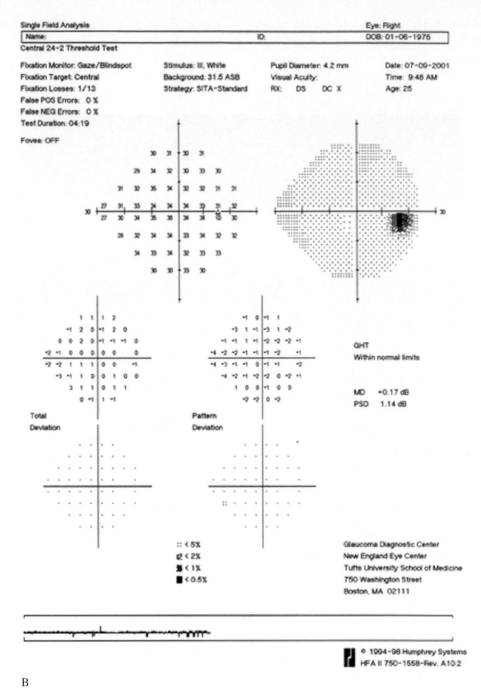

B

Figure 20-3A,B *(continued)*

IMAGING TECHNOLOGIES

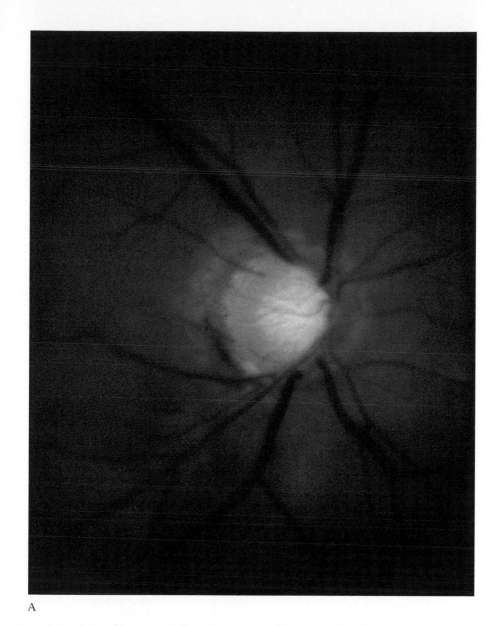

A

Figure 20-4A,B   SITA, glaucomatous eye   *A. ONH photograph of an eye with glaucoma*
B. SITA visual field showing a superior arcuate scotoma and an inferior nasal step.

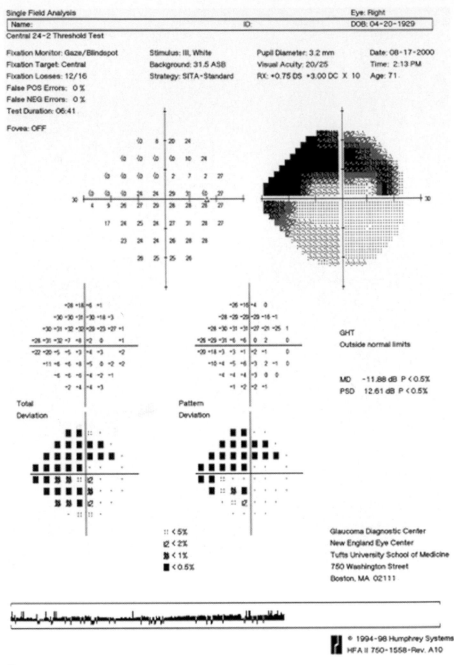

B

Figure 20-4A,B   *(continued)*

same or better test quality as the full threshold program.[2] Average test time is approximately 5 to 7 minutes per eye with SITA Standard. There is also a SITA Fast strategy, which requires approximately 50% less time than SITA Standard; however, there is a significant tradeoff in sensitivity for the reduction in testing time.

When to Use SITA SITA is quickly becoming the gold standard for clinical glaucoma care.

Short Wavelength Automated Perimetry (SWAP)

Short wavelength automated perimetry has better sensitivity than standard automated perimetry for glaucoma diagnosis at early stages of damage[3,4] (Figure 20-5A,B).

How SWAP Works A carefully chosen wavelength of blue light is used as the stimulus, and a specific color and brightness of yellow light is used for the background illumination. SWAP isolates and measures blue-yellow ganglion cell function. SWAP is thought to present earlier diagnosis because blue-yellow ganglion cells are selectively damaged in early glaucoma; however, the increased sensitivity of this test over standard achromatic perimetry may be a result of the reduction in the redundancy of the visual system achieved through the use of a blue target light on a yellow background.[5–7]

When to Use SWAP In glaucoma suspects, SWAP testing can be used on patients having one or more risk factors for glaucoma with normal achromatic perimetry. SWAP testing is appropriate for glaucoma and ocular hypertensive patients with mild to moderate field loss.

Limitations Patients having significant nuclear sclerotic cataracts or advanced achromatic visual

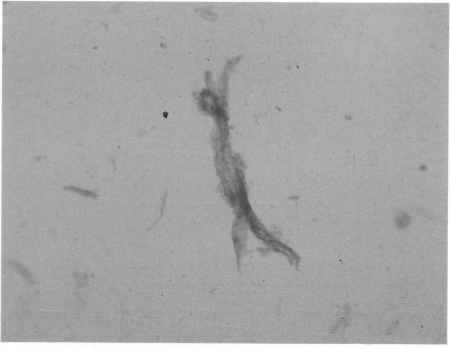

A

Figure 20-5A,B **Short wavelength automated perimetry (SWAP), normal eye** *A. Normal ONH photograph*

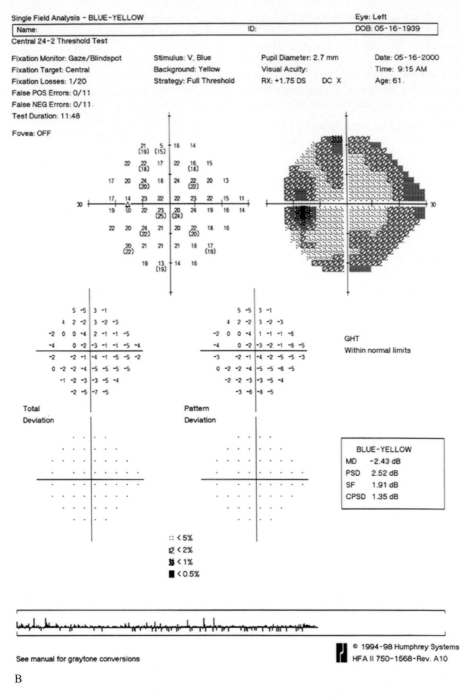

Single Field Analysis - BLUE-YELLOW   Eye: Left

Name: ID: DOB: 05-16-1939

Central 24-2 Threshold Test

Fixation Monitor: Gaze/Blindspot   Stimulus: V, Blue   Pupil Diameter: 2.7 mm   Date: 05-16-2000
Fixation Target: Central   Background: Yellow   Visual Acuity: Time: 9:15 AM
Fixation Losses: 1/20   Strategy: Full Threshold   RX: +1.75 DS   DC X   Age: 61
False POS Errors: 0/11
False NEG Errors: 0/11
Test Duration: 11:48

Fovea: OFF

GHT
Within normal limits

Total
Deviation

Pattern
Deviation

BLUE-YELLOW
MD   -2.43 dB
PSD   2.52 dB
SF   1.91 dB
CPSD 1.35 dB

:: < 5%
⧖ < 2%
🗙 < 1%
■ < 0.5%

© 1994-98 Humphrey Systems
HFA II 750-1568-Rev. A10

See manual for graytone conversions

B

Figure 20-5A,B   Short wavelength automated perimetry (SWAP), normal eye *(continued)* **B.** *Normal SWAP visual field.*

field loss may not be good candidates for blue-yellow testing, because nuclear sclerotic cataract confounds SWAP and the dynamic range of SWAP is exceeded with moderate to high degrees of achromatic visual field loss. Additionally, one obstacle to the interpretation of SWAP fields is the presence of greater long-term variability in normal subjects, which makes differentiation between random variations and true progression more difficult.[8,9]

Frequency Doubling Technology (FDT)

Frequency doubling technology perimetry (Welch Allyn, Skaneateles, NY, and Humphrey Systems, Dublin, CA) can serve as an effective initial visual field evaluation for detection of glaucomatous visual field loss. This small, tabletop unit is portable and can be easily used in the office or at off-site locations.

How FDT Works The frequency doubling illusion is the phenomenon that results when low spatial frequency grating patterns of black and white bars undergo rapid counterphase flicker, creating the perception that twice as many bars are visible to the patient as are actually present in the stimulus. Evidence has suggested that there is a selectively more rapid death of larger ganglion cells (M-cells) that project to the magnocellular layers of the lateral geniculate body than of other cell types in glaucoma.[10–12] This small subset of ganglion cells demonstrates a nonlinear response to the frequency-doubling stimuli delivered by FDT. This instrument detects glaucomatous visual field loss with greater than 90% sensitivity and specificity when compared to the HFA standard achromatic perimetry as the gold standard[13] (Figures 20-6 and 20-7).

When to Use FDT FDT is a good test for general glaucoma screening because it is quick, inexpensive, easily administered, and highly sensitive and specific. FDT is effective in detecting visual field loss in glaucoma. FDT can detect neurologic diseases, including anterior ischemic optic neuropathy, pseudotumor cerebri, and compressive optic neuropathies.

Limitations The current version of FDT shows 19 spots, each subtending 10 degrees of visual arc, in the N-30 glaucoma testing program. The number of spots is significantly fewer, with each spot covering a larger area, compared with the standard 24-2 Humphrey visual field program. In the 24-2 standard, there are 54 spots, each covering 4 degrees of arc. Newer FDT devices may incorporate more test spots, with each spot covering a smaller visual arc, in order to increase spatial resolution with this device. The dynamic range of FDT may actually be greater than that of the HFA gold standard achromatic perimetry.

Multifocal Electroretinography (mfERG)

Electroretinography objectively establishes the loss of retinal function. In multifocal electroretinography, focal responses are obtained from a large number of retinal patches, and topographic maps of dysfunctional areas are derived.

How mfERG Works All focal areas are independently and concurrently stimulated as the ERG signal is derived from the cornea by means of a contact lens electrode. The special mathematical scheme of multifocal stimulation permits precise extraction of the focal response contributions from the single ERG signal. No patient response is required. Using the Visual Evoked Response Imaging System (VERIS; Electro-Diagnostic Imaging, San Mateo, CA), the stimulus may consist of up to several hundred focal stimuli. Typically, 103 hexagonal patches displayed on a video monitor stimulate the central 50 degrees of the patient's visual field (Figure 20-8). In most cases, the focal stimulation consists of pseudorandomly presented flashes. The focal electrophysiologic response signals are organized and displayed topographically to produce functional maps of the retina, similar to those of visual field testing.

When to Use mfERG Although most of the ERG response originates in the outer layers of the retina (photoreceptors, bipolar cells), the mfERG can be used to objectively measure

FULL THRESHOLD N-30

Test Date/Time: 06/26/2001 12:57
FDT/VF Ver: 2.60 / 1.00
Test ID: 1019.2000835

Patient Name:
Age: 45
Patient ID:

LEFT EYE	RIGHT EYE

Test Duration: 5:06

Test Duration: 4:57

Threshold (dB)

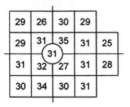

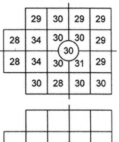

Total Deviation

30°

30°

Pattern Deviation

30°

30°

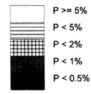

P >= 5%
P < 5%
P < 2%
P < 1%
P < 0.5%

MD: -0.05 dB
PSD: +3.11 dB

FIXATION ERRS: 0 / 6
FALSE POS ERRS: 0 / 8
FALSE NEG ERRS: 0 / 5

MD: -0.26 dB
PSD: +2.33 dB

FIXATION ERRS: 0 / 6
FALSE POS ERRS: 0 / 8
FALSE NEG ERRS: 0 / 5

Dx :

Notes :

FDT ViewFinder™

Welch Allyn®
FREQUENCY DOUBLING TECHNOLOGY

ZEISS Humphrey SYSTEMS

Figure 20-6   Frequency doubling technology (FDT), normal eye

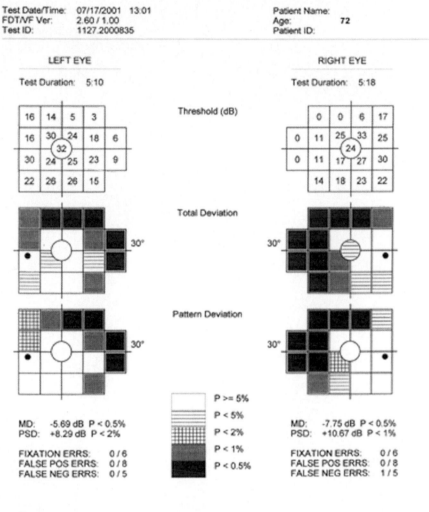

FULL THRESHOLD N-30

Test Date/Time: 07/17/2001 13:01
FDT/VF Ver: 2.60 / 1.00
Test ID: 1127.2000835

Patient Name:
Age: 72
Patient ID:

LEFT EYE

Test Duration: 5:10

Threshold (dB)

RIGHT EYE

Test Duration: 5:18

Total Deviation

Pattern Deviation

P >= 5%
P < 5%
P < 2%
P < 1%
P < 0.5%

MD: -5.69 dB P < 0.5%
PSD: +8.29 dB P < 2%

FIXATION ERRS: 0 / 6
FALSE POS ERRS: 0 / 8
FALSE NEG ERRS: 0 / 5

MD: -7.75 dB P < 0.5%
PSD: +10.67 dB P < 1%

FIXATION ERRS: 0 / 6
FALSE POS ERRS: 0 / 8
FALSE NEG ERRS: 1 / 5

Dx :

Notes :

FDT
ViewFinder™

WelchAllyn®
FREQUENCY
DOUBLING
TECHNOLOGY

Humphrey SYSTEMS

Figure 20-7   FDT, glaucomatous eye   *FDT of the same glaucomatous eye shown in Figure 20-4. The right eye shows a superior and inferior step defect.*

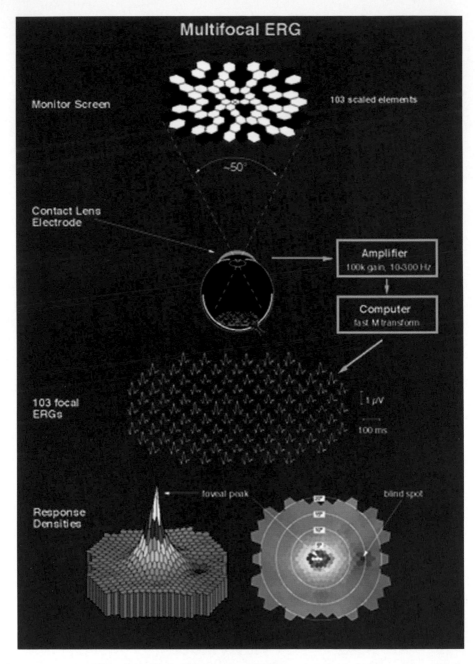

Figure 20-8   Multifocal electroretinography (mfERG)   *Schematic display of the mfERG showing stimulus array, the response trace array, and three-dimensional and two-dimensional plots. (Courtesy of Erich Sutter, PhD, Electro-Diagnostic Imaging, San Mateo, CA.)*

ganglion cell function. A portion of the response signal originates from ganglion cell fibers in the vicinity of the optic nerve head. This component is diminished in glaucoma patients. This technique does not require pupil dilation. Special paradigms are being developed and tested that enhance, isolate, and map this response component.

Limitations Currently, the mfERG is used experimentally and is not included in common clinical practice.

Visually Evoked Cortical Potential (VEP)

The visually evoked cortical potential (VECP, also abbreviated VEP or VER for visually evoked response) is an electrical signal generated by the occipital visual cortex in response to stimulation of the retina by either light flashes or patterned stimuli (Figure 20-9A,B). Pattern VEP is now preferred over flash VEP for the evaluation of the visual pathways, owing to its enhanced sensitivity in detecting axonal conduction defects.

How VEP Works The VEP measures the electrical response of the brain's visual cortex to patterned or flashed stimuli. The VER

potential is measured between electrodes on the scalp. One electrode, which measures the response itself, can be placed over or lateral to the external occipital protuberance (or inion) (see Figure 20-9B), located close to the primary visual cortex. Another electrode is placed at a reference location. The final electrode is used for grounding.

When to Use VEP The VEP is primarily used to identify visual loss secondary to diseases of the optic nerve and anterior visual pathways.

The multifocal technique described in the previous section can also be applied to the cortical response (mfVEP). In this instance, stimulus arrays are usually configured in a dartboard pattern whereby each sector contains a contrast reversing checkerboard stimulus. The difficulty with this method is that a reduction or absence of local responses is due in part to the convoluted cortical anatomy and does not always reflect loss of function. However, unilateral local loss of function can be demonstrated by comparison of the response maps from the two eyes. Recent studies have shown correlations between the VEP and visual field defects.

Limitations Similar to the mfERG, much more work remains to be done with mfVEP prior to general clinical adoption of this technique.

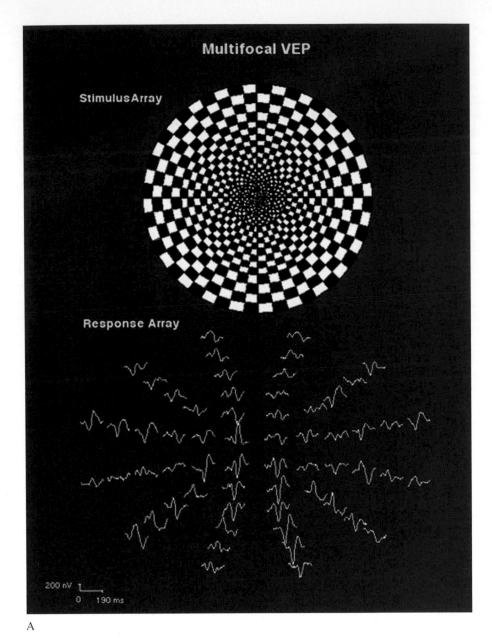

A

Figure 20-9A,B Multifocal visually evoked cortical potential (mfVEP) *A. Stimulus and response array of a normal mfVEP. (**A,B,** Courtesy of Erich Sutter, PhD, Electro-Diagnostic Imaging, San Mateo, CA.)*

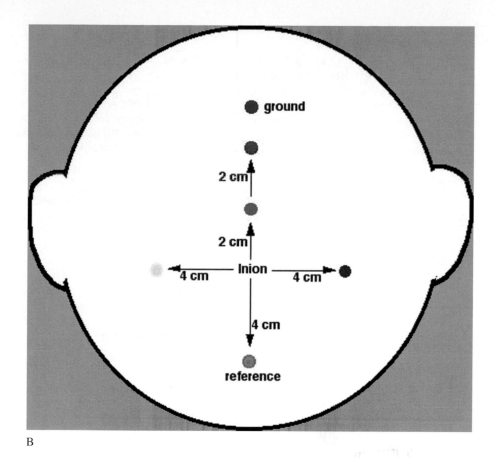

B

Figure 20-9A,B   Multifocal visually evoked cortical potential (mfVEP)   *(continued)*
B. Diagram of electrode placements above and lateral to the inion.

STRUCTURAL TESTS

Glaucoma can be measured through the assessment of optic nerve head cupping, retinal nerve fiber layer (NFL) defects, and possibly macular thickness. These are among the reliable signs of glaucoma and its progression.

The development of noninvasive, objective techniques that measure retinal structures most likely to suffer glaucomatous damage aids in the diagnosis of glaucoma and in the monitoring of progressive glaucomatous damage. Stereoscopic and NFL photography are among the simplest technologies that can be used for assessing glaucomatous structural damage; however, new computerized image analysis techniques have been developed for more objective and quantitative measurements of the retinal NFL and optic nerve head.

Photography

Stereoscopic optic nerve head photography is one of the most widely used optic nerve head imaging technologies. NFL photography, more difficult and less frequently used than optic nerve head photography, permits extended evaluation of the NFL following a patient examination. Specific retinal abnormalities associated with glaucoma include focal and diffuse NFL thinning. NFL losses in glaucoma correlate with visual field abnormalities.

How Stereoscopic Photography Works Stereo images can be produced using sequential (consecutive) or simultaneous photographic techniques. Sequential stereoscopic photography captures two consecutive images using a manual shift of the camera joystick. Simultaneous stereoscopic photography captures instantaneous stereo images with a single exposure to produce a split-frame image of two images on one or two 35-mm slides, depending on the system used (Figure 20-10A,B). The images can be viewed stereoscopically using a specialized viewing apparatus.

When to Use Stereoscopic Photography Stereoscopic optic nerve head photography should be used whenever available every 1 to 2 years to evaluate glaucoma suspects and glaucoma patients for progressive disease.

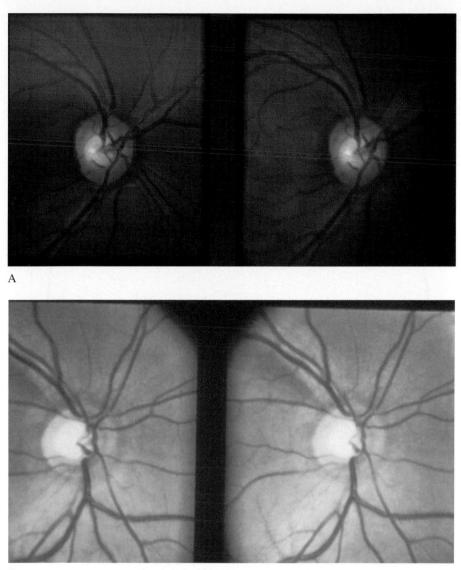

A

B

Figure 20-10A,B   Stereoscopic photography   *A. Stereo photograph of normal eye.*
B. Stereo photograph of an optic nerve; however, supranasally, there is a nerve fiber layer defect.

Limitations Stereoscopic optic nerve head photography does not offer an objective system for interpretation of the optic nerve.

How NFL Photography Works The NFL is composed of the axons from the ganglion cells, neuroglia, and astrocytes. Axons of the ganglion cells travel toward the optic nerve in an organized fashion (Figure 20-11). The NFL is best observed using a red-free, blue or green light. Green or blue wavelengths are highly

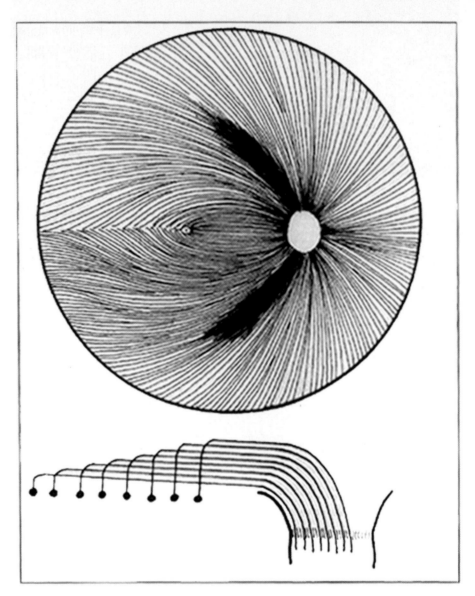

Figure 20-11 Nerve fiber layer (NFL) representation *Lower drawing represents the topography of the NFL where the distal ganglion cell axons project to the peripheral area of the optic disc rim. (Reprinted with permission from Schuman JS.* Imaging in Glaucoma. *Thorofare, NJ: SLACK, 1997.)*

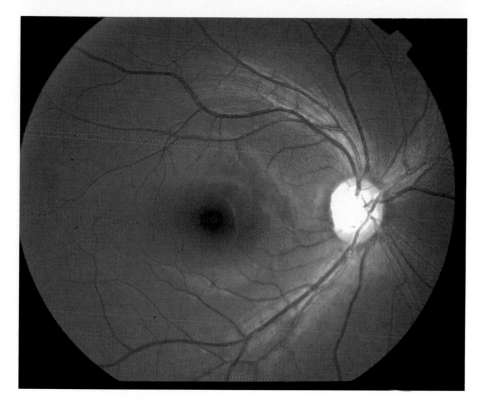

Figure 20-12   NFL photograph, normal eye

absorbed by the retinal pigment epithelium and choroid while the axon bundles reflect the light and appear as silvery striations (Figures 20-12 and 20-13).

When to Use NFL Photography   NFL examination is useful in distinguishing between glaucoma suspects and true glaucoma damage. Defects in the NFL may precede optic nerve head and visual field changes. Therefore, correlating NFL appearance with visual fields is an objective way of confirming a subjective finding in automated perimetry.

Limitations   Media opacity such as cataract, poorly focused photographs, and poor contrast because of a lightly pigmented fundus are among the factors that can cause difficulty in evaluating or photographing the NFL.

Scanning Laser Polarimetry (SLP)

Scanning laser polarimetry derives peripapillary NFL thickness from measurements of total ocular birefringence.

How SLP Works   The GDx (Laser Diagnostic Technologies, San Diego, CA) takes advantage of the properties of the interaction of polarized light with birefringent tissue to measure the thickness of the NFL. This technique is based on the principle that the birefringence of the NFL causes a change in the state of the polarized light, known as retardation. This retardation is linearly related to the thickness and optical properties of

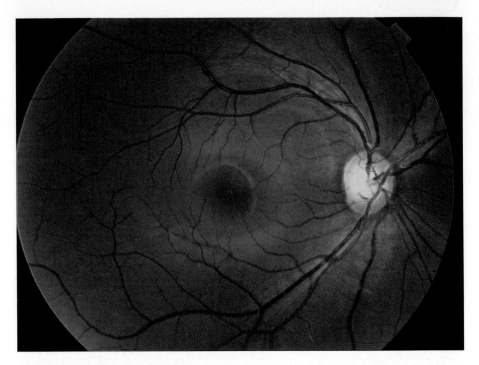

Figure 20-13   Color NFL photograph, normal eye

the NFL[14] (Figures 20-14 and 20-15). The 780-nm near-infrared diode polarized light source is focused onto one point of the retina. The polarized light penetrates the NFL and is partially reflected back from its deeper layers. The polarized state of the reflected light is analyzed digitally. A fixed compensation device neutralizes the average anterior segment birefringence. Retardation data at 65,536 individual retinal locations (256 by 256 pixels) covering 15 degrees is obtained from circular band of 1.5 to 2.5 disc diameters concentric to the disc. Each pixel is qualitatively illustrated as yellow and white for high retardation and dark blue for low retardation.

When to Use SLP   SLP may be useful in detecting glaucoma and following its progression.

Limitations   The cornea and lens represent significant sources of birefringence that may alter the retardance and lead to inaccurate measurements of NFL thickness. Additionally,

the magnitude of retardation represents a relative, rather than absolute, measure of RNFL thickness. Confounding of SLP NFL thickness measurements by nonretinal (e.g., corneal and lenticular) birefringence is an obstacle to the widespread utility of this technology. The user is required to define the measurement ellipse.

Confocal Scanning Laser Ophthalmoscopy (CSLO)

Confocal scanning laser ophthalmoscopy is a method for acquiring and analyzing real-time three-dimensional topographic images of the optic nerve head.

How CSLO Works   The Heidelberg Retina Tomograph (HRT; Heidelberg Engineering GmbH, Heidelberg, Germany), is the only currently available confocal scanning laser ophthalmoscope. It uses a confocal scanning system based on the principle of spot illumination and spot detection. In this system, one spot

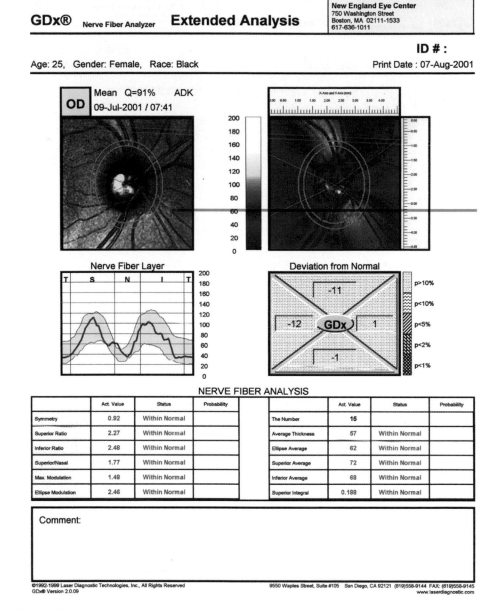

Figure 20-14 Scanning laser polarimetry (SLP), normal eye *SLP of a normal eye showing the CSLO image in the upper left corner and the birefringence representation in the upper right. The retardance (NFL thickness) data are shown in the middle left panel. The subject eye is shown in dark blue, while the 95% confidence interval for the normal range is illustrated in light blue. The "Deviation from Normal" chart is shown in the middle right panel. Nerve fiber analysis parameters are displayed at the bottom.*

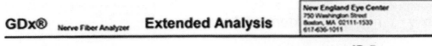

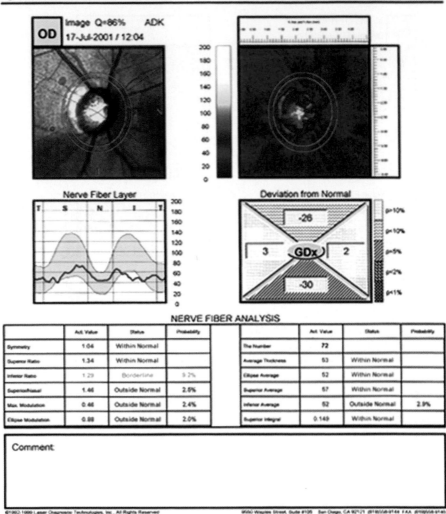

Figure 20-15   SLP, glaucomatous eye *SLP of the same glaucomatous eye shown in* **Figures** ***20-4*** *and* ***20-7***. *Note the general reduction in retardation illustrated in the "Nerve Fiber Layer" graph, and the deviation from normal represented in the middle right panel. Nerve fiber layer parameters that are borderline or outside of normal limits are highlighted.*

on the retina or optic nerve head is illuminated at a time, allowing only light originating from the illuminated area to pass through the aperture while scattered light and tissue planes that are out of focus do not. Thus, areas that do not lie close to the plane of focus are not illuminated and are not seen. This allows for high-contrast images. In addition, layer-by-layer (tomographic) imaging within the retina and optic nerve head is possible. HRT uses a diode laser of 670 nm to scan and analyze the posterior segment. A three-dimensional image is obtained from a series of optical sections at 16 to 64 consecutive focal planes. The information is displayed in two images—a topographic image and a reflectivity image (Figures 20-16A,B and 20-17A,B). The topographic image consists of 256 × 256 or 384 × 384 pixel elements, each of which is a measurement of height at its corresponding location. The optical transverse resolution is approximately 10 μm, whereas the longitudinal resolution is about 300 μm. In current clinical practice, three scans of each eye are taken and then averaged to create a mean topographic image. Images can be obtained through undilated pupil, but dilation will improve image quality in patients with small pupils and cataracts.[15] Reproducibility is best in undilated eyes.[16]

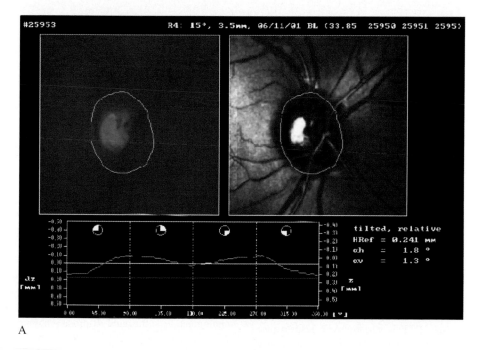

A

Figure 20-16A,B   Confocal scanning laser ophthalmoscopy (CSLO), normal eye *CSLO of a normal eye using the Heidelberg Retina Tomograph (HRT) I. **A.** Topographic image (left) and reflectivity image (right) showing the ONH image and contour graph. In the graph, the white line represents the reference plane at which there is a height of zero. The red line represents the height of the reference line between the cup and disk. The green line is the retinal height of the subject eye at the contour line showing the typical double hump feature at the superior and inferior poles. **B.** Topographic image with the cup represented in red, the sloping neural tissue in blue, and the rim in green. The ONH parameters and subject classification are listed on the right. The classification number for the HRT I is determined by an automated algorithm devised by Frederick Mikelberg based on the ONH and retinal parameters. The classification number for HRT II is derived from an algorithm developed by Wollstein et al at Moorfields Eye Hospital.*

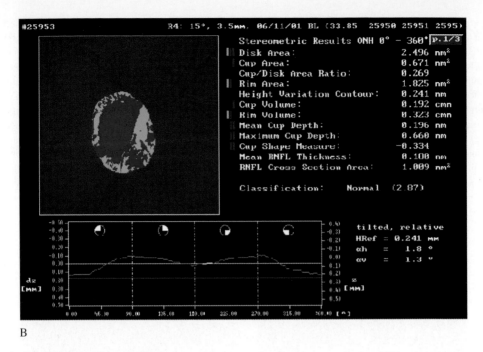

Stereometric Results ONH 0° - 360° P.1/3
Disk Area: 2.496 nm²
Cup Area: 0.671 nm²
Cup/Disk Area Ratio: 0.269
Rim Area: 1.825 nm²
Height Variation Contour: 0.241 nm
Cup Volume: 0.192 cmn
Rim Volume: 0.323 cmn
Mean Cup Depth: 0.196 nm
Maximum Cup Depth: 0.660 nm
Cup Shape Measure: -0.334
Mean RNFL Thickness: 0.100 nm
RNFL Cross Section Area: 1.009 nm²

Classification: Normal (2.87)

tilted, relative
HRef = 0.241 mm
αh   =   1.8 °
αv   =   1.3 °

B

Figure 20-16A,B *(continued)*

When to Use CSLO   CSLO may be useful in detecting glaucoma and following its progression.

Limitations   CSLO optic nerve head measurements require a reference plane to calculate many of the parameters: cup area, cup-to-disc ratio, cup volume, rim area, rim volume, retinal NFL thickness, and retinal NFL cross-sectional area. The reference plane used by the current software may change over time, especially in patients with glaucoma who have changing topography.[16] This variation can lead to inaccurate measurements. The user is required to define the optic nerve head border. Cup shape, cup volume below the surface, mean cup depth, maximum cup depth, and disc area are the parameters that are independent of the reference plane. Misalignment between the patient and the scanner in the horizontal plane is also a potential source of significant variability.

Optical Coherence Tomography (OCT)

Optical coherence tomography (Humphrey Systems, Dublin, CA) computes NFL thickness measurements from high-resolution cross-sectional images of the retina.

How OCT Works   OCT uses low-coherence light in an interferometer to perform high-resolution imaging. The operation of OCT is analogous to ultrasound B-mode imaging or radar except that light is used rather than acoustic or radio waves. OCT measurements of distance and microstructure are performed by measuring the time of flight of light reflected from different microstructural features within the eye. A sequence of longitudinal measurements (i.e., A-scans) is used to construct a false-color topographic image of tissue microsections

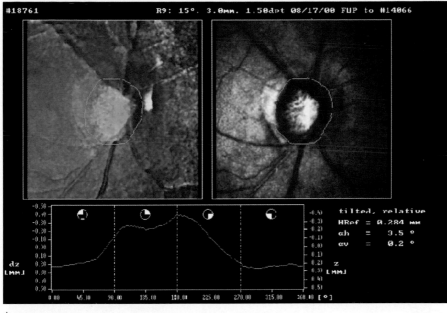

A

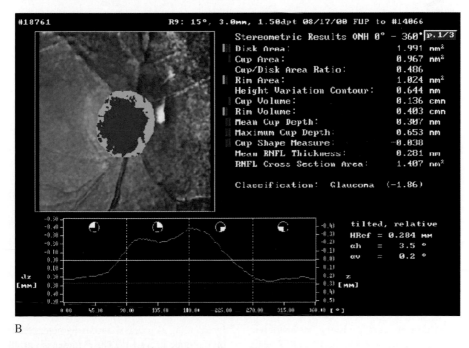

B

Figure 20-17A,B   CSLO, glaucomatous eye   *CSLO of the same glaucomatous eye shown in Figures 20-4, 20-7, and 20-15. A. Topographic and reflectivity images. B. ONH analysis and measured parameters.*

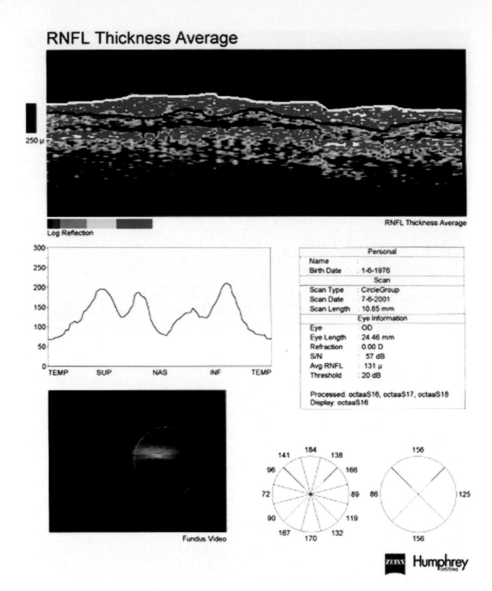

Figure 20-18 Optical coherence tomography (OCT), normal eye *OCT peripapillary circular scan of a normal eye. NFL thickness is graphed below the scan image. Average overall NFL thickness is shown in the right middle panel. NFL thickness by quadrant and clock hour is displayed on the bottom right. The bottom left image shows a video frame of the fundus during scanning.*

that appears remarkably similar to histologic sections (Figures 20-18 and 20-19). OCT has a longitudinal-axial resolution of about 10 μm and a transverse resolution of approximately 20 μm. In the clinical evaluation of glaucoma, OCT is used to create cylindrical retinal sections by scanning a circle 3.4 mm in diameter centered on the optic nerve.[17,18] The cylinder is unfolded and displayed as a flat cross-sectional image. OCT can be used to create a thickness map of the macula through a series of six radial scans, covering each clock hour, centered on the

---

IMAGING TECHNOLOGIES

Retinal Map

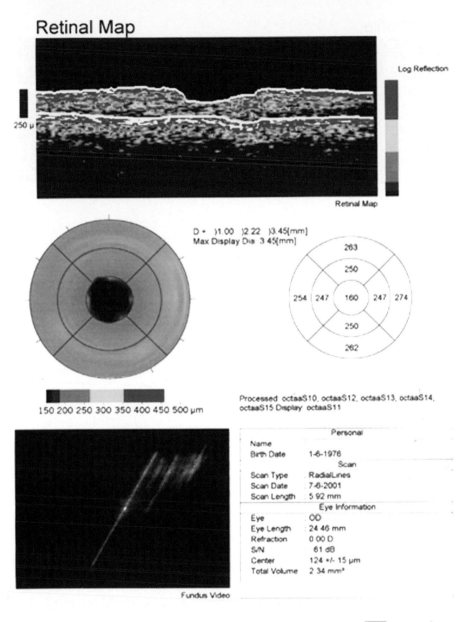

Log Reflection

250 μ

Retinal Map

D +)1.00)2.22)3.45[mm]
Max Display Dia 3 45[mm]

	263	
254	247	160	247	274
	250	
	282	

150 200 250 300 350 400 450 500 μm

Processed octaaS10, octaaS12, octaaS13, octaaS14,
octaaS15 Display octaaS11

Personal
Name
Birth Date   1-6-1978
                           Scan
Scan Type   : RadialLines
Scan Date   : 7-6-2001
Scan Length   : 5 92 mm
                     Eye Information
Eye   : OO
Eye Length   : 24 46 mm
Refraction   : 0 00 D
S/N   61 dB
Center   124 +/- 15 μm
Total Volume   2 34 mm³

Fundus Video

ZEISS Humphrey SYSTEMS

Figure 20-19   OCT, glaucomatous eye   *OCT peripapillary circular scan of the same glaucomatous eye shown in* **Figures 20-4, 20-7, 20-15,** *and* **20-17.** *Note the considerably thinner NFL thickness measurements.*

Scan Profile

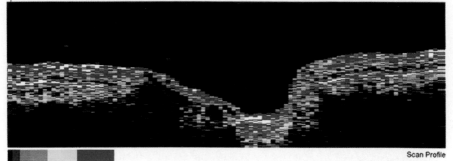

Log Reflection

Scan Profile

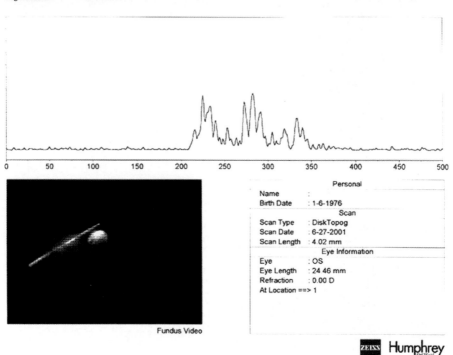

0	50	100	150	200	250	300	350	400	450	500

Fundus Video

Personal

Name :
Birth Date : 1-6-1976

Scan

Scan Type : DiskTopog
Scan Date : 6-27-2001
Scan Length : 4.02 mm

Eye Information

Eye : OS
Eye Length : 24.46 mm
Refraction : 0.00 D
At Location ==> 1

ZEISS Humphrey SYSTEMS

Figure 20-20 OCT, normal eye *OCT macular scan of a normal eye. The macula has a ring of tissue surrounding the fovea that is thicker than the fovea centralis, as can be seen in the macular thickness map. The map is displayed in false color, and the quantitative data are shown to its right.*

foveola; the optic nerve head can be mapped in a similar fashion, centering the radial scans on the ONH. (Figures 20-20 through 20-22). An automated computer algorithm makes the NFL thickness measurements with no user input. Unlike CSLO, OCT does not require a reference plane. The NFL thickness is an absolute cross-sectional measurement. The refractive state or the axial length of the eye does not affect OCT measurements. OCT measurements of NFL thickness are not dependent on tissue birefringence.

RNFL Thickness Average

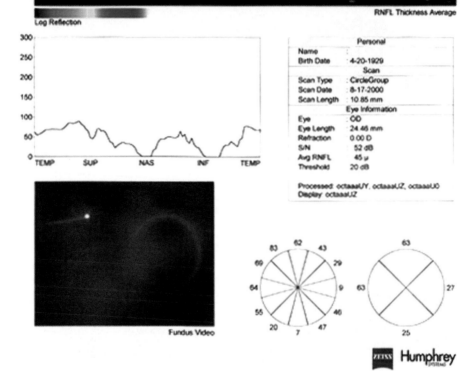

Figure 20-21 OCT, normal eye *OCT ONH scan of a normal eye. This scan profile illustrates the optic disc physical characteristics.*

When to Use OCT OCT may be useful in detecting glaucoma and following its progression.

Limitations OCT requires a nominal pupil diameter of 5 mm, although in practice most patients can undergo OCT scanning without dilation. Cortical and posterior subcapsular cataracts may limit the ability to perform OCT.[19]

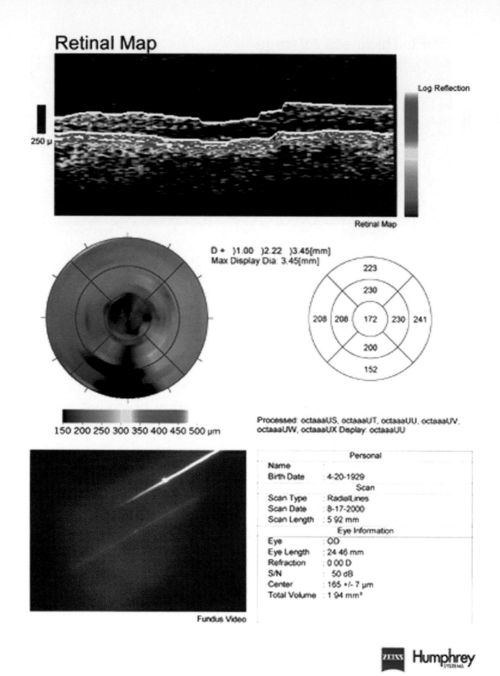

Figure 20-22 OCT, glaucomatous eye *OCT macular scan of another glaucomatous eye showing macular thinning.*

IMAGING TECHNOLOGIES

Retinal Thickness Analyzer (RTA)

Retinal thickness analyzer (Talia Technology, Mevaseret Zion, Israel) computes macular thickness and displays the measurement in two-dimensional and three-dimensional images.

How RTA Works Retinal thickness mapping with the RTA uses a green, 540-nm HeNe laser slit beam to image the retina. The distance between the laser's intersection with the vitreoretinal interface and the retina–retinal pigment epithelial interface is directly proportional to the retinal thickness (Figure 20-23). Nine scans with nine separate fixation targets are taken. The compositions of these scans cover the central 20 degrees (measuring 6 by 6 mm) of the fundus.

Unlike OCT and SLP, which measure the NFL, or CLSO or OCT, which measure optic nerve head contour, RTA measures macular thickness. Because the highest concentrations of retinal ganglion cells reside in the macula, and retinal ganglion cells are significantly thicker than their axons (which comprise the NFL), macular thickness may be a good measure of glaucoma. RTA and OCT may both be used for macular thickness assessment.

When to Use RTA RTA may be useful in detecting glaucoma and following its progression.

Limitations RTA requires a 5-mm pupil size and is limited by eyes with numerous floaters or significant media opacity. Because of the shorter wavelength of the light used for RTA, this technology is more sensitive to nuclear sclerotic cataract than OCT, CSLO, or SLP. Axial length and refractive error are needed to convert values into absolute thickness values.

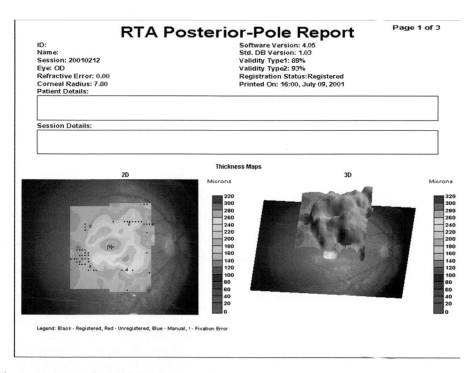

Figure 20-23 Retinal thickness mapping *Normal eye analyzed with the Retinal Thickness Analyzer (RTA). The two-dimensional and three-dimensional images are shown in false color.*

SUMMARY

The diagnosis of glaucoma and the assessment of its progression are dependent on the evaluation of the structure and function of the optic nerve and nerve fiber layer. Through the use of advanced technologies that provide objective, quantitative measures of ocular structure and refined evaluation of retinal function, such as those described earlier, clinicians may have a means of detecting glaucoma earlier and more accurately. The ultimate goal is the early diagnosis of glaucoma and its progression, with prompt and appropriate intervention in order to prevent loss of vision due to this disease.

ACKNOWLEDGMENT

Electrophysiologic testing information was contributed by Erich Sutter, PhD, at Smith-Kettlewell, San Francisco and Electro-Diagnostic Imaging, San Mateo, CA. Supported in part by NIH R29-EY11006, R01-EY13178, R01-EY11289.

REFERENCES

1. Bengtsson B, Heijl A, Olsson J, Rootzen H. A new generation of algorithms for computerized threshold perimetry, SITA. *Acta Ophthalmol Scand* 75:368–375, 1997.
2. Bengtsson B, Heijl A, Olsson J. Evaluation of a new threshold visual field strategy, SITA, in normal subjects. *Acta Ophthalmol Scand* 76:165–169, 1998.
3. Johnson CA, Adams AJ, Casson EJ, Brandt JD. Progression of early glaucomatous visual field loss as detected by blue-on-yellow and standard white-on-white perimetry. *Arch Ophthalmol* 111:651–656, 1993.
4. Sample PA, Taylor JD, Martinez GA, Lusky M, Weinreb RN. Short-wavelength color visual fields in glaucoma suspects at risk. *Am J Ophthalmol* 115:225–233, 1993.
5. Heron G, Adams AJ, Husted R. Central visual fields for short wavelength sensitive pathways in glaucoma and ocular hypertension. *Invest Ophthalmol Vis Sci* 29:64–72, 1988.
6. Sample PA, Boynton RM, Weinreb RN. Isolating the color vision loss in primary open angle glaucoma. *Am J Ophthalmol* 106:686–691, 1988.
7. Hart WM Jr, Silverman SE, Trick GL, et al. Glaucomatous visual field damage: Luminance and color-contrast sensitivities. *Invest Ophthalmol Vis Sci* 31:359–367, 1990.
8. Kwon YH, Park HJ, Jap A, Ugurlu S, Caprioli J. Test-retest variability of blue-on-yellow perimetry is greater than white-on-white perimetry in normal subjects. *Am J Ophthalmol* 126:29–36, 1998.
9. Blumenthal AZ, Sample PA, Zangwill L, et al. Comparison of long-term variability for standard and short-wavelength automated perimetry in stable glaucoma patients. *Am J Ophthalmol* 129:309–313, 2000.
10. Quigley HA, Dunkelberger GR, Baginski TA, Green WR. Chronic human glaucoma causes selectively greater loss of large optic nerve fibers. *Ophthalmology* 95:357–363, 1988.
11. Dondona L, Hendrickson A, Quigley HA. Selective effects of experimental glaucoma on axonal transport by retinal ganglion cells to the dorsal lateral geniculate nucleus. *Invest Ophthalmol Vis Sci* 32:1593–1599, 1991.
12. Chaturvedi N, Hedley-Whyte ET, Dreyer EB. Lateral geniculate nucleus in glaucoma. *Am J Ophthalmol* 116:182–188, 1993.
13. Quigley HA. Identification of glaucoma-related visual field abnormality with the screening protocol of frequency doubling technology. *Am J Ophthalmol* 125:819–829, 1998.

14. Weinreb RN, Shakiba S, Zangwill L. Scanning laser polarimetry to measure the nerve fiber layer of normal and glaucomatous eyes. *Am J Ophthalmol* 119:627–636, 1995.
15. Zeimer R, Asrani S, Zou S, et al. Quantitative detection of glaucomatous damage at the posterior pole by retinal thickness mapping. *Ophthalmology* 105:224–231, 1998.
16. Mikelberg F, Wijsman K, Schulzer M. Reproducibility of topographic parameters obtained with the Heidelberg retina tomograph. *J Glaucoma* 2:101–103, 1993.
17. Schuman JS, Pedut-Kloizman T, Hertzmark E, et al. Reproducibility of nerve fiber layer thickness measurements using optical coherence tomography. *Ophthalmology* 103:1889–1898, 1996.
18. Schuman JS, Hee MR, Puliafito CA, Wong C, Pedut-Kloizman T, Lin CP, Hertzmark E, Izatt JA, Swanson EA, Fujimoto JG. Quantification of nerve fiber layer thickness in normal and glaucomatous eyes using optical coherence tomography: A pilot study. *Arch Ophthalmol* 113:586–596, 1995.
19. Swanson E, Izatt, Hee M, et al. In vivo retinal imaging by optical coherence tomography. *Optics Letters* 18:1864–1866, 1993.

Chapter 21

BLOOD FLOW IN GLAUCOMA

Alon Harris, PhD
Clinton Sheets

Increases in intraocular pressure have long been associated with progression of visual field damage in patients with primary open-angle glaucoma. However, many patients continue to lose visual field despite lowering of intraocular pressure to target pressure, suggesting that other factors are involved.

Epidemiologic studies show that there is an association between blood pressure and risk factors for glaucoma, and our studies show that the autoregulatory mechanism is insufficient in glaucoma patients to compensate for lower blood pressure. In addition, studies show that

some normal-tension glaucoma patients present with reversible vasospasm.

As research has progressed, it has become more evident that blood flow is an important factor in studying both the vascular etiologies of glaucoma and its treatment. Abnormal blood flow in glaucoma has been shown to take place in the retina, optic nerve, retrobulbar vessels, and the choroid. No single device that is now available can accurately measure all of these areas, so a multi-instrument approach is used to better understand the circulation throughout the entire eye (Figure 21-1).

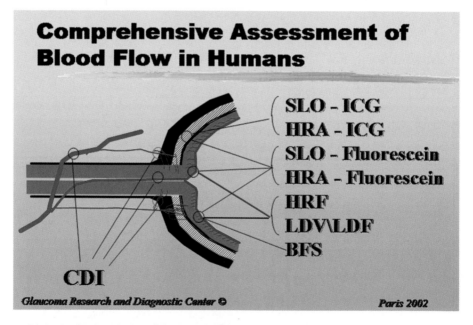

Figure 21-1 Instruments used to measure hemodynamics *Different technologies measure hemodynamics in specific ocular tissue beds.*

SCANNING LASER OPHTHALMOSCOPE (SLO) ANGIOGRAPHY

Scanning laser ophthalmoscope angiography builds upon fluorescein angiography, one of the first modern measurement techniques to gather empirical data about the retina. The SLO overcomes many of the limitations of traditional photographic or video angiography techniques by replacing the incandescent light source with a low-power argon laser beam to achieve better penetration through lens and corneal opacities (Figure 21-2). The laser beam frequency is chosen according to properties of the injected dye, either fluorescein or indocyanine green. As dye enters the eye, the reflected light exits the pupil where a detector measures the intensity of the light in real time. This is to create a video signal, which passes through a video timer and is directed toward an S-VHS recorder. The videos are then analyzed off-line to obtain measurements such as arteriovenous passage (AVP) time and mean dye velocity.

Fluorescein SLO Angiography

Purpose   Evaluation of retinal hemodynamics, specifically AVP time.

Description   Fluorescein dye is used in conjunction with a low-penetrating laser beam frequency to optimize visualization of retinal vessels. High clarity allows isolation of individual retinal vessels in both the superior and inferior

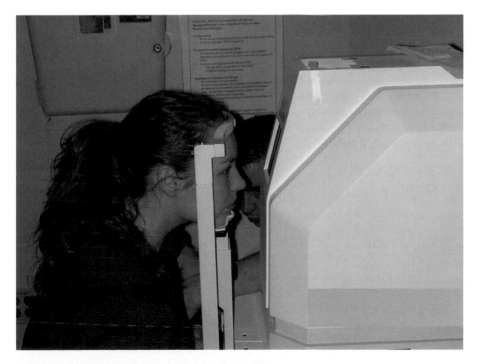

Figure 21-2   Scanning laser ophthalmoscope (SLO) angiography   *The SLO can use either fluorescein or indocyanine green dye to look at retinal or choroidal vessels.*

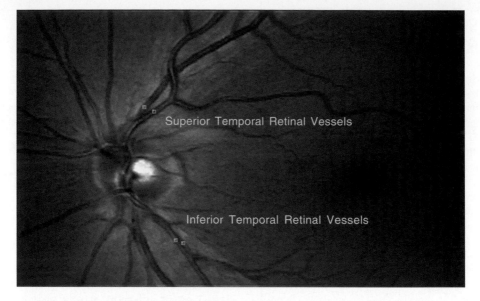

Figure 21-3 Fluorescein SLO angiography *Fluorescein SLO angiography provides high-clarity visualization of retinal vessels.*

hemiretinas. The light intensity of 5×5 pixel areas in adjacent retinal arteries and veins are plotted as the fluorescein dye perfuses the tissue (Figure 21-3). The AVP time equals the time differences in dye arrival between the artery and the vein (Figure 21-4).

Indocyanine Green SLO Angiography

Purpose Evaluation of choroidal hemodynamics, specifically comparing perfusion of the optic disk to the macula.

Description Indocyanine green dye is used in conjunction with a higher-penetrating laser beam

frequency to optimize visualization of the choroidal vasculature. Two areas adjacent to the optic disk and four areas surrounding the macula, each 25×25 pixels, are selected (Figure 21-5). Area dilution analysis (Figure 21-6) measures the brightness of these six areas and determines the time required to reach predefined levels of brightness (10% and 63%). Next, the six areas are compared relative to each other to determine their relative brightness. Relative comparisons are possible because there is no need to compensate for variations in optics, lens opacity, or movement as all data are being collected through an identical optical system, with all six areas filmed simultaneously.

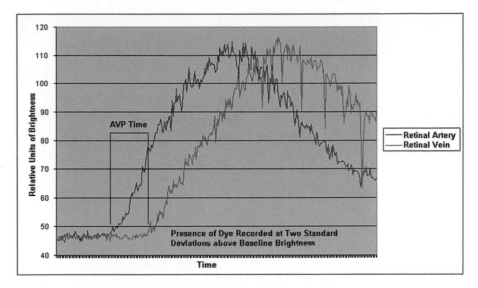

Figure 21-4   Arteriovenous passage (AVP) time   *AVP time equals the time differences in dye arrival between the isolated retinal artery and adjacent retinal vein.*

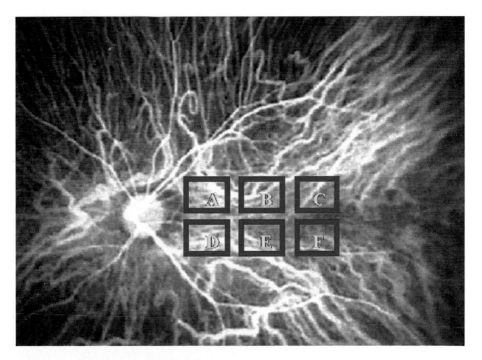

Figure 21-5   Indocyanine green SLO angiography   *Indocyanine green SLO angiography allows analysis of six areas of the choroid: two areas near the optic disk, and four areas centered around the macula.*

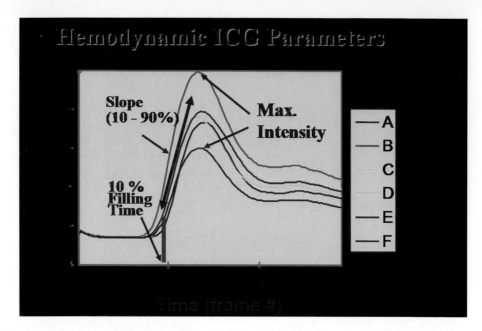

Figure 21-6 Area dilution analysis *Area dilution analysis measures the brightness of an area to determine the time required to reach predefined levels of brightness (10% and 63%). It also allows relative brightness comparisons to be made between the six areas.*

COLOR DOPPLER IMAGING (CDI)

Purpose Evaluation of retrobulbar vessels, specifically the ophthalmic, central retinal, and posterior ciliary arteries.

Description CDI is an ultrasound technique that combines B-scan gray-scale imaging with superimposed color representation of blood flow derived from Doppler-shifted frequencies and pulsed-Doppler measurements of blood velocities. A single, multifunction probe, generally 5 to 7.5 MHz, is used to perform all functions (Figure 21-7). Vessels are selected, and the shifts in returning sound waves are used to produce measurements of blood velocity based on the Doppler equation (Figure 21-8). The velocity data are graphed against time, and the peak and trough are identified as the peak systolic (PSV) and end diastolic (EDV) velocities (Figure 21-9). Pourcelot's resistive index is then calculated for a measure of downstream vascular resistance.

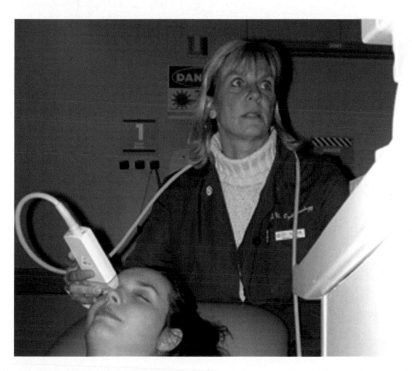

Figure 21-7 Color Doppler imaging (CDI) *CDI is performed by placing a single, multifunction probe (usually 5 to 7 MHz) over the closed eye.*

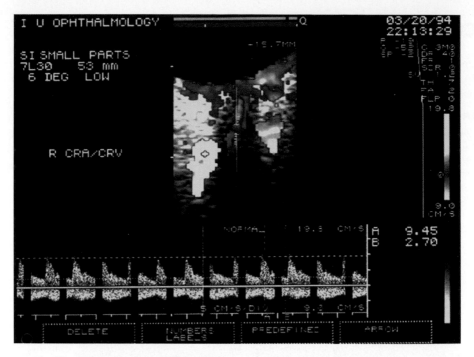

Figure 21-8 **CDI** *Specific retrobulbar vessels can be chosen with the CDI. These include the ophthalmic, central retinal, and posterior ciliary arteries.*

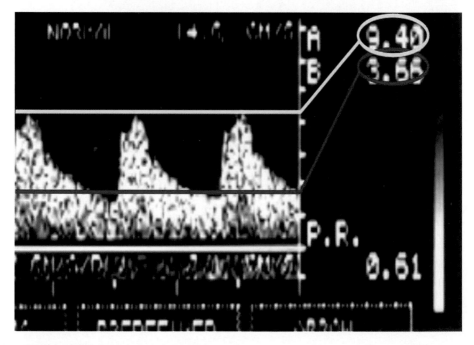

Figure 21-9 **CDI** *The peak systolic (PSV) and end diastolic (EDV) velocities are taken from the peak and trough of the velocity plot. Pourcelot's resistive index can then be calculated from these two values.*

PULSATILE OCULAR BLOOD FLOW (POBF)

Purpose   Estimation of choroidal blood flow during systole by real-time measurement of intraocular pressure.

Description   The POBF device uses a modified pneumotonometer interfaced with a microcomputer to measure intraocular pressure approximately 200 times per second (Figure 21-10). The tonometer is placed on the cornea for several seconds (Figure 21-11) and the amplitude of the intraocular pressure pulse wave is used to calculate the change in ocular volume. The pulsations in intraocular pressure are thought to be the ocular blood flow delivered during systole, assumed primarily to be to choroidal flow because it consists of about 80% of the eye's circulation (Figure 21-12). Glaucoma patients have been shown to have significantly reduced pulsatile ocular blood flow compared with healthy subjects.

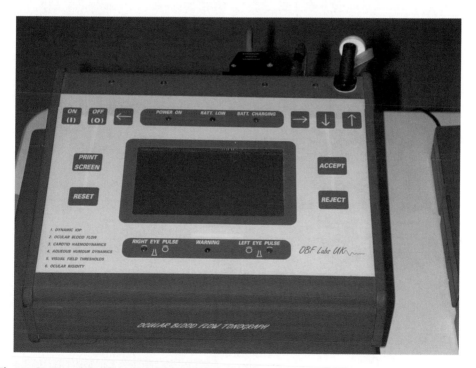

Figure 21-10   Pulsatile ocular blood flow (POBF)   *The POBF device provides real-time measurement of IOP approximately 200 times per second.*

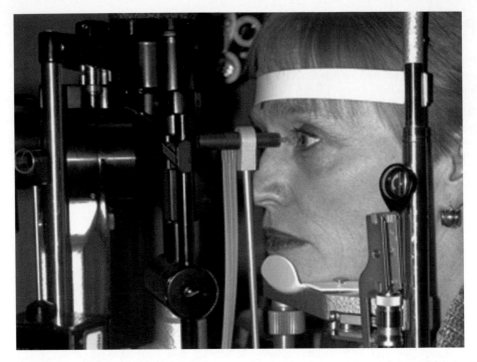

Figure 21-11 **POBF** *The POBF tonometer is placed on the cornea to record the amplitude of the intraocular pressure pulse wave.*

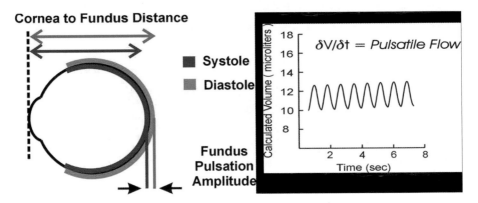

Figure 21-12 **POBF** *The intraocular pressure pulse wave is thought to correlate primarily with systolic choroidal blood flow.*

LASER DOPPLER VELOCIMETRY (LDV)

Purpose Evaluation of the maximum blood cell velocity present in larger retinal vessels.

Description LDV is a precursor to retinal laser Doppler flowmetry and Heidelberg retina flowmetry. This device aims a low-powered laser beam at large retinal vessels at the fundus and analyzes the Doppler shifts observed in light scattered by moving blood cells. The maximum velocity is used to derive the average blood cell velocity, which is then used to derive a calculated flow measurement.

RETINAL LASER DOPPLER FLOWMETRY

Purpose To evaluate blood flow in retinal microvessels.

Description Retinal laser Doppler flowmetry is the intermediate step between LDV and Heidelberg retina flowmetry. The laser beam is directed away from visible vessels to evaluate the blood velocity in microvessels. Only an approximation of blood velocity can be made because of the random directionality of capillaries. Volumetric blood flow can be calculated by using the frequencies in the Doppler-shifted spectra (which signify the velocities of blood cells) together with the signal amplitude at each frequency (which signify the proportion of the blood cells at each velocity).

HEIDELBERG RETINA FLOWMETRY (HRF)

Purpose To evaluate perfusion within peripapillary and optic disc capillary beds.

Description The Heidelberg retina flowmeter has expanded upon the abilities of laser Doppler velocimetry and retinal laser Doppler flowmetry. The Heidelberg retina flowmeter uses a 785-nm infrared laser beam to scan the fundus (Figure 21-13). This frequency was chosen because it reflects both oxygenated and deoxygenated red blood cells with equal intensity. The device scans the fundus to create a physical map of flow values in the retina without favoring arterial or venous blood (Figure 21-14). The interpretation of the flow maps has proven to be difficult. Analysis using software provided by the manufacturer leads to large variations in flow readings when the measurement location is changed, even minutely. Using pointwise analysis developed by the Glaucoma Research and Diagnostic Center, larger areas of the flow map can be examined and better described (Figure 21-15). A histogram of the unitless flow values is produced to describe the "shape" of the flow distribution within the retina, including perfused and avascular tissue.

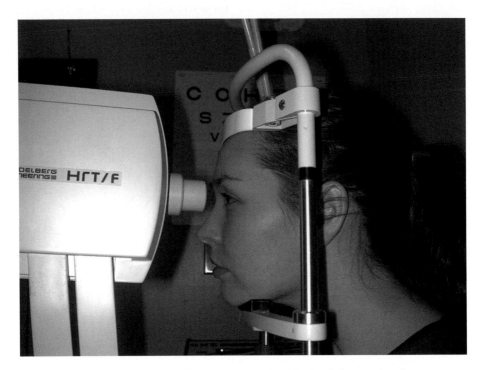

Figure 21-13   Heidelberg retinal flowmetry (HRF)   *The Heidelberg retina flowmeter uses the principles of retinal laser Doppler flowmetry.*

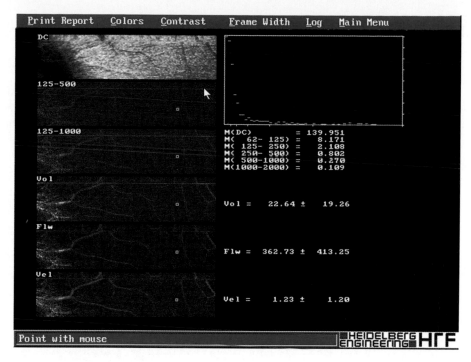

Figure 21-14　HRF　*The amplitudes of Doppler-shifted frequencies caused by moving blood cells are used to create a flow map of the peripapillary retina and optic disk.*

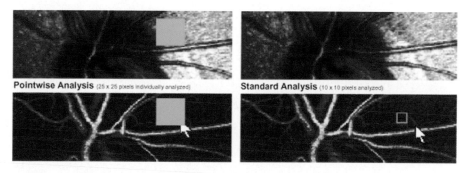

Figure 21-15　HRF　*Pointwise analysis of the HRF flow maps provides a more robust interpretation of flow map by providing a description of the varying degrees of perfused and avascular tissues.*

SPECTRAL RETINAL OXIMETRY (SRO)

Purpose   Evaluation of oxygen tension in the retina and optic nerve head.

Description   The spectral retinal oximeter uses the different spectrophotometric properties of oxygenated and deoxygenated hemoglobin to determine the oxygen tension of the retina and the optic nerve head. A bright flash of white light is delivered to the retina, and the reflected light passes through a 1:4 image splitter as it returns to the digital camera (Figure 21-16). The image splitter (Figure 21-17) creates four equally illuminated images, which are then filtered out to four different wavelengths (Figure 21-18). The brightness of each pixel is recalculated as an optical density. After removing camera noise and calibrating the images to optical density, the oxygen map is calculated.

The isobestic image is filtered at a frequency at which oxygenated and deoxygenated hemoglobin reflect identically. The oxygen-sensitive image is filtered at a frequency at which oxygenated hemoglobin reflection is maximized compared with deoxygenated hemoglobin reflection. The isobestic image is divided by the oxygen-sensitive image to create a map that expresses oxygen content in terms of an optical density ratio. In this image, the lighter areas represent more oxygen, and raw pixel values represent the oxygen level (Figure 21-19).

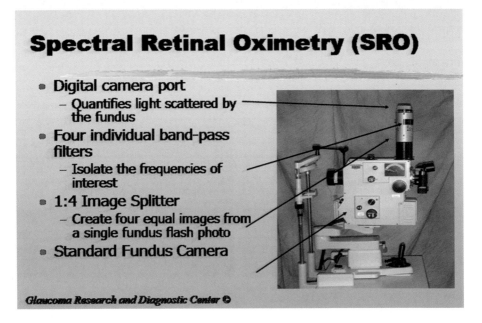

Figure 21-16   Spectral retinal oximetry (SRO)   *The spectral retinal oximeter uses the spectrophotometric properties of oxygenated and deoxygenated hemoglobin to determine the oxygen tension in the retina and optic nerve head.*

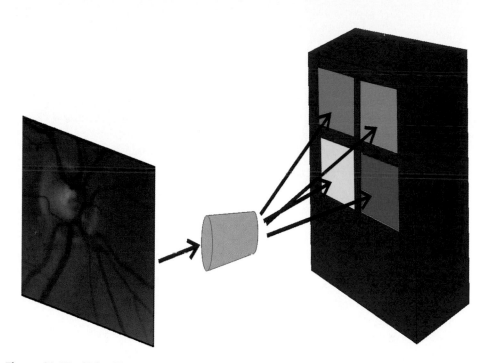

Figure 21-17 SRO *The image splitter transforms one image into four equally illuminated images.*

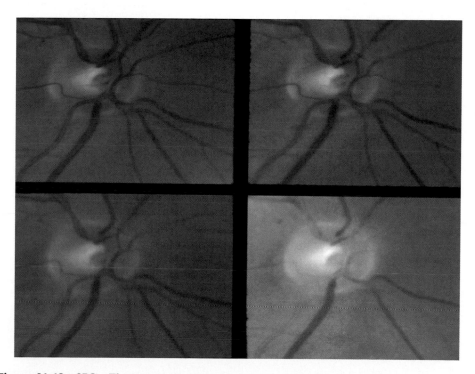

Figure 21-18 SRO *The images are filtered out to four different wavelengths.*

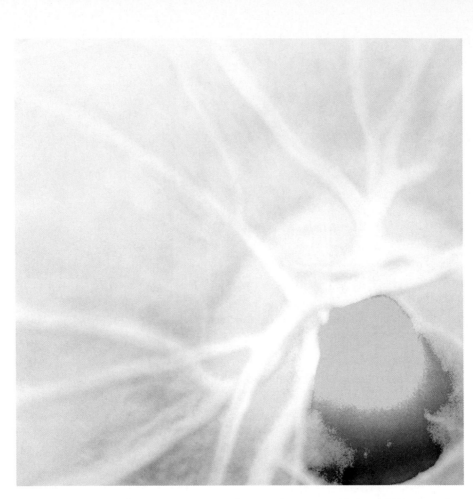

Figure 21-19 SRO *Differences in oxygenated versus deoxygenated hemoglobin are used to create an optical density map in which lighter areas represent higher oxygen concentration.*

SUMMARY

Many factors influence blood flow in humans: autonomic responses, metabolic demands, and myogenic reflexes, to name a few. The key to understanding these factors lies in our ability to measure their effects. As our technologies progress, we will be able not only to detect diseases in their infancies, but also to prevent and treat diseases much more effectively.

BIBLIOGRAPHY

Harris A, Kagemann L, Amin C, Migliardi R, Siesky B, Rechtman E, McCranor L. Test-retest reproducibility of retina and optic nerve oxymeter measurements in the human fundus. Presented at the American Glaucoma Society Conference, San Juan, Puerto Rico, March 2, 2002.

Harris A, Kagemann L, Cioffi G. Assessment of human ocular hemodynamics. *Surv Ophthalmol* 42(6):509–533, 1998.

Harris A, Kagemann L, Hopkins M, Amin C, Migliardi R, Siesky B, Rechtman E, McCranor L. Retina and optic nerve oximetry in humans: A first report of metabolic measurements. Presented at the American Glaucoma Society Conference, San Juan, Puerto Rico, March 1, 2002.

Harris A, Kagemann L, Jonescu-Cuypers C, Siesky B, Sheets C, Coleman A. Heidelberg retinal flowmetry: A comparison of pointwise, SLDF and HRF analysis software. IOVS; 2001, in press.

Orge F, Kagemann L, Chung HS, Zalish M, Zarfati D, Kopecki K, Nowacki EA, Arend O, Harris A. Validation of the first technique for non-invasive measurements of volumetric ophthalmic artery blood flow in humans. (ARVO Abstract) IOVS. 200; abstract no. 2044.

Zarfati D, Harris A, Garzozi HJ, Ishii Y, Jonescu-Cuypers CP, Martin B. A review of ocular blood flow measurement techniques. *Neuro-Ophthalmology* 24:401–409, 2001.

INDEX

Note: Page numbers followed by t *and* f *indicate tables and figures, respectively.*

block removal, 138*f*
complications of, 149*t*. *See also Specific complication*
conjunctiva ballooning in, 134*f*
description of, 132–140
post, 133*f*
postoperative care for, 144, 148
purpose of, 132
topical anesthetic agents in, 133*f*
topical steroids for, 144
traction suture placement in, 134*f*
with releasable sutures. *See* Beaujon technique
Trabeculitis, 257
Traction suture, placement of, 134*f*
Transpupillary cyclophotocoagulation, 176, 176*f*
Traumatic cataract, 308*f*
Traumatic glaucoma, 300–321
Traumatic hyphema, 300–309, 303*f*
angle recession in, 310–311, 311*f*
clinical examination of, 307
cyclodialysis cleft, 312, 313*f*
definition of, 300
eight-ball, 305*f*
epidemiology of, 300
hemorrhage in, 303*f*
history of, 307
management of, 307, 309
pathophysiology of, 306
small, 301*f*
total, 305*f*
Travoprost, 106*t*

U

Ultrasound biomicroscopy, 364–388
Unoprostone isopropyl, 106*t*
Uveitic glaucoma, 254–283
closed-angle mechanisms in, 258–261
diagnosis of, 262, 263*f*–264*f*
epidemiology of, 255, 255*t*
etiology of, 256–261
management of, 265–271
medical therapy for, 265–266
open-angle mechanisms in, 256–258
Uveitis, 57, 57*f*
bilateral anterior, 268*f*–269*f*
lens-associated, 293–294, 294*f*, 295*f*

V

Van Herick's technique, 32*f*–34*f*
Vannas scissors, 139*f*
Vessels, in optic nerve, 83
Visually evoked cortical potential (VEP), 403
Von Recklinghausen's disease, 202, 203*f*

X

Xylocaine 2%, 133*f*

Z

Zeiss goniolens, 38*f*
Zentmeyer's line, 236*f*